Biological Response Modifiers in the Treatment of Hematopoietic Neoplasia

HEMATOLOGY

Series Editors

Kenneth M. Brinkhous, M.D.
Department of Pathology
University of North Carolina
School of Medicine
Chapel Hill, North Carolina

Sanford A. Stass, M.D.
Hematopathology Program
The University of Texas System Cancer Center
M. D. Anderson Hospital and Tumor Institute
Houston, Texas

1. Prostaglandins and Leukotrienes: Blood and Vascular Cell Function, *Jonathan M. Gerrard*
2. Hematopoietic Stem Cells, *edited by David W. Golde and Fumimaro Takaku*
3. Bone Marrow Transplantation: Biological Mechanisms and Clinical Practice, *edited by Dirk W. van Bekkum and Bob Löwenberg*
4. Myelofibrosis: Pathophysiology and Clinical Management, *edited by S. M. Lewis*
5. Plasma Fibronectin: Structure and Function, *edited by Jan McDonagh*
6. The Acute Leukemias: Biologic, Diagnostic, and Therapeutic Determinants, *edited by Sanford A. Stass*
7. Hemostasis and Animal Venoms, *edited by Hubert Pirkle and Francis S. Markland, Jr.*
8. Hematopoiesis: Long-Term Effects of Chemotherapy and Radiation, *edited by Nydia G. Testa and Robert Peter Gale*
9. Coagulation and Bleeding Disorders, *edited by Theodore S. Zimmerman and Zaverio M. Ruggeri*
10. Disorders of the Spleen, *edited by Carl Pochedly, Richard H. Sills, and Allen D. Schwartz*
11. Red Blood Cell Membranes: Structure, Function, Clinical Implications, *edited by Peter Agre and John C. Parker*
12. Graft-vs.-Host Disease: Immunology, Pathophysiology, and Treatment, *edited by Steven J. Burakoff, H. Joachim Deeg, James Ferrara, and Kerry Atkinson*

13. Chronic Myelogenous Leukemia: Molecular Approaches to Research and Therapy, *edited by Albert B. Deisseroth and Ralph B. Arlinghaus*
14. Therapy of Hematopoietic Neoplasia, *edited by Emil J Freireich and Hagop Kantarjian*
15. Biological Response Modifiers in the Treatment of Hematopoietic Neoplasia, *edited by Moshe Talpaz, Razelle Kurzrock, and Jordan U. Gutterman*

Additional Volumes in Preparation

Biological Response Modifiers in the Treatment of Hematopoietic Neoplasia

edited by
Moshe Talpaz
Razelle Kurzrock
Jordan U. Gutterman
University of Texas
M.D. Anderson Cancer Center
Houston, Texas

Marcel Dekker, Inc. New York • Basel • Hong Kong

Library of Congress Cataloging-in-Publication Data

Biological response modifiers in the treatment of hematopoietic neoplasia / edited by Moshe Talpaz, Razelle Kurzrock, Jordan U. Gutterman.
p. cm. — (Hematology: v. 15)
Includes bibliographical references and index.
ISBN 0-8247-8627-0 (alk. paper)
1. Leukemia—Immunotherapy. 2. Lymphoma—Immunotherapy. 3. Hematopoietic system—Cancer—Immunotherapy. 4. Biological response modifiers. I. Talpaz, Moshe. II. Kurzrock, Razelle. III. Gutterman, Jordan U. IV. Series: Hematology (New York, N.Y.): v. 15.
[DNLM: 1. Biological Response Modifiers—therapeutic use. 2. Leukemia—therapy. 3. Lymphoma—therapy. W1 HE873 v. 15]
RC643.B544 1992
616.99'41906—dc20
DNLM/DLC
for Library of Congress 92-4640
CIP

This book is printed on acid-free paper.

MARCEL DEKKER, INC.
270 Madison Avenue, New York, New York 10016

Current printing (last digit):
10 9 8 7 6 5 4 3 2 1

PRINTED IN THE UNITED STATES OF AMERICA

Introduction to the Series

For most of this century, hematology has followed a pattern of major scientific discoveries, improved understanding of disease, and rapid application of new knowledge in the clinic. The rate of advance continues at an accelerating pace, so that all but the most zealous have difficulty in keeping up with the literature in even a limited area of specialized interest. As the explosive development of knowledge continues apace, it is a continuing challenge to keep abreast of significant new developments as they impact on clinical and laboratory hematology. The Hematology series is designed to help in this respect, by providing up-to-date and expert presentations on important subject areas in our field. It is hoped that these works, both individually and collectively, will become important volumes for updating information and for reference for the clinician, investigator, teacher, and student, and in this manner contribute to the advancement of hematology.

This volume on therapy of hematopoietic malignancies and other hematologic disorders is the fifteenth in this series and the first on molecular medicine. It deals with the use of trace physiological polypeptides normally available in the body, growth factors and cytokines, as therapeutic agents. Availability of these proteins became possible only in the last few years, with the cloning of the genes and the production of the proteins by recombinant DNA technology. These proteins are secreted in sizable amounts by bacteria, yeast, and mammalian cells transduced with a specific cloned gene. The list of proteins thus produced is a long one, including interferons, interleukins, and multiple growth factors. The rationale for the use of these agents may be relatively straightforward as with replacement therapy for erythropoietin deficiency in the anemia of renal failure. For the proteins used in the treatment of malignancy or its complications, the rationale is based on modifications in function of a remarkably complex cellular network, which yields products that are cytotoxic or antiproliferative in their action, or that operate through the immune system or in other ways. The potential for these biological agents in tumor therapy appears enormous.

This volume presents a stimulating and comprehensive assessment of the field, ranging from a delightful historical chapter on the importance of semisolid cell culture media for growing hematopoietic cells and the identification of these new factors, one by one, to the use of these new agents in combination therapy with traditional drugs for treating leukemias and lymphomas. The basic knowledge in this whole field is expanding rapidly, and several of these new growth factors and cytokines are currently undergoing clinical trials. With these developments, a revolution in hematologic science and practice is underway. The authors clearly present both the present state of the art and the implications for the future, which makes for exciting reading.

KENNETH M. BRINKHOUS

Preface

The rapid developments in the laboratory and clinical research of hematologic malignancies mandate periodic updated reviews of the field. This is particularly true for new therapeutic approaches derived from the intensive exploitation of recombinant DNA engineering. This technique provides a means to generate novel agents with growth regulatory and immunotherapeutic properties. Such molecules are in the process of revolutionizing the practice of hematology. In this book, we attempt to summarize the emerging biologic therapies from the perspective of clinical and laboratory investigators who have carried out pioneering work in the field. Each topic begins with a chapter that covers some of the biologic rationale for the usage of the specific therapeutic concept in the clinic, followed by a contemporary review of the clinical results of this therapy.

This book was put together particularly for those hematologists/oncologists who are increasingly aware of biologic therapies and would like to complement their knowledge with a more comprehensive, in-depth review of biologic therapies. We hope they will find the topics discussed useful in addressing this particular niche.

MOSHE TALPAZ
RAZELLE KURZROCK
JORDAN U. GUTTERMAN

Contents

Contributors

Giuseppe Avvisati, M.D., Ph.D. Department of Human Biopathology, La Sapienza University, Rome, Italy

Linda M. Bavisotto, M.D. Division of Hematology, Department of Medicine, University of Washington, Seattle, Washington

Ernest C. Borden, M.D. Departments of Medicine, Microbiology, and Pediatrics, Medical College of Wisconsin, Milwaukee, Wisconsin

Migeil Bronchud, D.M. Division of Medical Oncology, Oncological Hospital, Barcelona, Spain

Elihu H. Estey, M.D. Department of Hematology, University of Texas, M.D. Anderson Cancer Center, Houston, Texas

Zeev Estrov, M.D. Department of Clinical Immunology and Biological Therapy, University of Texas, M.D. Anderson Cancer Center, Houston, Texas

Carlo Gambacorti-Passerini, M.D.* Department of Human Oncology, University of Wisconsin, Madison, Wisconsin

*On leave from the Istituto Nazionale Tumori, Milan, Italy.

Jordan U. Gutterman, M.D. Department of Clinical Immunology and Biological Therapy, University of Texas, M.D. Anderson Cancer Center, Houston, Texas

Friedhelm Herrmann, M.D., Ph.D. Department of Hematology and Oncology, University of Freiburg Medical Center, Freiburg, Germany

Hagop Kantarjian, M.D. Department of Hematology, University of Texas, M.D. Anderson Cancer Center, Houston, Texas

Adi Kimchi Department of Molecular Genetics and Virology, Weizmann Institute of Science, Rehovot, Israel

Razelle Kurzrock, M.D., F.A.C.P. Department of Clinical Immunology and Biological Therapy, University of Texas, M.D. Anderson Cancer Center, Houston, Texas

Albrecht Lindemann, M.D. Department of Internal Medicine, Hematology/Oncology, University of Freiburg Medical Center, Freiburg, Germany

Eva Lotzová, Ph.D. Section of Natural Immunity, Department of General Surgery, University of Texas, M.D. Anderson Cancer Center, Houston, Texas

Vera Malkovska, M.D., M.R.C.P., M.R.C. Path. Department of Medicine, University of Wisconsin, Madison, Wisconsin

Franco Mandelli, M.D. Section of Hematology, Department of Human Biopathology, La Sapienza University, Rome, Italy

Håkan Mellstedt, M.D., Ph.D. Department of Oncology, Karolinska Hospital, Stockholm, Sweden

Roland Mertelsmann, M.D., Ph.D. Department of Medicine I, University of Freiburg Medical Center, Freiburg, Germany

Wolfgang Oster, M.D. Department of Clinical Research, Behringwerke AG, Marburg, Germany

Anders Österborg, M.D., Ph.D. Department of Oncology, Karolinska Hospital, Stockholm, Sweden

Felicia Mechtild Rosenthal, M.D. Department of Internal Medicine I, University of Freiburg Medical Center, Freiburg, Germany

Leo Sachs, Ph.D. Department of Molecular Genetics and Virology, Weizmann Institute of Science, Rehovot, Israel

Cherylyn A. Savary, Ph.D. Section of Natural Immunity, Department of General Surgery, University of Texas, M.D. Anderson Cancer Center, Houston, Texas

Paul M. Sondel, M.D., Ph.D. Departments of Pediatrics and Human Oncology, University of Wisconsin, Madison, Wisconsin

Gary Spitzer, M.D. Departments of Medical Oncology and Hematology, and Bone Marrow Transplantation, St. Louis University Medical Center, St. Louis, Missouri

Moshe Talpaz, M.D. Department of Clinical Immunology and Biological Therapy, University of Texas, M.D. Anderson Cancer Center, Houston, Texas

Meir Wetzler, M.D. Department of Clinical Immunology and Biological Therapy, University of Texas, M.D. Anderson Cancer Center, Houston, Texas

Biological Response Modifiers in the Treatment of Hematopoietic Neoplasia

I

INTERFERONS

1

Scientific Aspects of Interferon Therapy in Hematologic Malignancies

Adi Kimchi

Weizmann Institute of Science, Rehovot, Israel

The growth of mammalian cells is normally regulated by extracellular signals, often generated by soluble polypeptide factors. During the past few years it has become evident that in addition to the well-studied growth factors there exists a second group of polypeptides (cytokines) that inhibits cellular proliferation. As such, these negative factors could turn out to be useful in a suppressing tumor cell growth. Several families of growth inhibitory polypeptides have been purified thus far to homogeneity and molecularly cloned, including interferons (IFNs), tumor necrosis factors (TNFs), and transforming growth factor β (TGF-β). The different IFNs were the first to be cloned and produced in commercial quantities and were therefore the first cytokines applied in tumor therapy. However, the clinical trials were performed without any basic knowledge of the complex network of intracellular elements that mediate inhibitory responses and without considering the status of these elements in the tumor cells. It was already clear at the beginning of the 1980s that the presence of functional high-affinity receptors on the surface of cells is necessary but not sufficient for assuring that the ligand-receptor interaction step results in an efficient cell growth arrest. Negative growth responses therefore depend on the presence of additional active forms of postreceptor elements that need to be studied and identified. The latter enable maximizing the efficiency of response during cytokine-mediated tumor therapy and exclude individuals that carry resistant tumor cells. Based on such molecular information it should be possible to choose potential responders and design the best protocols for therapy, that is, which cytokine or combination of cytokines to use in each individual case.

A major difficulty in identifying elements that lie along the growth suppressive pathways of IFN stems from the fact that IFNs exert a wide range of biologic effects on cells in addition to their cytostatic properties. The barrier is therefore to select from among the various postreceptor molecular changes those that specifically transduce antimitogenic signals.

One of the main observations that initiated the molecular mode of action study in our laboratory was the interaction between IFN and the expression of the c-*myc* nuclear oncogene, a tumor-related gene whose product is located in the nucleus. A few years ago we and others noticed that some leukemic cell types, among them "Daudi" cells, which are derived from a patient with Burkitt's lymphoma, responded to exogenous IFN-α by selective reduction in the steady-state levels of the c-*myc* messenger RNA (mRNA), implying that IFN selectively and rapidly reduced the expression of this gene (1–6). In contrast, other cell types, such as HL-60 (a promyelocytic leukemia cell line) and U-937 (a monocytic leukemia cell line), failed to respond to IFN by reduction of c-*myc* mRNA despite the presence of active IFN receptors and that such cells displayed other IFN-initiated responses, such as induction of 2′,5′-oligo A-(2,5-A)-synthetase and HLA genes (1). In other words, there was heterogeneity with regard to whether c-*myc* was downregulated by IFN. It was also noticed that all cells that responded to IFN by a specific cell cycle arrest displayed reduction in c-*myc* expression before the growth arrest (1). These observations raised the following questions:

1. Does the downregulation of c-*myc* mediate at least part of the antiproliferative effects of interferon?
2. What are the molecular mechanisms that lead to this reduction in c-*myc* expression?
3. Why are some cell lines resistant, and what is the molecular basis of resistance in these phenotypes?
4. Is this resistance one of the critical steps in the multistage process of carcinogenesis?

To try to answer the first question, a direct approach of genetic manipulation was taken and a derivative form of the c-*myc* gene that no longer responds to IFN was introduced into sensitive cells to determine whether this specific genetic deregulation altered the growth responses. These gene transfer experiments were first performed in fibroblasts (7,8) and were then further extended to the M1 myelomonocytic cells that are sensitive to IFN-α and β (5,9). In the latter cell system the authentic promoters of c-*myc* were exchanged with the SV40 early promoter so that the construct driving the coding region of c-*myc* was no longer sensitive to IFN. Analysis on gels showed that the exogenous c-*myc* transcripts failed to be inhibited by IFN, whereas the endogenous transcripts continued to be inhibited. In this way a situation was created in which cells exposed to IFN no longer showed downregulation of c-*myc* protein (9).

A detailed examination of the individual c-*myc*-transfected clones for antimitogenic responses to IFN revealed that these cells have completely lost their ability to be growth arrested at the G_0/G_1 phase of the cell cycle (9). However, the transfection with deregulated *myc* did not rescue other growth responses to IFN, thus generating a new partially resistant phenotype. Based on these studies it has been concluded that the downregulation of c-*myc* mediates part of the antiproliferative effects of IFN, and therefore the suppressive elements that communicate between the cell surface receptors and the c-*myc* gene should be further investigated.

The first step toward the elucidation of the molecular mechanisms of c-*myc* inhibition included nuclear run experiments that showed selection reduction in c-*myc* transcription (1,5,6). Recent studies using both the first and second single-stranded exon probes illustrated that both were equally reduced, thus suggesting that IFNs selectively reduced the initiation rate of c-*myc* transcription in M1 myelomonocytic cells (10). Transfection of sensitive hematopoietic cells with reporter genes driven by c-*myc* promoters and upstream sequences identified a negative region that was responsible for the inhibitory effects of IFN on c-*myc* expression. By DNase I protection footprinting analysis two close sites of interaction with nuclear proteins have been identified within the IFN-responsive, negative cis-acting domains. These negative sequences differ from the consensus IFN-responsive element associated with the upregulation of IFN-induced genes (11), thus implying that IFN-induced pathways diverge and only some of them transduce the growth inhibitory signals.

Why do so many leukemic cells fail to respond to IFN by c-*myc* reduction despite the presence of normal cell surface receptors and that they can induce 2,5-A synthetase? There are two possibilities. Either the DNA regulatory elements of c-*myc* are somehow deregulated, or the *trans*-acting elements are not present or become inactivated in the resistant phenotype. To try to address this problem, the technique of somatic cell hybridization was used and hybrids were prepared between resistant and sensitive cells of Burkitt's lymphoma: Daudi, Raji, and P3HR1. In Burkitt's lymphoma, as in other leukemic cell lines, a heterogeneity in response is observed. Thus far 80% of the cells screened have expressed a resistant phenotype. Following exposure to IFN of these resistant cells (such as Raji cells) there was no downregulation of c-*myc* and even a slight stimulation was always observed (5). The remaining 20% of Burkitt's lymphoma cells, such as Daudi and P3HR1, express a sensitive phenotype. If the resistant cells are fused with one or the other sensitive cell to make two independently isolated hybrids, both of them express a sensitive phenotype that reduce c-*myc* in response to IFN. This means that sensitivity is dominant and the failure to reduce c-*myc* results from loss or inactivation of elements that can be complemented by fusion with the sensitive cell (5). Because the experiments used Burkitt lymphoma cell lines that carry different mutations in the first noncoding exon of c-*myc*, it is possible to perform very detailed nucleotide mapping analysis and follow c-*myc* mRNA transcripts arising from the resistant and the sensitive parental cell lines. It was thus found that transcripts from resistant cell lines are reduced in the cell hybrid with the same efficiency as transcripts coming from the sensitive parental cell line (5). This means there are no changes in *cis*: the negative *cis*-acting elements of c-*myc* in the resistant cells are intact. The changes here are in *trans*, and work is ongoing in an attempt to clone and isolate the gene that is missing or inactivated in the resistant phenotype and then to convert resistance back to sensitivity by gene transfer.

Very little is known about the transcytoplasmic coupling proteins that transduce the signals from the membrane receptor to the nuclear compartment. Studies have begun to investigate whether protein kinase C is involved in the negative signaling system of IFN. Daudi and the M1 myelomonocytic cells were depleted of protein kinase C (PKC) by treatment for 24 h with the phorbol ester phorbol myristic acid (PMA), which results in an approximate 90% reduction in PKC activity in cells. These depleted cells were then exposed to IFN-α to determine whether there were changes in the cell cycle responses. It was found that if cells are treated with phorbol ester, cell cycle responses are lost (12). Normally the cells respond by transition to the G_0/G_1 phase of the cell cycle; depletion of PKC abrogates the cell cycle responses. This must be a specific effect on the cell cycle responses because depletion of PKC activity does not interfere with the induction of 2,5-A-synthetase activity. Thus every response in the cell is not being abrogated, but specifically those relating to the cell cycle. Surprisingly, the depletion of PKC activity did not interfere with downregulation of c-*myc* by IFN. Taken together, these experiments suggest the existence of two independent pathways that transduce the negative signals of IFN. One involves c-*myc* reduction and is PKC independent, and the other requires active PKC and its putative target is not yet identified. Each of these two pathways is necessary but not sufficient by itself for mediating the cell cycle responses to IFN (Fig. 1).

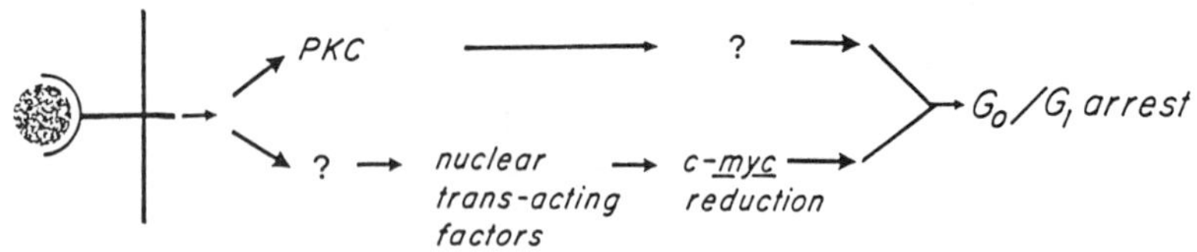

FIGURE 1 Cellular pathways that mediate the suppressive effects of IFN on cell growth.

We have isolated a series of IFN-resistant cell variants (either to IFN-α + β or to IFN-γ) from M1 myeloid cells and from Daudi cells. All these mutants displayed genetic deregulations at the postreceptor level, and first classification was aimed at distinguishing between defects that prevented reduction of c-*myc* and others distal to c-*myc* or in the PKC pathway. All the IFN-resistant M1 clones continued to respond normally to the cytostatic effects of TGF-β, thus confirming the suggestion, first based on the molecular information already mentioned, that different pathways are used by each of these two cytokines to exert G_0/G_1 arrest. The IFN-resistant mutants were then used to analyze the issue of terminal cell division during cell differentiation.

We reported in the past that IFN-β is produced during differentiation of several cell lineages of the hematopoietic system and functions in a typical autocrine mode of action (13–15). Recently we focused on the M1 myeloid cells that in response to interleukin-6 (IL-6) undergo differentiation to mature monocytes and enter terminal cell division. We found that IL-6-treated M1 cells produced murine IFN-β mRNA and protein and responded to it as monitored by induction of the 2,5-A-synthetase gene. Addition of anti-IFN-β antibodies to the IL-6-treated cells prevented the entry into G_0/G_1 on day 3, referring a functional role to the endogenous IFN in the complex process of terminal cell division. Another approach in this issue was to analyze growth and differentiation of the *myc*-transfected and of the IFN-resistant M1 clones after exposure to IL-6. The constitutive expression of c-*myc* protein in the *myc* clones that were treated by IL-6 led to transient expansion in the limited growth capacity of the cells and to a complete loss of the G_0/G_1 arrest (9). Differentiation was not prevented, however, thus suggesting that this subtle defect along one of the IFN pathways dissociates between terminal cell division and morphologic differentiation. A similar expansion in proliferative activity was detected when the different IFN-resistant clones were exposed to IL-6. These extra cycles of division were followed by an unusual G_2 type of growth arrest, while morphologic differentiation went on normally.

Taken together, the in vitro model of terminal differentiation further suggests that loss or inactivation of elements that belong to the receptor signal-transducing machinery of a growth inhibitor, such as IFN, provides a growth advantage to differentiating cells and may be as important in the formation of tumors, like the well-studied oncogene gain of function. Moreover, unlike the dominant nature of oncogene activation, some of the genetic deregulations we have already studied with respect to IFN were recessive over the wild-type allele and could be complemented by fusion with sensitive cells. The isolation of the normal counterparts of ''recessive oncogenes'' has therefore an important therapeutic benefit in the long term concerning the issue of gene therapy, and our work has provided the tools for identifying and isolating these genes in the future. In addition, the molecular work on the mode of action of IFN provides the basis for the development of prognostic tests that will discriminate between tumor cells that are sensitive or resistant to IFN before starting clinical trials. Instead of the empiric approach that was used with respect to IFN therapy in leukemia and lymphoma, we suggest developing protocols of treatments designed in each individual case according to the molecular information provided on the tumor cells of each patient.

REFERENCES

1. Einat M, Resnitzky D, Kimchi A. Nature 1985; 313:597–600.
2. Jonak GJ, Knight E Jr. Proc Natl Acad Sci U S A 1984; 81:1747–50.
3. Knight E Jr, Anton ED, Fahey D, Friedland BK, Jonak GJ. Proc Natl Acad Sci U S A 1985; 82:1151–4.
4. Dani CH, Mechti NM, Piechaczyk M, Lebleu B, Jeanteur PH, Blanchard JM. Proc Natl Acad Sci U S A 1985; 82:4896–9.
5. Kimchi A, Resnitzky D, Ber R, Gat G. Mol Cell Biol 1988; 8:2828–36.
6. Yarden A, Kimchi A. Science 1986; 234:1419–21.
7. Einat M, Kimchi A. Oncogene 1988; 2:485–91.
8. Einat M, Resnitzky D, Kimchi A. Proc Natl Acad Sci U S A 1985; 82:7608–12.
9. Resnitzky D, Kimchi A. Cell Growth & Differentiation 1991; 2:33–41.
10. Yarden A, Lacaze T, Berissi H, Kimchi A. TGF-β and interferon use different molecular mechanisms to reduce c-*myc* expression in M1 myeloid cells. 1991; submitted.
11. Friedman RL, Stark GR. Nature 1985; 314:637–9.
12. Tiefenbrun N, Kimchi A. Oncogene 1991; 6:1001–07.
13. Friedman-Einat M, Revel M, Kimchi A. Mol Cell Biol 1982; 2:1472–80.
14. Yarden A, Shure-Gottlieb H, Chebath J, Revel M, Kimchi A. EMBO J 1984; 3:969–73.
15. Restnitzky D, Yarden A, Zipori D, Kimchi A. Cell 1986; 46:32–40.

2

Therapy of Hairy Cell Leukemia

Razelle Kurzrock, Moshe Talpaz, and Jordan U. Gutterman

University of Texas, M. D. Anderson Cancer Center, Houston, Texas

I. BACKGROUND

Bouroncle and colleagues first described hairy cell leukemia (HCL) in 1958 (1) but referred to it as leukemic reticuloendotheliosis. The typical morphology of the malignant cells led Schrek and Donnelly (2) to designate them, in 1966, as "hairy" cells, an appellation that rapidly gained wide acceptance.

HCL is a rare lymphoproliferative disorder representing <2% of adult leukemias (3); only 500–600 new cases are diagnosed annually in the United States. There is a strong predilection for occurrence in men, with <20% of patients being women. The median age at onset is 50 years, and although we have seen an occasional patient in their 20s or 30s, HCL has never been reported in children or teenagers. The etiology of this malignancy is not known, but there is no apparent genetic predisposition or association with toxins. The majority of patients survive longer than 5 years, and up to 10% have very mild manifestations and require no treatment. Even so, most individuals eventually require therapy for symptomatic splenomegaly or bone marrow failure (4).

Many patients present with cytopenias, although a fraction have the leukemic phase of the disease. Symptoms include easy bruising, fatigue, and infection. Splenomegaly is probably a nearly universal occurrence, and about one-fifth of patients have symptoms related to an enlarged spleen. Mediastinal, abdominal, and retroperitoneal adenopathy may be noted in more than half the cases, but

TABLE 1 Criteria for Treating Hairy Cell Leukemia

Hematologic parameters
Hemoglobin < 10 g/dl
Platelets < 100 × 10^9 L^{-1}
Neutrophils < 1.0–1.5 × 10^9 L^{-1}
Leukemia phase (white blood cells > 10 × 10^9 L^{-1} with >50% hairy cells)
Physical parameters
Symptomatic splenomegaly
Complications
Recurrent or serious infections
Autoimmune problems

Source: Adapted from Ref. 5.

peripheral adenopathy is uncommon. The marrow shows the presence of hairy cells. These are atypical mononuclear cells with prominent irregular cytoplasmic projections giving the appearance of hairs. Cytochemical staining for tartrate-resistant acid phosphatase (TRAP), immunoglobulin gene rearrangements, and B cell surface markers are positive. The last findings confirm the B cell origin of HCL (reviewed in Ref. 5).

Infection is the most frequent complication of this illness and may be secondary to neutropenia, monocytopenia, or disturbed T cell activity. There is also a bleeding diathesis. This is most likely related to thrombocytopenia, although defective platelet function may play a role. About one-quarter of patients develop an autoimmune syndrome with vasculitis and/or arthritis. Bony involvement with lytic lesions also occurs, albeit rarely.

Many patients with HCL have some degree of fibrosis in the marrow. It is therefore sometimes difficult to aspirate the marrow, and the clinical picture may be mistaken for myelofibrosis. The correct diagnosis is critical because HCL is a treatable disease and myelofibrosis is not.

II. THERAPY

Approximately 90% of HCL patients require treatment at some time during the course of the disease. Criteria for initiating therapy are outlined in Table 1. In general, chemotherapy-based regimens tend to aggravate myelosuppression and immunosuppression. Chlorambucil, the most commonly prescribed conventional drug, reverses anemia and thrombocytopenia but does little for granulocytopenia. Splenectomy was therefore the mainstay of therapy until the mid-1980s. At that time, interferon-α (IFN-α) and 2′-deoxycoformycin (DCF) were first noted to have a dramatic antitumor effect in HCL patients. Recently, a third agent, 2-chlorodeoxyadenosine (2CDA), has also been shown to have major antileukemic activity in this disease.

A. Splenectomy

Approximately half the patients undergoing splenectomy have normalization of counts. A rise in platelet counts occurs within days of surgery, and normalization of other counts is seen within 6 months. Although there is an improvement in blood counts, one large series suggests that the number of infectious episodes is not altered (6). Splenectomy is a logical approach for palliation because the spleen is the favored site of malignant cell proliferation. Eventually, however, 50% of these patients require other therapy because of recurrence of cytopenias. Patients with packed marrows (marrow cellularity $\geq$ 85%) before splenectomy often need additional treatment after a median of only 6 months postsplenectomy, and removal of the spleen seems to do little to alter the course.

B. Interferon-α

In 1984, Quesada and colleagues (7) showed that interferon-α is an effective therapy for HCL. These results have been confirmed by many other investigators (8–28) (reviewed in Ref. 5). It is clear that several different types of recombinant IFN-α, as well as the nonrecombinant molecules, are very active. IFN-β also has activity against HCL (29,30), but IFN-γ is not an effective agent (31). Very low dose IFN-α therapy (2×10^5 U/m^2 three times per week) has been noted to have activity in HCL but is inferior to standard dose therapy in inducing remissions (32–35). The standard doses are 3 million units, administered intramuscularly or subcutaneously, three times per week for at least 6–12 months. Responses often occur slowly, with normalization of platelet counts taking 2 months and normalization of hemoglobin and neutrophils taking up to 4–5 months. It should be noted that blood counts may fall transiently during the first month or two of therapy. Recovery of immune effector functions accompanies blood count increases, as demonstrated by normalization of monocytes and restoration of natural killer (NK) and T lymphocyte activity. In addition, there is a significant decrease in infectious episodes.

The majority of responses are partial remissions, with some hairy cells generally remaining in the bone marrow. The complete remission (CR) rate varies in different series from <5% to >40% (36,37). It should be noted that most patients who have achieved a partial remission have normal blood counts and can live normal lives despite a few residual hairy cells in the bone marrow. IFN-α is effective as initial therapy in patients with an intact spleen, as well as in those who have progressed postsplenectomy. Anecdotal descriptions of response in the uncommon T cell variant of HCL have also been published (38). Another rare HCL variant reacts positively with Leu-1 (CD5) monoclonal antibody (generally absent in HCL but present in chronic lymphocytic leukemia (CLL)) and has been reported to have a lower response rate (about 30%) to IFN-α (39). A small number of patients (approximately 5–10%) are IFN resistant because of the development of neutralizing antibodies to the recombinant preparations (40,41). In some cases, this resistance can be overcome by using partially pure IFN-α products (Kurzrock, unpublished data).

The optimum duration of therapy for HCL is not known. Patients seem to have ongoing improvement even after months or years of therapy, but the pace of improvement is slow after 1 year. The incidence of CRs, however, may be increased if 24 months, rather than 12 months, of treatment is administered, and the median time to CR is about 16 months (42). Recurrence of disease is common if therapy is discontinued within the first year, and relapse may take place at times ranging from several months to several years after treatment is stopped. Patients with a low posttreatment platelet count ($<160 \times 10^9\ L^{-1}$) may be at higher risk for relapse within the next year (40). In leukemic patients relapsing after chemotherapy, disease resistence is distressingly common; in contrast, HCL recurrence is almost universally sensitive to reinduction by IFN-α, with the response in second remission equal to or better than that after first remission.

IFN-α therapy is generally well tolerated at the doses used for HCL. Mild flu-like symptoms occur during the first week or two, but tachyphylaxis generally develops rapidly thereafter. Occasional neurologic depression may occur and some patients develop a chronic fatigue syndrome during prolonged therapy. Mild elevation in liver enzymes can be seen in 20–30% of patients and is reversible after stopping treatment.

The mechanism by which IFN-α induces remissions in HCL is not clear. Possible mechanisms include a direct antiproliferative effect, indirect effects through modulation of cytotoxic effector cells, suppression of HCL cell response to B cell growth factor (43), and promotion of differentiation of pluripotent lymphomyeloid stem cells to myelomonocytic cells (44). In addition, a defect in mononuclear cell production of endogenous IFN-α has been demonstrated and may explain, in part, the salutary effects of exogenous IFN-α (45). These cells are also defective in TNF-α production (46), and both IFN-α and TNF-α production are restored by successful IFN-α treatment.

C. 2′-Deoxycoformycin

There are two other experimental drugs that have shown substantial activity in HCL: pentostatin (2′-deoxycoformycin) and 2-chlorodeoxyadenosine. DCF was isolated from the culture broth of *Streptomyces antibioticus* and inhibits adenosine deaminase, an enzyme that catalyzes the deamination of adenosine and deoxyadenosine in the purine salvage pathway and is probably important in normal hematopoiesis. In 1984, Spiers and colleagues (47) showed that this drug could elicit dramatic responses in HCL. These results have been confirmed by several other investigators (reviewed in Refs. 5 and 48), and overall the response rate is ≥75%, most responses being CRs. A trial alternating DCF and IFN-α therapy for a total of 14 months has also been performed (49). All patients had >95% clearing of bone marrow leukemic infiltrate, and remissions were durable after a median follow-up of 27 months.

There is no significant impact of previous therapy on responsiveness to DCF, and this agent is also very active in IFN-resistant patients (50–52). Indeed, we have used DCF to treat 15 patients who were resistant to IFN-α, either because of antibody development or because of primary cellular resistance. A total of 14 patients responded with complete or nearly complete remissions. Relapses have not occurred, and the median duration of remission without maintenance therapy has not been reached after a median follow-up of over 1.5 years.

The major toxicities of DCF include nausea and vomiting, skin rash, conjunctivitis, lethargy, and myelosuppression. The last may be of some concern in patients with severe pancytopenia at initiation of therapy. Renal insufficiency is rare and generally reversible. We currently use doses of 4 mg/m^2 of DCF administered intravenously every 2 weeks for 24 weeks (12 courses). Fewer courses may be preferable since the average number of courses to CR is 6. At these doses, side effects in the majority of patients are mild.

One drawback of DCF may be long-term immunosuppression: this molecule induces T cell lymphopenia for prolonged periods after therapy (53). Further, some patients develop localized herpes zoster (53). This issue has not been studied in detail, however, and in our study, which has been ongoing for 3 years, opportunistic infections have not been a problem.

D. 2-Chlorodeoxyadenosine

Another new drug that has created much interest is 2CDA. 2CDA is an adenosine deaminase-resistant purine analog, but unlike DCF, it does not inhibit adenosine deaminase. It has potent lymphotoxicity. The first trial of this molecule revealed that durable CRs could be induced in 11 of 12 patients after a single course (54). Relapses were not observed after a median follow-up of 15.5 months (longest follow-up = 3.8 years). A course consisted of 4 mg/m^2 given by continuous 24 h infusion daily for 7 days. There was minimal myelosuppression, and the only constitutional side effect was fever. Although the fever was treated with antibiotics, no organisms were cultured, and it was hypothesized that temperature elevation may be due to cytokine release from the destroyed hairy cells. Preliminary results in a larger group of patients treated at our institution confirm these remarkable results. The long term effects are not yet elucidated, however.

E. Granulocyte Colony-Stimulating Factor

The colony-stimulating factors are hematopoietic growth factors that induce the proliferation, differentiation, and activation of various blood cells. Recently, Glaspy et al. treated four neutropenic, hairy cell leukemia patients with granulocyte colony-stimulating factor (G-CSF). Increasing doses to a maximum of 5 μg/kg/day were given for 5–6 weeks. The patients had significant improvement in their neutrophil counts (55). In an attempt to abort the period (several weeks to months) of neutropenia and susceptibility to infections that hairy cell leukemia patients suffer from until the beneficial effects of therapy take hold, these physicians gave an additional six patients a combination of G-CSF and consensus interferon-α. G-CSF, 3 μg/kg/day SC, was administered until the neutrophil count was $>5 \times 10^9$ L^{-1} for 2 weeks; interferon-α was then added and the G-CSF continued for 3 months. This strategy was successful in immediately reversing the neutropenia (56), and G-CSF may hence be a reasonable supportive measure during initial treatment with interferon or deoxycoformycin.

III. SUMMARY

The cardinal features of HCL are (1) cytopenias, (2) splenomegaly, and (3) mononuclear cells of B cell origin with cytoplasmic projections and a positive TRAP stain. The most common complication is infection. In the past, the mainstay of therapy has been splenectomy, and this procedure is still often suggested as a first-line approach (57). However, research during the last decade has resulted in three new, highly effective therapies for HCL—IFN-α, DCF, and 2CDA. IFN-α is currently approved for this indication. About 90% of patients have a durable hematologic recovery, and complete remission rates range from <5% to >40% in different series. It should be noted that patients with partial remissions generally have normal or nearly normal blood counts and can live indefinitely without disease-related problems, despite a few remaining hairy cells in the bone marrow. DCF and 2CDA are potent agents with very high remission rates and only minor or no side effects. These two drugs have the advantage that most of the remissions are CRs and maintenance is not required. Their disadvantage may relate to long-term immunosuppression because of T cell cytotoxicity. In the case of 2CDA, the newest of the three agents, the relatively short follow-up of most patients precludes identification of late (>2 year) toxicities. However, the requirement for only a 1 week course of therapy may ultimately elevate 2CDA to the treatment of choice for hairy cell leukemia. Although the majority of HCL patients are middle-aged or older men, a question that has been raised by several of our younger patients relates to the effects of these drugs on fertility. Some of our IFN-treated patients have fathered normal children, but in general this issue has been ignored. At present it seems that about 10% of patients never require treatment, and for the other 90% (Table 1), any one of these three therapies is a reasonable management option. Because all three agents are highly effective even in patients with tremendously enlarged spleens, we no longer perform splenectomy on our HCL population. As mentioned earlier, however, several other centers still recommend splenectomy for cytopenic patients in whom the disease is predominantly splenic (low hairy cell infiltrate in the bone marrow in the presence of a large spleen) (57,58). In regard to prognosis, our goal is a normal life expectancy for these patients. To achieve this objective, newly diagnosed patients must be carefully monitored and supported until their cytopenias resolve. Infections are the major cause of morbidity and mortality, and in addition to the danger of Gram-negative sepsis early in the course of the disease, persistent fevers and night sweats without an obvious source should alert the physician to the possibility of disseminated atypical mycobacterial infection (59). In this regard, G-CSF can quickly reverse neutropenia, and preliminary results suggest that it is a useful supportive measure (55,56). The question of susceptibility to late opportunistic infections or malignancy has not been answered. In one study, second malignancies were found in 15 of 172 patients (8.7%) followed for 10 years (60); it is unclear if this statistic represented an increase in the cancer rate, however, especially since four of the tumors were skin (three basal and one squamous) cancers, most of the patients were middle-aged or elderly men, and age-matched control subjects were not analyzed.

The discovery of the profound antitumor effects of IFN-α in HCL represented the first time that a cytokine was shown to have major anticancer activity. The impact of this discovery reached far beyond its relevance to a relatively rare disease. First, it culminated in the worldwide licensing of recombinant IFN-α, and with time, this agent has demonstrated activity against a wide range of malignancies as well as against viral infections. Further, the success of IFN-α as a single agent in the management of HCL heralded the establishment of a fourth modality of treatment, that is, biologic therapy for human cancer.

ACKNOWLEDGMENTS

The authors thank Mrs. Gayle Cannon for her expertise in the preparation of this manuscript. Research supported, in part, by Hoffmann-La Roche, Inc. Research conducted, in part, by the Clayton Foundation for Research. Dr. Gutterman is a Senior Clayton Foundation Investigator.

REFERENCES

1. Bouroncle BA, Wiseman BK, Doan CA. Leukemic reticuloendotheliosis. Blood 1958; 13:609–30.

2. Schrek R, Donelly WJ. "Hairy" cells in blood in lymphoreticular neoplastic disease and "flagellated" cells of normal lymph nodes. Blood 1966; 27:199–211.
3. Damasio EE, Pagnucco G, Federico M, et al. Hairy cell leukemia. A therapeutical update. Haematologica (Pavia) 1989; 74:205–18.
4. Golomb HM, Catovsky DC, Golde DW. Hairy cell leukemia. A clinical review based on 71 cases. An Intern Med 1978; 89:677–83.
5. Doane LL, Ratain MJ, Golomb HM. Hairy cell leukemia. Current management. Hematol Oncol Clin North Am 1990; 4:489–502.
6. Golomb HM, Hadad LJ. Infectious complications in 127 patients with hairy cell leukemia. Am J Hematol 1984; 16:383–401.
7. Quesada JR, Reuben J, Manning JT, Hersh EM, Gutterman JU. Alpha interferon for induction of remission in hairy cell leukemia. N Engl J Med 1984; 310:15–8.
8. Foon KA, Maluish AE, Abrams PG, et al. Recombinant leukocyte A interferon therapy for advanced hairy cell leukemia. Therapeutic and immunologic results. Am J Med 1986; 80:351–6.
9. Ratain MJ, Golomb HM, Vardiman JW, Vokes, EE, Jacobs RH, Daly K. Treatment of hairy cell leukemia with recombinant alpha 2 interferon. Blood 1985; 65: 644–8.
10. Thompson JA, Fefer A. Interferon in the treatment of hairy cell leukemia. Cancer 1987; 59:605–9.
11. Worman CP, Catovsky D, Cawley J, Bevan PC, Bottomley JM, Nethersell ABW. The U.K. experience with human lymphoblastoid interferon in HCL: a report of the first 50 cases. Leukemia 1987: 1:320–2.
12. Thompson JA, Fefer A. The treatment of hairy cell leukemia with recombinant alfa interferon: a multi-institutional study. Invest New Drugs 1987; 5:5–8.
13. Quesada JR, Hersh EM, Manning J, et al. Treatment of hairy cell leukemia with recombinant α-interferon. Blood 1986; 68:493–7.
14. Masuda M, Takanashi M, Motoji T, Oshimi K, Mizoguchi H. Effect of recombinant interferons on hairy cell leukemia progenitors. Int J Cell Cloning 1989; 7:120–8.
15. Fridrik MA, Wahl G, Herbinger W, et al. Morphological and immunological changes of hairy cell leukemia during a α-2-interferon therapy. Blut 1989; 58:261–4.
16. Ozer H, Golomb HM, Zimmerman H, Spiegel RJ. Cost-benefit analysis of interferon alfa-2b in treatment of hairy cell leukemia. J Natl Cancer Inst 1989; 81:594–602.
17. Ehmann WC, Silber R. Recombinant alpha-2 interferon for treatment of hairy cell leukemia without prior splenectomy. Am J Med 1986; 80:1111–4.
18. Golomb HM, Jacobs A, Fefer A, et al. Alpha-2 interferon therapy of hairy-cell leukemia: a multicenter study of 64 patients. J Clin Oncol 1986; 4:900–5.
19. Skotnicki AB, Wolska-Smolen T, Blicharski J, Zdunczyk A, Sasiadek U, Pituch-Noworolska A. Human recombinant interferon-alpha-2 in the treatment of patients with hairy cell leukemia. Cancer Detect Prev 1988; 12:511–22.
20. Romeril KR, Carter JM, Green GJ, et al. Treatment of hairy cell leukaemia with recombinant alpha interferon. Med J 1989; 102:186–8.
21. Flandrin G, Castaigne S, Sigaux F, Degos L. Results of treating 53 hairy cell leukemia patients with α-interferon. Leukemia 1987; 1:326–8.

22. Thompson JA, Rubin E, Fefer A. The treatment of hairy cell leukemia with α2b-interferon: experience with 27 patients treated more than one year. Leukemia 1987; 1:328–30.
23. Glaspy JA, Jacobs AD, Golde DW. The UCLA experience with type I interferons in hairy cell leukemia. Leukemia 1987; 1:323–6.
24. Holmes R, Schwarz MA, Whiteside MG, Firkin FC. Treatment of hairy cell leukemia with increasing doses of recombinant alpha A interferon. Aust N Z J Med 1988; 18:557–62.
25. Golomb HM, Fefer A, Golde DW, et al. Report of a multi-institutional study of 193 patients with hairy cell leukemia treated with interferon-alfa2b. Semin Oncol 1988; 15:7–9.
26. Gibson J, Cameron K, Gallagher K, et al. Clinical response of hairy-cell leukaemia to interferon-α: results of an Australian study. Med J Aust 1988; 149:293–6.
27. Golomb HM, Ratain MJ, Fefer A, et al. Randomized study of the duration of treatment with interferon alfa-2b in patients with hairy cell leukemia. J Natl Cancer Inst 1988; 80:369–73.
28. Aderka D, Michalevicz R, Daniel Y, et al. Recombinant interferon alpha-c for advanced hairy cell leukemia. Cancer 1988; 61:2207–13.
29. Michalevicz R, Aderka D, Frisch B, Revel M. Interferon-beta induced remission in a hairy cell leukemia patient resistant to interferon-alpha. Leuk Res 1988; 12:845–51.
30. Wiernik PH, Schwartz B, Dutcher JP, Turman N, Adinolfi C. Successful treatment of hairy cell leukemia with β-ser interferon. Am J Hematol 1990; 33: 244–8.
31. Quesada JR, Alexanian R, Kurzrock R, Barlogie B, Saks S, Gutterman JU. Recombinant interferon gamma in hairy cell leukemia, multiple myeloma, and Waldenstrom's macroglobulinemia. Am J Hematol 1988; 29:1–4.
32. Thompson JA, Kidd P, Rubin E, Fefer A. Very low dose alpha-2b interferon for the treatment of hairy cell leukemia. Blood 1989; 73:1440–3.
33. Gastl G, Werter M, DePauw B, et al. Comparison of clinical efficacy and toxicity of conventional and optimum biological response modifying doses of interferon alpha-2C in the treatment of hairy cell leukemia: a retrospective analysis of 39 patients. Leukemia 1989; 3:453–60.
34. Moormeier JA, Ratain MJ, Westbrook CA, Vardiman JW, Daly KM, Golomb HM. Low-dose interferon alfa-2b in the treatment of hairy cell leukemia. J Natl Cancer Inst 1989; 81:1172–4.
35. Hasselbalch H, Braide I, Lisse I, et al. Recombinant interferon-alpha-2b treatment of hairy-cell leukaemia: experience with a low-dose schedule. Eur J Haematol 1988; 41:438–44.
36. Lauria F, Foa R, Raspadori D, et al. Treatment of hairy-cell leukaemia with α-interferon (α-IFN). Eur J Cancer Clin Oncol 1988; 24:195–200.
37. Castaigne S, Sigaux F, Degos L, Flandrin G. Hairy cell leukemia: follow-up after completion of alpha interferon treatment. Nouv Rev Fr Hematol 1989; 31:321–5.
38. Hasselbalch H, Hippe E. Further evidence of the efficacy of interferon for T-cell hairy cell leukaemia. Eur J Haematol 1988; 40:188–9.

39. Lauria F, Raspadori D, Foa R, et al. Reduced hematologic response to alpha-interferon therapy in patients with hairy cell leukemia showing a peculiar immunologic phenotype. Cancer 1990; 65:2233–6.
40. Berman E, Heller G, Kempin S, Gee T, Tran L-L, Clarkson B. Incidence of response and long-term follow-up in patients with hairy cell leukemia treated with recombinant interferon alfa-2a. Blood 1990; 75:839–45.
41. Bekisz JB, Zur Nedden DL, Enterline JC, Zoon KC. Antibodies to interferon-α_2 in patients treated with interferon-α_2 for hairy cell leukemia. J Interferon Res 1989; 9:S1–7.
42. Quesada JR, Lepe-Zuniga JL, Gutterman JU. Mid-term observations on the efficacy of α-interferon in hairy cell leukemia and status of the interferon system of patients in remission. Leukemia 1987; 1:317–9.
43. Genot E, Billard C, Sigaux F, et al. Proliferative response of hairy cells to B cell growth factor (BCGF): in vivo inhibition by interferon-α and in vitro effects of interferon-α, -β, and -γ Leukemia 1987; 1:590–6.
44. Michalevicz R, Revel M. Interferons regulate the in-vitro differentiation of multilineage lymphomyeloid stem cells in hairy cell leukemia. Proc Natl Acad Sci U S A 1987; 84:2307–11.
45. Lepe-Zuniga JL, Quesada JR, Baron S, Reuben J, Gutterman JU. Alpha interferon production in patients with hairy cell leukemia: correlations with disease activity and remission status. Hematol Pathol 1987; 1:157–65.
46. Aderka D, Levo Y, Ramot B, et al. Reduced production of tumor necrosis factor by mononuclear cells in hairy cell leukemia patients and improvement following interferon therapy. Cancer 1987: 60:2208–12.
47. Spiers ASD, Parekh SJ, Bishop MB. Hairy cell leukemia. Induction of complete remission with pentostatin. J Clin Oncol 1984; 2:1336–42.
48. Cheson BD, Martin A. Clinical trials in hairy cell leukemia. Ann Intern Med 1987; 106:871–8.
49. Martin A, Nerenstone S, Urba WJ, et al. Treatment of hairy cell leukemia with alternating cycles of pentostatin and recombinant leukocyte A interferon: results of a phase II study. J Clin Oncol 1990; 8:721–30.
50. Blick M, Lepe-Zuniga JL, Doig R, Quesada JR. Durable complete remissions after 2′-deoxycoformycin treatment in patients with hairy cell leukemia resistant to interferon alpha. Am J Hematol 1990; 33:205–9.
51. Ho A, Thaler J, Mandelli F, et al. for the European Organization for Research and Treatment of Cancer Leukemia Cooperation Group. Response to pentostatin in hairy-cell leukemia refractory to interferon-alpha. J Clin Oncol 1989; 7:1533–8.
52. Durrleman S, Grem JL, Cheson BD. 2′-Deocycoformycin after failure of alpha-interferon in hairy cell leukemia. Eur J Haematol 1989; 43:297–302.
53. Urba WJ, Baseler MW, Kopp WC, et al. Deoxycoformycin-induced immunosuppression in patients with hairy cell leukemia. Blood 1989; 73:38–46.
54. Piro LD, Carrera CJ, Carson DA, Beutler E. Lasting remissions in hairy cell leukemia induced by a single infusion of 2-chlorodeoxyadenosine. Engl J Med 1990; 322:1117–21.

55. Glaspy J, Baldwin GC, Robertson PA, et al. Therapy for neutropenia in hairy-cell leukemia with recombinant human granulocyte colony stimulating factor. Ann Intern Med 1988; 109:789–95.
56. Glaspy J, Ambersley J, Narachi M, Wyres M, Golde DW. Treatment of hairy cell leukemia with granulocyte colony stimulating factor and alpha interferon (abstract). Proc Am Soc Clin Oncol 1990; 9:213.
57. Golomb HM, Ratain MJ, Vardiman JW. Sequential treatment of hairy cell leukemia: a new role for interferon. Important Adv Oncol 1986; 2:311–21.
58. Lill MCC, Golde DW. Treatment of hairy-cell leukemia. Blood Rev 1990; 4:238–44.
59. Bennett C, Vardiman J, Golomb HM. Disseminated atypical mycobacterial infection in patients with hairy cell leukemia. Am J Med 1986; 80:891–6.57.
60. Jacobs RH, Vokes EE, Golomb HM. Second malignancies in hairy cell leukemia. Cancer 1985; 56:1462–7.

3

Interferon Action in Myeloproliferative Disorders: Mechanisms of Response and Resistance to Therapy

Moshe Talpaz, Zeev Estrov, Meir Wetzler, and Razelle Kurzrock

University of Texas, M. D. Anderson Cancer Center, Houston, Texas

Interferons have been subjects of intense study since their discovery by Isaacs and Lindemann (1). These studies unraveled a multitude of activities exerted by interferons, including antiviral, antiproliferative, and immunomodulatory actions (2). Recently, interferons have been shown to possess clinical activity against several hematologic neoplasias and to a lesser extent against some solid tumors (3–6). The actual mode of action of interferons against these malignancies remains largely unknown. A direct growth inhibitory effect gained most attention as the likely mode of action in hematologic malignancies. Accordingly, the antiproliferative effect of interferons on normal and neoplastic hematopoietic tissues was studied extensively. Interferons inhibit normal myeloid progenitor cells, as well as chronic myelogenous leukemia (CML) progenitor cells, and it appears that the level of inhibition is similar (7), although slightly increased inhibition of CML progenitor cells was suggested by one group of investigators (8). The inhibition of myeloid progenitor cells is dose dependant up to 50,000 U/ml, and similar inhibition was observed with interferon-γ as well (8). Perhaps the most important information from these studies is that CML cells, although they undergo neoplastic transformation, are not less sensitive to the inhibitory effects of interferon than normal hematopoietic progenitors.

Because a direct growth inhibitory effect of interferon fails to provide a proper explanation for the selective effect of interferon against chronic myelogenous leukemia, it is likely that it is a necessary but, by itself, insufficient mechanism of action. Accordingly, other interferon mechanisms of action in CML have been proposed as well. Defects of CML progenitor cell ability to adhere to bone marrow stroma were recently demonstrated and corrected in vitro by the addition of interferon (9,10). Defects in the surface molecule LFA-3 were also described by a different group of investigators and again were demonstrated to be corrected with the addition of interferon-α (IFN-α) (11). The bone marrow stroma regulates progenitor cell growth by constitutive production of growth inhibitory molecules, such as transforming growth factor β (12), and it is suggested that the CML myeloid progenitor cell escapes this regulation because of its impaired adhesiveness, which is rectified by interferon.

A totally different mechanism that has recently been proposed involves deranged responsiveness to hematopoietic growth factors by the abnormal myeloproliferative stem cell. Multiple models with certain similarities to myeloproliferative disorders have been generated by transfecting growth factor genes into myeloid precursor cells. Increased sensitivity to myeloid growth factors was noted in some of these models (13). In various systems, interferons were recently shown to interfere with the effect of various growth factors either by modulating the receptor to these growth factors or by altering growth factor-induced cellular signal transduction (14–17). It is plausible to consider such an effect as an underlying mechanism to the aforementioned selective effect of interferon.

In conclusion, the mode of action of interferon in myeloproliferative disorders remains unknown, and at least three different direct activities of interferons on the transformed cell may be associated with the clinical effect. On the assumption that one of these direct effects takes place when interferon is administered in patients with myeloproliferative disorders, we embarked on studying the mode of action of interferon in situations of interferon sensitivity and resistant CML.

The direct effect of IFN-α is mediated by binding to a specific high-affinity cellular receptor (18). The response heterogeneity in CML provided us with the opportunity to study the IFN-α effect in responsive and resistant CML. Receptor binding affinity and receptor downregulation following therapy were studied in peripheral blood myeloid cells from patients with sensitive and resistant disease and failed to identify binding defects as the underlying cause for the development of therapy resistance (18). These studies were pursued by studies of the interferon-inducible enzyme 2′,5′-oligoadenylate synthetase (2′,5′-A), which was induced in seven of nine responders versus none of three nonresponding patients. Furthermore, in two patients with an initial response to therapy followed by the emergence of IFN-α-resistant disease, 2′,5′-A was induced during the responsive phase but not during the resistant phase (19).

These findings suggest potential defects in the interferon-responsive pathways downstream from receptor binding in the resistant disease. However, re-

TABLE 1 Gene Induction After Interferon-α Therapy in CML Ph[1] Patients

		% Induced			
Response	Patient	ISG-54	ISG-15	2′,5′-A-synthetase	6-16
IFN sensitive	8	100	100	100	100
IFN resistant	18	100	94	100	100

cently we extended our initial work and examined the induction of 2′,5′-A mRNA in CML Ph[1] (Philadelphia chromosome) cells following therapy with IFN-α. Surprisingly, multiple species of 2′,5′-A mRNA were induced in all patients either as IFN-α responders or as nonresponders (20). Further studies of 2′,5′-A mRNA expression, 2′,5′-A protein, and 2′,5′-A enzymatic activity must be conducted to assess whether any defects in this system are associated with the development of cellular resistance.

In recent years, several interferon-inducible genes have been identified, some with defined functions (2′,5′-A, interferon-associated protein kinase P67; major histocompatibility complex (MHC) class I; and metallothionein II), whereas others with still unknown functions have been cloned and sequenced, including interferon-stimulated genes (ISGs) 15, 54, and 56 and genes denoted 6-16, 6-26, and 9-27 (21–28). Studies of cell lines sensitive and resistant to IFN-α have demonstrated a spectrum of defects in various inducible genes (29–34), but when we extended this work to IFN-α-sensitive and IFN-α-resistant CML following in vivo therapy with IFN-α, we failed to identify any defect in the induction of ISG-15, ISG-54, or 6-16, in addition to the similar observation with the 2′,5′-A gene (Table 1 and Fig. 1) (20). It is therefore likely that "clinical resistance" to interferon bears no resemblance to the in vitro cellular resistance. A possible explanation of this resistance is with the increased proliferative capacity of the Ph[1] cells, perhaps driven by autocrine growth factors, that negates the inhibitory effects of the interferon. Support for the notion of altered growth characteristics of the malignant clone comes from recent work which shows that in vitro CML progenitor cells from either interferon-sensitive or IFN-resistant CML are equally sensitive to the inhibitory effect of IFN-α regardless of the clinical response. However, progenitor cells from the resistant phase exhibit a reduced response to exogenous growth factors and a relative autonomous growth pattern in the methylcellulose colony assay (Fig. 2) (35). This work suggests that a putative growth factor produced by the malignant clone or by bone marrow accessory cells provides the transformed clone with relatively autonomous growth and renders it less sensitive to growth inhibitory molecules. In parallel,

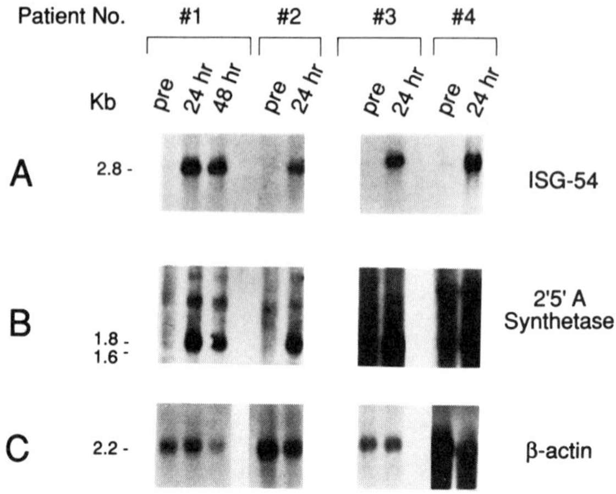

FIGURE 1 Northern blot of RNA collected from CML patients before therapy and 24 ± 48 h after therapy. Blots were hybridized with probes for ISG-54 (A), 2′,5′-A-synthetase (B), and β-actin (C). Patients 1 and 3 are interferon-α-resistant patients, whereas patients 2 and 4 are interferon-sensitive patients.

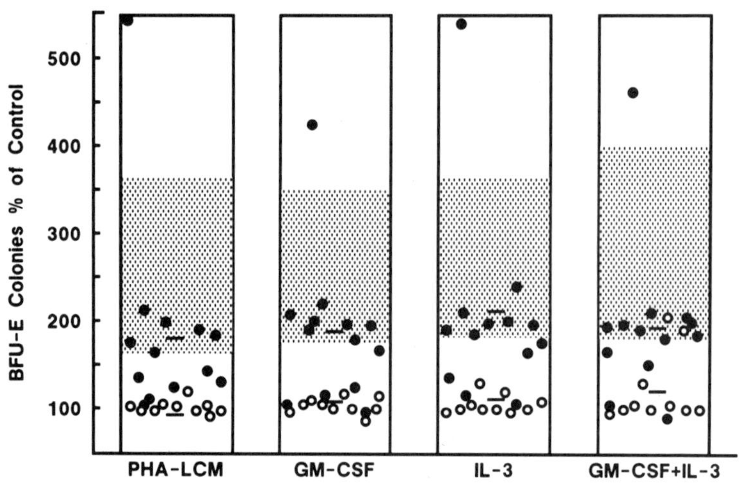

FIGURE 2 Growth pattern of BFU-E colonies from IFN-sensitive (•) and IFN-resistant (○) CML patients. Results obtained from 23 patients are depicted. The data are presented as the percentage of the mean number of colonies obtained from each patient in the presence of fetal calf serum and erythropoietin without exogenous colony-stimulating factor. The mean number of BFU-E colonies in control dishes ranged from 89 to 224. The shaded areas represent the range of the mean number of colonies ± SD (standard deviation, presented as percentage of control) from five normal BM samples. (PHA-LCM: phytohaemaglutinin-leukocyte conditioned medium; GM-CSF: granulocyte-macrophage colony stimulating factor; BFU-E: burst forming units erythroid.)

we also demonstrated detectable levels of interleukin-1β in a high proportion of cell lysates from interferon-resistant patients and patients in accelerated disease but in only a minority of patients with interferon-responsive CML (Table 2) (36,37). Further extension of this work shows the possible involvement of bone marrow stroma in the very advanced stages of the disease. In myeloid and undifferentiated blastic crisis, we noted constitutive growth factor expression (IL-1β, IL-6, and granulocyte-macrophage colony stimulating factor, GM-CSF) not seen in the chronic phase of the disease (Table 3). This work provides circum-

TABLE 2 Constitutive Expression of Interleukin-1β among Interferon-α-Sensitive and IFN-α-Resistant Patients

	IFN sensitive	IFN resistant	
IL-1 mRNA$^+$	4	12	
			$p < 0.05$
IL-1 mRNA$^-$	10	6	
IL-1 protein > 50	3	12	
			$p < 0.01$
IL-1 protein < 50	10	4	

TABLE 3 Growth Factor Expression in CML Ph^1 Bone Marrow Culture Adherent Layers

Patient	Blastic crisis morphologic characterization	Growth factor expression[a] IL-1β	IL-6	GM-CSF
A	Undifferentiated	++++	++++	++++
B	Undifferentiated	++	++	−
C	Undifferentiated	+	+	−
D	Myeloid	+	+	−
E	Myeloid	−	−	−
F	Mixed	+	+	−
G	Lymphoid	−	−	−
H	Lymphoid	−	−	−
I	Lymphoid	−	−	−
J	Lymphoid	−	−	−
N	Chronic	−	−	−

[a](++++) Maximal increased expression according to densitometric reading as shown in Figs. 2 and 3; (+++) from 75 to 51% of the maximum; (++) from 21 to 50% of the maximum; (+) from 1 to 20% of the maximum.

stantial evidence of the escape mechanism acquired by a malignant clone from control by growth inhibitory cytokines. Upon further confirmation, such overproduction of growth factors in a subset of patients may serve as a useful prognostic marker for disease progression and perhaps as a target for therapeutic intervention.

Finally, although the focus of this chapter is the direct antitumor activities of interferons in myeloproliferative disorders, immune-mediated mechanisms, such as activation of cytotoxic immune cells, may also play a role in the clinical activity of interferon in this disease (38). This needs to be studied further as well.

REFERENCES

1. Isaacs A, Lindemann J. Viros interference. 1. The interferon. Proc R Soc Lond [Biol] 1957; 147:258.
2. Borden EC, Fall LA. Interferons: biochemical, cell growth, inhibitory, and immunological effects. Prog Hematol 1981; 135:1.
3. Goepfert J, Sessions RB, Gutterman JU, et al. Leukocyte interferon in patients with juvenile laryngeal papillomatosis. Ann Otol Rhinol Laryngol 1982; 91:431.
4. Quesada JR, Reuben J, Manning JT, et al. Alpha interferon for induction of remission in hairy cell leukemia. N Engl J Med 1984; 310:15.
5. Gutterman JU, Blumenschein GR, Alexanian R, et al. Leukocyte interferon-induced tumor regression in human metastatic breast cancer, multiple myeloma, and malignant lymphoma. Ann Intern Med 1980; 93:399.
6. Foon KA, Sherwin SA, Abrams PG, et al. Treatment of advanced non-Hodgkin's lymphoma with recombinant leukocyte A interferon. N Engl J Med 1984; 311: 1148.
7. Oladipupo-Williams CK, Svet-Moldavskaya I, Vilcek J, Ohnuma T, Holland JF. Inhibitory effects of human leukocyte and fibroblast interferons on normal and chronic myelogenous leukemic granulocytic progenitor cells. Oncology 1981; 38:356–60.
8. Clarkson B, Strife A. Discordant maturation in chronic myelogenous leukemia. In: Deisseroth AB, Arlinghaus RB, eds. Chronic myelogenous leukemia: molecular approaches to research and therapy. New York: Dekker, 1991; 3–90.
9. Gordon MY, Dowding CR, Riley GP, Goldman JM, Greaves MF. Adhesive defects in chronic myeloid leukemia. Curr Top Microbiol Immunol 1989; 149:151–5.
10. Osterholz J, Dowding, C, Goldman JM. Interferon-alpha enhances the binding of CFU-GM from the marrow of patients with chronic myeloid leukemia (CML) to preformed stroma in long-term bone marrow culture (abstract). Blood 1989; 74:320a.
11. Upadhyaya G, Guba SC, Emerson ST, et al. Interferon-alpha restores the deficient expression of the cytoadhesion molecule LFA-3 by chronic myelogenous leukemia progenitor cells. J Clin Invest.
12. Wetzler M, Kurzrock R, Taylor K, et al. Constitutive and induced expression of growth factors in normal and chronic phase CML Ph^1 bone marrow stroma. Cancer Res 1990; 50:5801–5.

13. McCubrey JA, Steelman LS. Viral models for understanding chronic myelogenous leukemia. In: Deisseroth AB, Arlinghaus RB, eds. Chronic myelogenous leukemia: molecular approaches to research and therapy. New York: Dekker, 1991; 134–52.
14. Pfeffer LM, Donner DB, Tamm I. Interferon-alpha down-regulates insulin receptors in lymphoblastoid (Daudi) cells. Relationship to inhibition of cell proliferation. J Biol Chem 1987; 262:3665–70.
15. Pfeffer LM, Tamm I. Interferon-beta inhibition of concanavalin A-stimulated calcium uptake and exchange in HeLa cells. J Interferon Res 1986; 6:551–6.
16. Fish EN, Banerjee K. Growth control: characterizations of the antagonism between growth factors and interferon (abstract). J Interferon Res 1989; 9:2–7.
17. Pfeffer LM, Eisenkraft BL, Nanus DM, Albino AP. IFNα inhibits the proliferation of a subset of renal carcinoma cell lines and down-regulates epidermal growth factor receptors (abstract). J Interferon Res 1989; 9:2–9.
18. Maxwell B, Talpaz M, Gutterman JU. Down-regulation of peripheral blood cell interferon receptors in chronic myelogenous leukemia patients undergoing human interferon (HuIFN) therapy. Int J Cancer 1985; 36:23–8.
19. Rosenblum M, Maxwell B, Talpaz M, Kelleher P, McCredie K, Gutterman JU. In vivo sensitivity and resistance of chronic myelogenous leukemia cells to alpha interferon: correlation with receptor binding and induction of 2′5′ oligoadenylate synthetase. Cancer Res 1986; 46:4848–52.
20. Talpaz M, Chernajovsky Y, Troutman-Worden K, et al. Interferon stimulated genes in interferon-sensitive and -resistant chronic myelogenous leukemia (CML) patients. Submitted.
21. Levy D, Larner A, Chaudhuri A, Babiss LE, Darnell JE Jr. Interferon-stimulated transcription: isolation of an inducible gene and identification of its regulatory region. Proc Natl Acad Sci U S A 1986; 83:8929–33.
22. Larner AC, Chaudhuri A, Darnell JE Jr. Transcriptional induction by interferon. New protein(s) determine the extent and length of the induction. J Biol Chem 1986; 261:453–9.
23. Kelly JM, Porter ACG, Chernajovsky Y, Gilbert CS, Stark GR, Kerr IM. Characterization of a human gene inducible by α- and β-interferons and its expression in mouse cells. EMBO J 1986; 5:1601–6.
24. Rutherford MN, Hannigan GE, Williams BRG. Interferon-induced binding of nuclear factors to promoter elements of the 2-5A synthetase gene. EMBO J 1988; 7:751–9.
25. Rice AP, Kerr SM, Roberts WK, Brown RE, Kerr IM. Novel 2′,5′-oligoadenylates synthesized in interferon-treated, vaccinia virus-infected cells. J Virol 1985; 56:1041–4.
26. McMahon M, Stark GR, Kerr IM. Interferon-induced gene expression in wild-type and interferon-resistant human lymphoblastoid (Daudi) cells. J Virol 1986; 57:362–6.
27. Hovanessian AG, Galabru J, Svab J, Robert N. Characterization of the double-stranded RNA dependent protein kinase with a specific monoclonal antibody. In: Friedman RM, Merigan T, Sreevalsan T, eds. Interferons as cell growth inhibitors and antitumor factors. Proceedings of UCLA Symposia. Vol. 50. New York: Alan R. Liss, 1986; 35–48.

28. Reich N, Evans B, Levy D, Fahey D, Knight E Jr, Darnell JE Jr. Interferon-induced transcription of a gene encoding a 15-kDa protein depends on an upstream enhancer element. Proc Natl Acad Sci U S A 1987; 84:6394–8.
29. Dron M, Tovey MG, Eid P. Isolation of Daudi cells with reduced sensitivity to interferon. III. Interferon-induced proteins in relation to the phenotype of interferon resistance. J Gen Virol 1985; 66:787–95.
30. Dron M, Tovey MG. Isolation of Daudi cells with reduced sensitivity to interferon. I. Characterization. J Gen Virol 1983; 64:2641–7.
31. Hannigan GE, Gewert DR, Williams BRG. Characterization and regulation of α-interferon receptor expression in interferon-sensitive and -resistant human lymphoblastoid cells. J Biol Chem 1984; 259:9456–60.
32. Affabris E, Romeo G, Belardelli F, et al. 2-5A synthetase activity does not increase in interferon-resistant Friend leukemia cell variants treated with α/β interferon despite the presence of high-affinity interferon receptor sites. Virology 1983; 125:508–12.
33. Reid TR, Race ER, Wolff BH, Friedman RM, Merigan TC, Basham TY. Enhanced in vivo therapeutic response to interferon in mice with an in vitro interferon-resistant B-cell lymphoma. Cancer Res 1989; 49:4163–9.
34. Silverman RH, Watling D, Balkwill FR, Trowsdale J, Kerr IM. The $ppp(A2'p)_nA$ and protein kinase systems in wild-type and interferon-resistant Daudi cells. Eur J Biochem 1982; 126:333–41.
35. Estrov Z, Kurzrock R, Wetzler M, et al. Suppression of chronic myelogenous leukemia colony growth by IL-1 receptor antagonist and soluble IL-1 receptors: a novel application for inhibitors of IL-1 activity. Blood 1991; 78(6):1476–84.
36. Wetzler M, Kurzrock R, Estrov Z, et al. Constitutive expression of IL-1β correlates with interferon-α resistance in CML. Blood 1991; 76:335a.
37. Wetzler M, Kurzrock R, Lowe D, Kantarjian H, Gutterman JU, Talpaz M. Alteration in bone marrow stromal growth factor expression—a possible mechanism of disease progression in chronic myelogenous leukemia (abstract). AACR Proc 1990; 31:179.
38. Lotzova E. Role of natural killer cells in defense against leukemia: therapeutic considerations. Nat Immun Cell Growth Regul 1988; 7:170–9.

4

Therapy of CML and Myeloproliferative Disorders with Interferons

Moshe Talpaz, Hagop Kantarjian, Razelle Kurzrock, and Jordan U. Gutterman

University of Texas, M.D. Anderson Cancer Center, Houston, Texas

I. INTRODUCTION

Myeloproliferative disorders are hematopoietic stem cell disorders that include chronic myelogenous leukemia (CML), polycythemia vera, agnogenic myeloid metaplasia, and essential thrombocythemia and are characterized by the following:

1. Deranged growth leading to expansion of myeloid progeny, such as expansion of the granulocytic series in CML; however, unlike acute leukemias, terminal differentiation is maintained.
2. A progressive clinical course that reflects the underlying genetic instability in the involved stem cell; in CML, this progression is mainifested by the preordained regular transition from the chronic phase to the blastic phase, whereas in the other myeloproliferative disorders, such changes occur but with a much lower frequency.

II. CLINICAL AND LABORATORY FEATURES OF CML

CML accounts for about 25% of adult leukemias and has an incidence of 1 case per 100,000 persons per year (1,2).

In the early benign stage, patients are asymptomatic or complain of unexplained fatigue. Physical examination often reveals splenomegaly and slight hepatomegaly. Blood tests reveal leukocytosis and occasional thrombocytosis (3,4). The bone marrow is hypercellular with granulocytic hyperplasia. Other characteristic laboratory abnormalities include a low or undetectable neutrophil alkaline phosphatase (5) and high serum vitamin B_{12} levels (6). In about 90% of patients, karyotype studies of bone marrow demonstrate a shortened chromosome 22, the Philadelphia (Ph^1) chromosome.

The benign phase of CML can be easily controlled by oral chemotherapeutics, such as busulfan or hydroxyurea. However, these therapies fail to alter the progressive course of the disease and these patients are at constant risk of developing a blastic phase. Although the duration of the benign phase varies considerably from patient to patient, the average risk of blastic transformation is 25%/year after the second year of the benign phase (7–9). The phenotype of the blasts can be myeloid, lymphoid, erythroid, megakaryocytic, promyelocytic, or undifferentiated (10–16). Myeloid and lymphoid blast crises are the most frequent phenotypes, constituting about 65 and 25% of cases, respectively.

III. INTERFERONS IN CML

Interferon activity was discovered by Isaacs and Lindenmann in 1957 (17), but subsequently it was found to consist of a complex group of naturally occurring proteins produced by eukaryotic cells in response to viruses, antigens, and mitogens (18). These proteins exhibit pleiotropic biologic activities, including potent antiproliferative, immunomodulatory, antiviral, and differentiation-inducing effects (19). Interferons are currently classified according to various biochemical and antigenic properties into three groups: interferon-α (IFN-α), interferon-β (IFN-β), and IFN-γ. IFN-α and IFN-β are acid stable and are produced primarily by leukocytes and fibroblasts, respectively. In contrast, IFN-γ is an acid-labile, structurally distinct molecule produced mainly by T lymphocytes (20).

Since 1981, we have conducted a series of clinical trials with interferons in Ph^1 CML. The interferons that have been investigated include partially pure IFN-α, recombinant IFN-α (rIFN-α), rIFN-γ, and combinations of α and γ interferons. More recent studies evaluated combinations of chemotherapy and interferon, as well as autologous bone marrow transplantation and interferons.

A. Interferon-α

In the first studies, the role of partially pure alpha interferon-α (Finnish Red Cross, Helsinki, Finland) was examined in CML. IFN-α given at doses of 3–9 X 10^6 U/day was effective in normalizing excessive white blood cells and platelets in patients with benign-phase CML Ph^1 (21). This led subsequently to a larger study of 51 CML patients. The responses to interferon among these pa-

TABLE 1 Response Criteria for Interferon Therapy in CML

Hematologic remission	WBC count	Splenomegaly	Cytogenetic remission	Percentage Ph^1 of bone marrow
Complete	$<9 \times 10^3$ per μl normal morphology	None	Complete	0
Partial	$<20 \times 10^3$ per μl and $>50\%$ decline	Persistence	Partial	≤35
Failure	$>20 \times 10^3$	Persistence	Minor	35–95
			None	100

tients also required the establishment of response criteria (Table 1), which are now widely accepted.

Of 51 patients, 36 (71%) achieved complete hematologic remission. Other laboratory indices of disease activity, such as elevated lactate dehydrogenase levels, elevated levels of serum and vitamin B_{12}, and increased bone marrow cellularity, normalized as well. In a smaller fraction of the patients (41%), we noted cytogenetic responses with various degrees of Ph^1 chromosome suppression. Furthermore, in 7 patients a complete suppression of the Ph^1 clone was noted on at least one test, and partial suppression (≤35% Ph^1 chromosome) was seen in 3 additional patients (22,23).

A multivariate regression model derived from a population of chemotherapy-treated patients identified three prognostic groups with distinct clinical outcome among patients with chronic-phase CML Ph^1 (24). This model was applied to the interferon-treated patients and demonstrated that low-risk patients are more likely to respond hematologically and cytogenetically, whereas patients with high-risk features are less likely to respond (Table 2).

Studies with recombinant interferon-α followed the initial studies. Recombinant interferon-α_{2a} (Roferon; Hoffmann-LaRoche, Nutley, NJ) was administered at an initial dose of 5×10^6 U/m^2 intramuscularly (IM) daily (25) and demonstrated a response rate of 75% (34 of 45 patients studied) in early CML Ph^1 (≥ 1 year from diagnosis). In this study, 11 patients (23%) achieved complete cytogenetic response on at least one test. Partial cytogenetic responses were seen in 3 additional patients (23).

Confirmatory studies were carried out by several additional groups and essentially demonstrated similar activities. Niederle et al. reported on 40 of 59 CML Ph^1 patients treated with rIFN-α_{2b} at 4×10^6 U/m^2/daily. Of these patients 33% also had cytogenetic responses (26). Alimena et al. studied 63 CML Ph^1 patients in the benign phase treated at doses between 2 and 5×10^6 U/m^2 IM daily. Hemotologic responses were seen in 68% of the patients, and 37 (56%) also had various degrees of cytogenetic responses (27). The Cancer and Leuke-

TABLE 2 Results of Partially Purified Interferon-α Therapy in 51 Patients with Benign-Phase CML

Category	Number of patients in risk category (%)[a]							
	Total		Low		Intermediate		High	
Complete hematologic remission	36 (71)		18 (82)		10 (62)		7 (64)	
Philadelphia chromosome status, %								
100	15 (29)		4 (18)		3 (19)		7 (64)	
35–95	11 (21)	41%	10 (46)	66%	1 (6)	44%	—	0
5–34	3 (6)		1 (6)		2 (13)		—	
0	7 (14)		3 (14)		4 (25)		—	
Partial hematologic remission	5 (10)		2 (9)		3 (19)		—	
Resistant disease	10 (20)		2 (9)		3 (19)		4 (36)	
Total	51 (100)		22 (100)		16 (100)		11 (100)	

[a]Pretreatment characteristics to determine risk category were not available for two patients: one had resistant disease and died in accelerated phase, and one achieved complete hematologic remission but no Ph[1] suppression.

mia Group B (CALGB) studied 128 patients, all newly diagnosed and previously untreated. Patients were treated with rIFN-α_{2b} (Intron) at 5 × 10^6 U/m^2 daily. Of 47 evaluable patients, 27 (57%) achieved complete hematologic remission; 40% of the patients also exhibited various degrees of chimerism (28,29).

The commonly used doses of IFN-α in these studies ranged from 2 to 5 × 10^6 U/M^2 daily. However, only one study (27) formally examined the association between dose of therapy and response and demonstrated a higher response rate in the higher dose-treated group (Table 3) and also a high response rate among patients treated with 5 × 10^6 U/m^2 of rIFN-α_{2b} after failing a lower dose of 2 × 10^6 U/m^2. It therefore appears that the effective dose of IFN-α in CML is considerably higher than in hairy cell leukemia. Furthermore, high doses of IFN-α are associated with a higher incidence of hematologic remissions. It is not known, however, whether further escalation of the IFN-α dose beyond 5 × 10^6 U/m^2 will also increase the frequency of cytogenetic responses.

A hematologic response rate between 50 and 70% was consistently seen in patients who were treated within a short period from diagnosis (<1 year). The question of whether patients with long-standing disease will respond as well was addressed by us, and we have noted (Table 4) that in patients with disease du-

TABLE 3 Response of CML Patients According to Disease Status, Schedule, and Dose of IFN Treatment[a]

Patient	IFN dose	No. patients evaluable	No. of responders (%) Total	CHR	PHR
CP, untreated	R1	13	5 (38.5)	5 (38.5)	1 (7)
IT	R2	14	8 (57)	7 (50)	3 (37)
	R1 R2	8	6 (75)	3 (37)	3 (37)
CP, pretreated	R1	20	4 (20)	3 (15)	1 (5)
IT	R2	16	11 (69)	7 (37.5)	4 (25)
	R1 R2	13	9 (77)	4 (30)	5 (38.5)
AP	R2	9	3 (33)	1 (11)	2 (22)
IT					
CP, untreated	R1	4	3 (75)	3 (75)	—
DT	R1 R2	4	4 (100)	4 (100)	—

[a]R1 = 2×10^6 IU/m^2 IFN dose; R2 = 5×10^6 IU/m^2 IFN dose. CP, chronic phase; AP, accelerated phase; IT, intermittent treatment; DT, daily treatment. Patients assigned to R1 and subsequently crossed to R2 owing to nonresponse.

Source: From Alimena G, et al. Interferon alpha-2b as therapy for Ph-positive chronic myelogenous leukemia: a study of 82 patients treated with intermittent or daily administration. Blood 1988; 72:642.

ration of greater than 1 year there was a dramatic decline in response rate, whereas complete and partial cytogenetic responses were not seen at all in this group of patients.

1. Complete Cytogenetic Responses with Interferon-α

In the interferon-α studies, we noticed a small, albeit consistent fraction of the treated patients who achieved a complete cytogenetic response. In a recent analysis of 96 patients who were treated with either partially pure IFN-α (51 patients) or the recombinant inferferon-α_{2a} (45 patients), 18 (19%) achieved a complete cytogenetic response on at least one test. Of those, 11 (12% of the total patient population) have had ongoing complete remission for periods ranging from 6^+ to 48^+ months (median 30^+ months) (23).

Although cytogenetic responses were seen before with intensive chemotherapy regimens (30–37), these were not durable, and virtually all patients relapsed within a median period of 6 months. Studies with IFN-α are therefore the first to demonstrate a durable complete cytogenetic remission.

We conducted Southern blot analysis of DNA extracted from chronic myelogenous leukemia (CML) patients in complete cytogenetic response. This DNA was hybridized to a breakage cluster region (bcr) probe from chromosome 22, which corresponds to the breakage area in the Ph^1 chromosome. No residual

TABLE 4 Hematologic and Cytogenetic Responses Among Ph[1] CML Patients Treated with Recombinant Interferon α_{2a}.

	Disease duration			
	≤1 year		>1 year	
Number of patients studied	45		16	
Complete hematologic remission	34	(75%)	4	(25%)
Philadelphia chromosome status				
No cytogenetic response	11	(44%)	1	(25%)
>35–95%	9		3	
>5–<35%	3	(31%)	–	(0%)
0%	11		–	
Partial hematologic remission	2	(4%)	1	(6%)
Resistant disease	9	(21%)	11	(69%)

population of abnormal cells was detected by this assay. However, the level of sensitivity of this assay was not superior to cytogenetic analysis although it was useful in monitoring patients with Ph bcr-rearranged CML, as well as patients on interferon therapy in whom low bone marrow cellularity and low proliferative activity of the myeloid precursors result in a low yield of analyzable metaphase (38).

A polymerase chain reaction (PCR) assay can selectively amplify in vitro specific DNA segments. In the case of CML Ph[1], oligoprimers corresponding to the abl and the bcr components of the *bcr-abl* gene have been constructed and allow the in vitro amplification of a c-DNA of *bcr-abl* mRNA. Two types of RNA are formed by the Ph[1] rearrangement. This provided a means to detect one Ph[1]-positive cell in 10^5–10^6 cells (39). A group of 18 patients in complete cytogenetic response following therapy with IFN-α were subjected to PCR and then hybridized to a bcr probe (40). Evidence for residual disease was demonstrated in 17 of the patients, and in 1 patient no residual disease could be detected. The significance of these findings is not clear at this point, and they will have to be compared with the clinical outcome. This is highlighted by the case of a patient who achieved a complete cytogenetic response and was taken off therapy with IFN-α. During the 15 month follow-up since therapy cessation, she has had no evidence of either cytogenetic or clinical relapse although residual disease could have been demonstrated by PCR analysis before therapy discontinuation.

Further studies of "true" minimal residual disease will focus on the nature of the remaining cells to determine whether they are clonogenic with proliferative potential or whether they represent a population of "mature" nondividing cells that carry the genotype but have lost the malignant potential.

2. Survival of IFN-α-Treated Patients

Although several controlled studies comparing the effects of interferon to those of standard therapies are currently in progress, none has been followed for a sufficient period to provide information on survival outcome. However, two single-arm studies at the M. D. Anderson Cancer Center (MDACC) have been followed now for a period exceeding 7 years. The overall survival of patients in these studies (51 patients treated with IFN-α and 45 treated with rIFN-α_{2a}) has been 62 months and does not differ between the two studies ($P > 0.2$ by the log arithmic rank test) (Fig. 1). This survival exceeds the MDACC experience of 39 months of median survival among patients treated with various chemotherapies (23).

This survival may in part be affected by changes in referral patterns, earlier diagnosis, and improvement in supportive care and thereby preclude assessment of change in survival outcome with interferon therapy at this point. However, the dismal 10 year survival of patients with CML on chemotherapy ($\leq 5\%$) is less likely to be affected by patient selection because even low-risk patients are unlikely to survive 10 years. If, at that point, we are able to demonstrate a substantial number of patients alive in remission, this will provide strong support to the notion that IFN-α affects survival of CML Ph^1 patients.

B. Interferons in Combination with Other Treatment Modalities in CML

Shortly after the demonstration of IFN-α activity in CML, several groups initiated studies combining IFN-α and chemotherapy either as maintenance therapy after chemotherapy-induced remission or in combination with chemotherapy. Bergsagel et al. (41) examined the ability of rIFN-α_2b to maintain remission induced by busulfan. The starting dose of IFN in this study was 2×10^6 U/m^2 three times weekly. This dose was escalated in some patients. In six of eight patients studied, remission was maintained for $3^+ - 24^+$ months.

To examine if IFN-α can maintain remission induced by intensive chemotherapy, patients at the M. D. Anderson Cancer Center were given one to three cycles of intensive chemotherapy with daunorubicin, vincristine, cytarabine, and prednisone (DOAP) followed by IFN-α maintenance (42). Of the 32 patients studied in the benign phase of CML Ph^1, 28 (86%) had Ph^1 suppression with intensive chemotherapy; 21 (66%) of them have Ph^1 suppression to $<35\%$. This effect was transient in the majority of the patients, but cytogenetic remission was maintained in 8 patients (31%) for 12^+ months, for a range of $21^+ - 42^+$ months.

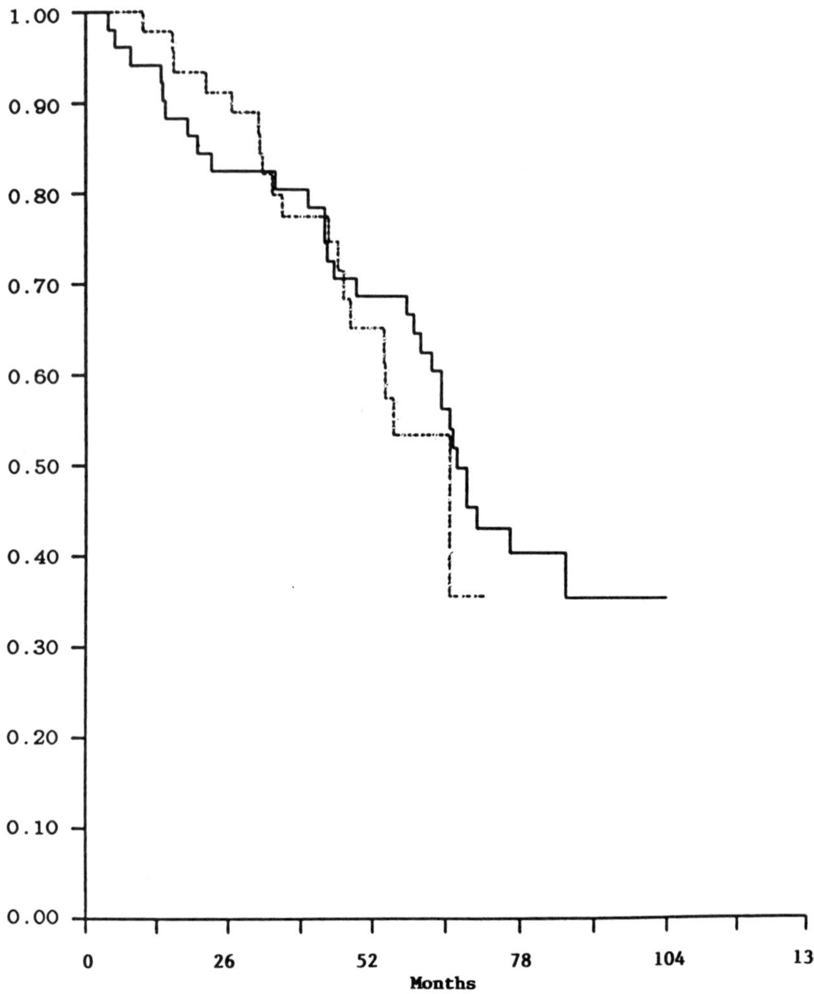

FIGURE 1 Kaplan-Meier estimate of the probability of survival of patients treated with interferon-α (IFN-α) ——— or recombinant IFN-α (rIFN-α_{2a}), ------ ($P > 0.20$).

Concomitant administration of IFN-α with various chemotherapies was recently studied by several investigators. The combination of IFN-α, low-dose Ara-C (cytarabine), and hydroxyurea was studied by Ma and Arthur (43). They noted 2 complete and 2 partial cytogenetic responses in 8 patients with early (≤1 year) CML Ph^1, and 3 minor cytogenetic responses of 5 patients with long-standing CML. Similar observations were seen by Guilhot et al. (44), who noted complete and partial cytogenetic responses (0–10% Ph^1) in 3 of 12 patients with early CML and in 3 of 10 previously treated CML patients.

At MDACC, we studied the combination of rIFN-α_{a2} and low-dose Ara-C in patients with advanced stages of CML Ph[1] either in the long-standing benign phase or in the accelerated phase of the disease (45). The results compare favorably with the results of IFN-α in a similar patient population. Furthermore, suppression of secondary clones was noted in 5 of 16 patients with clonal evolution treated with the combination. Overall, the combination therapy studies have not accrued a sufficient number of patients, nor have they been followed for a long enough period to conclude whether the addition of chemotherapy improves the outcome.

C. Interferon-α and Bone Marrow Transplantation in the Management of CML Ph[1]

A small percentage of patients who undergo allogeneic bone marrow transplantation exhibit disease relapse. This problem, however, is more common among patients who are transplanted in the accelerated phase, or blastic crisis phase, of the disease. Since it is plausible that IFN-α may be more active in minimal residual disease, two groups of investigators examined the role of IFN-α after transplantation.

Higano et al. (46) demonstrated that among patients with relapse after transplant, reinduction of complete cytogenetic remission was achieved in 1 and partial cytogenetic response in 3. These patients were managed with considerably lower doses of interferon than those commonly used in the management of CML. In an Italian study of patients who relapsed after allogeneic bone marrow transplantation with T cell-depleted marrow, cytogenetic improvements were seen only in patients with confined cytogenetic relapse (2 of 14 of whom achieved complete cytogenetic response).

In a different approach (47) IFN-α was administered in patients after *autologous* bone marrow transplantation at MDACC. All the patients were resistant to IFN-α at the time they were studied. In preliminary data, we noted reestablishment of IFN-α sensitivity in three patients, one with an ongoing cytogenetic response for 12^+ months.

The addition of interferons in vitro to bone marrow cultures to improve the recovery of cells with normal karyotype was examined by McGlave et al. (48). They treated bone marrow cultures from eight CML patients with IFN-γ, reinfusing the marrow to the patients. Three patients developed complete cytogenetic response, and four patients developed partial cytogenetic responses following autologous bone marrow transplantation with the cultured marrow.

All these studies support a role for IFN-α in conjunction with autologous and allogeneic bone marrow transplantation. However, the vast heterogeneity in the clinical outcome of patients undergoing these procedures will require identification of patient subsets (early disease and cytogenetic relapse only) who are likely to benefit from the addition of IFN-α to therapy. Future goals should include studies in patients with a high risk of relapse (T cell-depleted mismatched transplant and transplant in accelerated phase and blast crisis) in whom interferon should probably be started shortly after hematopoietic recovery from transplant.

D. Interferon-γ in CML

Although IFN-γ is structurally distinct from IFN-α, it suppresses in vitro hematopoietic progenitor cells in a fashion similar to that of IFN-α (49–51). We therefore carried out a study of rIFN-γ (Genentech, South San Francisco, CA) at doses of 0.25–0.5 mg/m^2/day IM (5–10 $\times$ 10^6 U/m^2) in patients with benign-phase Ph^1-positive CML (52). Of 30 patients entered in the study, 26 were evaluable; 6 patients have achieved a complete hematologic response and 4 a partial hematologic response. Cytogenetic improvement has been seen in 5 patients, with emergence of 10–45% diploid cells in the bone marrow. Control of thrombocytosis was achieved in all 4 patients with baseline platelet counts of $>1 \times 10^6$ per μl. In these patients, the median pretherapy platelet count was 12×10^6 per μl; the median posttherapy nadir counts were 450×10^3 per μl. Fever and flulike symptoms were the most common side effects, with partial tachyphylaxis often developing after about 1 week. The majority of patients tolerated therapy with minimal change in performance status.

To determine the prevalence of cross-resistance, we treated patients who failed one interferon species with an alternative species. A group of 14 patients who failed IFN-α were subsequently treated with rIFN-γ: 2 patients achieved a complete hematologic remission, and 2 achieved a partial hematologic remission. Conversely, 12 patients who failed rIFN-γ were subsequently treated with rIFN-α. Of these patients 2 achieved a complete hematologic remission and 1 a partial hematologic remission. From these results, it is apparent that patients who are resistant to IFN-γ can respond to IFN-α, and vice versa. On the basis of these data and the documented in vitro synergistic antiproliferative activity of the two interferons, we also carried out studies combining the two interferons, but preliminary data failed to demonstrate increased activity of the combination.

IV. INTERFERON FOR THE MANAGEMENT OF ESSENTIAL THROMBOCYTHEMIA, POLYCYTHEMIA VERA, AND OTHER PHILADELPHIA CHROMOSOME-NEGATIVE MYELOPROLIFERATIVE DISORDERS

Myeloproliferative disorders, such as essential thrombocythemia, polycythemia vera, and agnogenic myeloid metaplasia, display a pathophysiologic resemblance to CML Ph^1 (53), all sharing the salient features of clonal expansion of a pluripotent hematopoietic stem cell, deranged growth of various components of the myeloid system, and a preordained progression toward an acute leukemia phenotype.

Patients with essential thrombocythemia, polycythemia vera, and agnogenic myeloid metaplasia have a much lower risk of disease transformation than patients with CML Ph[1] but may be at risk from complications related to the increased number of platelets or red blood cells, such as thromboembolic complications or hemorrhagic diathesis, which occasionally mandate expeditious therapy (54–57).

The initial observation that IFN-α causes a dramatic decline in platelet count among patients with long-standing Ph[1] CML complicated with thrombocytosis (58) was pursued by studies on the role of IFN-α in essential thrombocythemia. In a cumulative experience in >100 patients, a response rate of 88% was observed. Typically, the patients showed a prompt response to IFN-α. The average time for a 50% reduction in the platelet counts was between 2 and 3 weeks (59–66). Patients with elevated white blood cell counts also demonstrate a decline in this cell population. The duration of response varies considerably. Gradual increases in platelet counts was noted in studies that incorporated dose reduction with maintenance therapy. However, durable and ongoing remissions were noted as well. Gisslinger et al. noted that remissions were maintained as long as therapy continued. Rapid relapse (within 1 month) was noted when therapy was discontinued in a subset of patients after 1 year of therapy (62).

The mechanisms of action of IFN-α in this condition remain unknown but could consist of platelet precursor inhibition and, alternatively, accelerated peripheral blood platelet clearance. The latter option is supported by the finding of α-IFN-induced, immune-mediated thrombocytopenia (67) and by the fact that in Ph[1] CML we noted that frequently a response was confined to the platelets, whereas the white blood count (WBC) continued to increase (58), an observation suggestive of a selective antiplatelet effect rather than general suppression of bone marrow hematopoietic precursors by the IFN-α.

Polycythemia vera is another condition that may respond to IFN-α. Thus far only anecdotal reports point to the activity of IFN-α in this condition (68), whereas patients with agnogenic myeloid metaplasia had either marginal responses (69) or no response at all (M. Talpaz, unpublished results).

In a series of studies over the last 9 years, we have demonstrated that IFN-α and, to a lesser extent, IFN-γ have antileukemic activity in CML. The key observations in these studies were that IFN-α induces hematologic remission in 60–70% of patients with early benign phase and, more importantly, that varying degrees of Ph chromosome suppressor occur in about 40% of the patients, some of whom had complete cytogenetic responses.

The effect of IFN-α on survival cannot be fully assessed because of the uncontrolled nature of the studies thus far. However, emerging patterns include a higher activity of IFN-α in patients with favorable prognoses; a clinical outcome that compares favorably with that of the commonly used chemotherapeutic agents; and the discovery of a subset of patients who may experience a sustained complete cytogenetic and clinical remission.

Complete cytogenetic response should become the objective of interferon therapy. The implementation of several concepts may maximize Ph chromosome suppression in future studies. Refinement of single-agent therapy is unlikely to significantly change therapy outcome, but various combinations of interferon and chemotherapies may be superior to interferon alone. Also, the development of biologic therapies for the management of minimal residual disease after allogeneic and autologous transplants may further improve therapy outcome in CML.

Understanding the mechanisms leading to the deranged growth of the malignant clone, as well as the growth arrest of the residual "normal" stem cells, is likely to yield therapies geared at improving the suppression of the malignant clone and restoring the normal stem cells. Potential therapies may include diverse biologic agents, both growth inhibitory and growth stimulatory. Therapies directed toward the enhancement of the bone marrow cellular immune response may also be applicable for the management of minimal residual disease.

REFERENCES

1. Koeffler HP, Golde DW. Chronic myelogenous leukemia—new concepts. N Engl J Med 1981; 304:1201.
2. Young JL Jr, Percy CL, Asire AJ, et al. Cancer incidence and mortality in the United States, 1973–77. National Cancer Institute Monograph No. 57. Bethesda, Md: NCI, Surveillance, Epidemiology, and End Results Program, 1978.
3. Spiers ASD, Bain BJ, Turner JE. The peripheral blood in chronic granuloctytic leukaemia: study of 50 untreated Philadelphia-positive cases. Scand J Haematol 1977; 18:25–38.
4. Mason JE Jr, DeVita VT, Canellos GP. Thrombocytosis in chronic granulocytic leukemia: incidence and clinical significance. Blood 1974; 44:483.
5. Rosner F, Schreiber ZR, Parise F. Leukocyte alkaline phosphatase: fluctuations with disease status in chronic granulocytic leukemia. Arch Intern Med 1972; 130:892.
6. Gilbert HS, Krauss S, Pasternack B, Pasternack B, Herbert V, Wasserman LR. Serum vitamin B_{12} content and unsaturated vitamin B_{12}-binding capacity in myeloproliferative disease: value in differential diagnosis and indicators of diagnosis and indicators of disease activity. Ann Intern Med 1976; 71:719–29.
7. Minot GR, Buckman TE, Isaacs R. Chronic myelogenous leukemia: age, incidence, duration, and benefit derived from irradiation. JAMA 1924; 82:1489–94.
8. Inbal A, Akstein E, Barak I, Meytes D, Many A. Cyclic leukocytosis and long survival in chronic myeloid leukemia. Acta Haematol (Basel) 1983; 69:353–7.
9. Sokol JE, Cox EB, Baccarini M, et al., and the Italian Cooperative CML Study Group. Prognostic discrimination in "good risk" chronic granulocytic leukemia. Blood 1984; 63:789–99.
10. Rosenthal S, Canellos GP, DeVita V Jr, Gralnick HR. Characteristics of blast crisis in chronic granulocytic leukemia. Blood 1977; 49:705.

11. Rosenthal S, Canellos GP, Whang-Peng J, Gralnick HR. Blast crisis of chronic granulocytic leukemia. Morphologic variants and therapeutic implications. Am J Med 1977; 63:542.
12. Rosenthal S, Canellos GP, Gralnick H. Erythroblastic transformation of chronic granulocytic leukemia. Am J Med 1977; 63:116.
13. Breton-Gorius J, Reyes F, Bernant JP, Tulliez M, Dreyfus B. The blast crisis of chronic granulocytic leukaemia: megakaryoblastic nature of cells as revealed by presence of platelet-peroxidase—a cytochemical ultrastructural study. Br J Haematol 1978; 39:295.
14. Griffin JD, Todd RF, Ritz J, et al. Differentiation patterns in the blastic phase of chronic myeloid leukemia. Blood 1983; 61:85.
15. Ekblom M, Borgstrom G, Willebrand E, Gahmberg CG, Vuopio P, Andersson LC. Erythroid blast crisis in chronic myelogenous leukemia. Blood 1983; 62:591–6.
16. Bain B, Catovsky D, O'Brien M, Spiers ASD, Richards GH. Megakaryoblastic transformation of chronic granulocytic leukaemia. An electron microscopy and cytochemical study. J Clin Pathol 1977; 30:235–42.
17. Isaacs A, Lindemann J. Virus interference. 1. The interferon. Proc R Soc Lond [Biol] 1957; 147:258–67.
18. Steward WEI, ed. The interferon system. New York: Springer-Verlag, 1979.
19. Borden EC, Fall LA. Interferons: biochemical, cell growth, inhibitory, and immunological effects. Prog Hematol 1981; 350:1.
20. Vilcek J, Gray PW, Rinderknecht E, Sevastopoulos CG. Interferon-gamma: a lymphokine for all seasons. Lymphokines 1985; 11:1.
21. Talpaz M, McCredie KB, Mavligit GM, Gutterman JU. Leukocyte interferon-induced myeloid cytoreduction in chronic myelogenous leukemia. Blood 1983; 62:689–92.
22. Talpaz M, Kantarjian HM, McCredie KB, Keating MJ, Trujillo J, Gutterman J. Clinical investigation of human alpha interferon in chronic myelogenous leukemia. Blood 1987; 69:1280–8.
23. Talpa M, Kantarjian H, Kurzrock R, Trujillo JM, Gutterman JU. Interferon-alpha produces sustained cytogenetic responses in chronic myelogenous leukemia. Ann Intern Med 1991; 114:532–8.
24. Kantarjian HM, Smith TL, McCredie KB, et al. Chronic myelogenous leukemia: a multivariate analysis of the associations of patient characteristics and therapy with survival. Blood 1985; 66:1326–35.
25. Talpaz M, Kantarjian HM, McCredie KB, Trujillo JM, Keating MJ, Gutterman JU. Hematologic remission and cytogenic improvement induced by recombinant human interferon alpha in chronic myelogenous leukemia. N Engl J Med 1986; 314:1065-9.
26. Niederle N, Doberauer C, Kloke O, Osieka R, Schweers C, Schmidt CG. Treatment of chronic myelogenous leukemia with recombinant interferon alpha (IFN-α2b). Proc Am Soc Clin Oncol 1986; 5:236.
27. Alimena G, Morra E, Lazzarino M, et al. Interferon alpha-2b as therapy for Ph^1-positive chronic myelogenous leukemia: a study of 82 patients treated with intermittent or daily administration. Blood 1988; 72:642–7.
28. Ozer H, Mich R, Testa J, et al. Subcutaneous α-interferon (α-IFN) shows substantial activity in untreated chronic phase myelogenous leukemia (CML) (Abstract). Proc Am Soc Clin Oncol 1988; 7:177.

29. Ozer H. Biotherapy of chronic myelogenous leukemia with interferon. Semin Oncol 1988; 15:14–20.
30. Clarkson B. Chronic myelogenous leukemia: is aggressive treatment indicated? J Clin Oncol 1985; 3:135.
31. Brodsky I, Fuscaldo KE, Kahn SB, Conroy JF, Lamping CG. Chronic myelogenous leukemia. A clinical and experimental evaluation of splenectomy and intensive chemotherapy. Semin Hematol 1975; 8:143.
32. Smalley RV, Vogel J, Huguley CM Jr, Miller D. Chronic Vilcek granulocytic leukemia: cytogenetic conversion of the bone marrow with cycle-specific chemotherapy. Blood 1977; 50:107.
33. Cunningham I, Gee T, Dowling M, et al. Results of treatment of Ph^{1+} chronic myelogenous leukemia with an intensive treatment regimen (L-5 protocol). Blood 1979; 53:375.
34. Goto T, Nishikori M, Arlin Z, et al. Growth characteristics of leukemic and normal hematopoietic cells in Ph^{1+} chronic myelogenous leukemia and effects of intensive treatment. Blood 1982; 59:793.
35. Kantarjian HM, Vellekoop L, McCredie KB, et al. Intensive combination chemotherapy (ROAP 10) and splenectomy in the management of chronic myelogenous leukemia. J Clin Oncol 1985; 3:192–200.
36. Hester JP, Waddell CC, Coltman CA Jr, et al. Response of chronic myelogenous leukemia patients to COAP-splenectomy. Cancer 1984; 54:1977–82.
37. Sharp JC, Joyner MV, Wayne AW, et al. Karyotypic conversion in Ph^1-positive chronic myeloid leukaemia with combination chemotherapy. Lancet 1979; 1:1370.
38. Yoffe G, Blick M, Kantarjian H, Spitzer G, Gutterman J, Talpaz M. Molecular analysis of interferon-induced suppression of Philadelphia chromosome in patients with chronic myeloid leukemia. Blood 1987; 69:961–3.
39. Lee MS, Chang KS, Freireich EJ, et al. Detection of minimal residual bcr/abl transcripts by a modified polymerase chain reaction. Blood 1988; 72:893–7.
40. Dhingra K, Kurzrock R, Kantarjian H, Gutterman JU, Talpaz M. Polymerase chain reaction (PCR) for minimal residual disease in 20 CML patients in complete cytogenetic response induced by interferon therapy (abstract). Blood 1989; 74:235a.
41. Bergsagel DE, Haas RH, Messner HA. Interferon alpha 2 in treatment of chronic granulocytic leukemia. Semin Oncol 1986; 13:29.
42. Kantarjian H, Talpaz M, Keating M, et al. Therapy of Philadelphia chromosome (Ph)-positive chronic myelogenous leukemia with initial intensive chemotherapy (DOAP) followed by maintenance with human leukocyte alpha interferon (abstract). Blood 1986; 67:224a.
43. Ma DDF, Arthur CK. Treatment of chronic myeloid leukemia (CML) using alpha-interferon (IFN), and low dose cytosine arabinoside (ara-C) (abstract). Blood 1989; 74:363a.
44. Guilhot F, Tanzer J, Brizard A, Huret JL, Dreyfus B. Combination of alpha2a interferon and chemotherapy in Ph^+ chronic myelogenous leukemia (CML) updated results. Proc Am Soc Clin Oncol 1989; 8:203.
45. Kantarjian H, Keating M, McCredie K, Gutterman J, Freireich A, Talpa M. Treatment of advanced stages of Philadelphia-chromosome (Ph)-positive chronic my-

elogenous leukemia (CML) with alpha interferon (IFN-A) and low-dose cytosine arabinoside (ara-C) (abstract). Blood 1989; 74:235a.

46. Higano CS, Raskind W, Durnam D, Singer JW. Alpha interferon (IF) induces cytogenetic remission in patients who relapse with chronic myelogenous leukemia (CML) after allogeneic bone marrow transplantation (BMT) (abstract). Blood 1989; 74:83a.
47. Kantarjian H, Talpaz M, Spinolo J, et al. High doses of cyclophosphamids, BCNU and etoposide induce cytogenetic responses in most patients with advanced stages of Philadelphia chromosome-positive chronic myelogenous leukemia (CML) (abstract). Blood 1989; 74:2273a.
48. McGlave P, Miller W, Arthur D, et al. Ph^1 mosaicism after autologous transplantation (ABMT) for CML with gamma interferon treated bone marrow (abstract). Blood 1989; 74:281a.
49. Klimpel GR, Fleischmann WF Jr, Klimpel KD. Gamma interferon (IFN-gamma) and IFN-alpha/beta suppress murine myeloid colony formation (CFUOC): magnitude of suppression is dependent upon level of colony-stimulating factor CSF). J Immunol 1982; 129:76.
50. Raefsky EL, Platanias LC, Zoumbos NC, Young NS. Studies of interferon as a regulator of hematopoietic cell proliferation. J Immunol 1982; 135:2507.
51. Broxmeyer HE, Williams DE, Lu L, et al. The suppressive influences of human tumor necrosis factor on bone marrow hematopoietic progenitor cells from normal donors and patients with leukemia: synergism of tumor necrosis factor and interferon-gamma. J Immunol 1986; 136:4487.
52. Kurzrock R, Talpaz M, Kantarjian H, et al. Therapy of chronic myelogenous leukemia with recombinant interferon-gamma. Blood 1987; 70:943–7.
53. Jandl JJ. Chronic myeloproliferative disorders. In: Jandl JJ ed. Blood, textbook of hematology. Boston: Little, Brown, 1987; 671.
54. Kessler CM, Klein HG, Havlik RJ. Uncontrolled thrombocytosis in chronic myeloproliferative disorders. Br J Haematol 1982; 50:157–67.
55. Hehlmann R, Jahn M, Baumann B, Kopcke W. Essential thrombocythemia: clinical characteristics and course of 61 patients. Cancer 1988; 61:2487–96.
56. Silverstein MN. Primary or hemorrhagic thrombocythemia. Arch Intern Med 1968; 122:18–22.
57. Wu KK. Platelet hyperaggregability and thrombosis in patients with thrombocythemia. Ann Intern Med 1978; 88:7–11.
58. Talpaz M, Mavligit G, Keating M, Walters RS, Gutterman JU. Human leukocyte interferon to control thrombocytosis in chronic myelogenous leukemia. Ann Intern Med 1983; 99:789.
59. Talpaz M, Kurzrock R, Kantarjian H, O'Brien S, Gutterman JU. Recombinant interferon-alpha therapy of Philadelphia chromosome-negative myeloproliferative disorders with thrombocytosis. Am J Med 1989; 86:554.
60. Giles FJ, Gray AG, Brozovic M, et al. Alpha-interferon therapy for essential thrombocythaemia. Lancet 1988; 1:70.
61. Velu T, Delwiche F, Gangji D, et al. Therapeutic effect of human recombinant interferon-alpha-2c in essential thrombocythaemia. Oncology 1985; 42:10–4.

62. Gisslinger H, Linkesch W, Fritz E, Ludwig H, Chott A, Radaszkiewicz TH. Long-term interferon therapy for thrombocytosis in myeloproliferative diseases. Lancet 1989; 1:634.
63. May D, Wandl UB, Niederle N. Treatment of essential thrombocythaemia with interferon alpha-2b. Lancet 1989; 1:96.
64. Bellucci S, Harousseau JL, Brice P, Tobelem G. Treatment of essential thrombocythaemia by alpha2a interferon. Lancet 1988; 2:960.
65. Kasparu H, Reisner R, Bernhart M, et al. Recombinant alpha-2b interferon in the treatment of essential thrombocythaemia. Blut 1987; 55:284.
66. Gugliotta L, Macchi S, Catani L, et al. Recombinant α-2a interferon (α-IFN) in the treatment of essential thrombocythaemia. Preliminary report. Haematological (Pavia) 1987; 72:277–9.
67. McLaughlin P, Talpaz M, Quesada J, et al. Immune thrombocytopenia following alpha-interferon therapy in patients with cancer. JAMA 1985; 254:1353.
68. Silver RT. Recombinant interferon-alpha for treatment of polycythemia vera. Lancet 1988; 2:403.
69. Parmeggiana L, Ferrant A, Rodhain J, Michaux JL, Sokal G. Alpha interferon in the treatment of symptomatic myelofibrosis with myeloid metaplasia. Eur J Haematol 1987; 39:228–32.

5

Interferon Treatment of Multiple Myeloma: An Emerging Dilemma for the 1990s

Giuseppe Avvisati and Franco Mandelli

La Sapienza University, Rome, Italy

I. INTRODUCTION

Multiple myeloma (MM) is a generalized hematologic malignancy originating from the uncontrolled proliferation of a single clone of plasma cells, which in 99% of the cases secretes large quantities of monoclonal immunoglobulins and/or light chains and frequently produce bone destruction, bone marrow failure, hypercalcemic renal failure, and recurrent infections.

Since the introduction in the therapy of MM of alkylating agents, the median survival duration of this aggressive and debilitating disease has improved from 7 months (1) to about 3–4 years (2). However, this improvement in survival duration was so far independent of the aggressive nature of the induction treatment adopted (2). Moreover, once the relapse occurs or the disease becomes resistant or is primarily resistant (with patients clearly progressing on induction therapy), the course of MM is rapidly fatal (3).

During the past years, several attempts have been made to identify MM patients with a worse prognosis. As a consequence, different staging systems (4–6) as well as different prognostic variables (7–10) have been proposed to recognize those MM patients with a more aggressive disease. The results of these studies revealed that MM patients with stage III disease, renal failure, high β_2-serum globulin, high labeling index, low platelet count, and low interleukin-2 serum levels have a very short survival duration (4–10), influencing the overall median survival duration. Therefore, to improve the prognosis of MM, several new investigational approaches are under study, particularly in high-risk patients. These approaches include high-dose traditional induction chemotherapy (11,12), followed or not by bone marrow transplantation (allogeneic or autologous) procedures (13–17) or peripheral stem cell infusion (18) associated or not with the use of biologic response modifiers.

Nevertheless, the disease is still uncurable, and taking into account the high median age observed in MM patients, these aggressive investigational therapeutic approaches are applicable only to a minority of MM patients. Therefore, keeping in mind the suggestion of using a gentle approach in refractory patients (19) and extending this therapeutic concept to other categories of patients (i.e., those with stable disease or those older than 50–60 years), future clinical research must provide a more realistic therapy for myeloma patients.

As interferon (IFN) treatment has thus far proven to be a gentle and, in some circumstances, efficacious therapeutic approach for myeloma patients, it is our opinion that IFN therapy should be more widely used as first-line treatment of this malignancy.

The aim of the present review is to summarize the results thus far obtained with both chemotherapy and IFN in the treatment of newly diagnosed, relapsing, refractory, or resistant MM patients.

II. INDUCTION TREATMENT OF PREVIOUSLY UNTREATED MM PATIENTS

A. The Problem of the Best Chemotherapeutic Approach

Many therapeutic approaches using alkylating agents in association with prednisone or in combinations of three or more drugs have been investigated in MM. However, large randomized studies comparing the standard treatment (oral melphalan plus prednisone) versus more complex combination regimens have failed to show any statistical significant improvement, especially in overall survival duration, in favor of the combination therapeutic regimens (20–26). Unfortunately, because of the differences in these studies in the selection of patients, the duration of treatment, and the criteria for evaluating the response to treatment, a metaanalysis of the overall results obtained by pooling these studies cannot be made.

1. Conventional Alkylating Chemotherapy

The association of the alkylating agent melphalan with prednisone is still the standard first-line therapy in MM. This simple therapeutic schedule gives an objective response and a median survival duration ranging from 35 to 61% and from 19 to 39 months, respectively (20–30).

TABLE 1 Results of Induction Treatment with IFN Alone in MM

Number of patients			
Evaluable	Responders	% Response	Reference
4	4	100	32
11	3	27	33
3	1	23	34
12	3	25	35
74	10	14	36
18	2	11	37
14	7	50	38
17	1	6	39
56	18	36	40

The intermittent administration of melphalan is probably better than the continuous in terms both of response and of survival duration. The other alkylating agent comparable to melphalan in its efficacy in MM is cyclophosphamide (31).

2. Multidrug Combination Chemotherapy

Several combination chemotherapeutic modalities have been proposed during the last decade in the hope of improving the results obtained with the simple association of melphalan and prednisone. Thus far, however, the majority of these studies have not provided any statistically significant evidence in favor of the more aggressive combination treatments for an improvement in the response rate or the survival duration (2,24–26).

B. Interferon Alone as Induction Treatment

The first study dealing with the use of IFN in previously untreated MM patients was reported in 1979 by Mellstedt et al. (32). The induction treatment consisted of a daily dosage of 3 megaunits of human leukocyte IFN-α administered intramusclarly to four previously untreated MM patients. The result was astonishing: all patients demonstrated a durable response lasting from 3 to 19 months.

Shortly after this study, Osserman et al. (33), in a phase II trial sponsored by the American Cancer Society, reported a response in 3 of 11 previously untreated MM patients using a daily intramuscular administration of 3 megaunits of human leukocyte IFN-α. The increasing availability of IFN and the results obtained by Mellstedt et al. (32) encouraged several investigators to utilize this biologic agent in the treatment of MM. Since then, several other studies have been published. Table 1 summarizes the results of these clinical studies in which IFN has been used as single induction agent for treating newly diagnosed MM patients.

Recently, the myeloma group of central Sweden (MGCS) reported the results of a randomized trial comparing the administration of the human leukocyte IFN-α in 74 patients with MM versus the administration of melphalan and prednisone (MP) in 53 MM patients (36). The overall result of this study is in favor of chemotherapy (44% of responses versus 14% in the IFN group). However, the IgA and BJ (Bence-Jones) myeloma have a response rate similar to that observed in the MP group. Moreover, the overall survival duration was similar in both groups because the response to second-line therapy was more favorable in the previously IFN-treated group.

In a more recent study, Ludwig et al. (37) randomized 42 previously untreated patients to receive recombinant IFN:α_{2c} or the polychemotherapy vincristine, melphalan, cyclophosphamide, prednisone (VMCP) as induction treatment. In the IFN group, 6 of 18 evaluable patients obtained a response, but 17 of 19 patients who received the VMCP as treatment achieved a response. In this study patients unresponsive to IFN were crossed to VMCP. Despite the low response rate observed in the IFN-treated group, the survival duration of both groups was identical.

Finally, a new pilot study of the MGCS has confirmed the efficacy of the natural IFN-α in the treatment of IgA MM, obtaining a response rate of 41% in 37 newly diagnosed MM patients (40).

These studies yield a wide response rate, ranging from 20 to 100%, with an overall response rate of about 30%. This response rate, even though clearly inferior to that of conventional chemotherapy, deserves further investigation to identify those patient characteristics predictive of a better response to IFN, as already observed in IgA and BJ myeloma (36,40).

C. Studies Combining IFN with Chemotherapy During Induction

The results obtained with IFN as a single agent in inducing a response in previously untreated MM patients associated with in vitro evidence of a synergism between IFN and chemotherapy (41–44) prompted some investigators to evaluate the association of IFN with chemotherapy as induction treatment of MM.

Using the MP + IFN induction regimen, Cooper et al. demonstrated in a pilot study a response rate of 75% in previously untreated MM patients (45).

This very high response rate was confirmed by a successive pilot study by the ECOG cooperative group. In this study the induction treatment consisted of VBMCP + IFN and the response rate was 80%. Noteworthy in the ECOG study was the observation of 30% complete remissions defined as the disappearance of the M component from the serum and/or from the urine associated with the absence of plasma cells in the bone marrow (46).

Recently, Alexanian et al. treated 54 newly diagnosed MM patients with IFN-α_{2b} and dexamethasone, obtaining a response rate of 57%; this response rate was significantly higher than the 25% obtained in similar patients treated previously with IFN alone ($P = 0.02$) (47).

At present five prospective randomized trials are comparing chemotherapy (CT) alone versus CT + IFN. The preliminary results from three of these studies have confirmed the higher response rate of the CT + IFN arm compared to the response rate observed in the CT arm (48–50).

In particular, in the study of Scheithauer et al. (48), the response rate of the combined IFN-α_{2c} + VMCP was 65% versus the 35% response obtained with VMCP polychemotherapy not associated with IFN. Similarly, the Swedish study demonstrated a response rate of 66% in the MP + IFN-treated group versus 48% ($P = 0.02$) in the MP-treated group (49). Moreover, from this Swedish study it was evident that stage II MM and IgA MM respond significantly better to MP + IFN than to MP alone. Furthermore, in this study stage II patients have a statistically significant increase in survival. A third study comparing VMCP alone versus VMCP + IFN confirmed a better response rate in the VMCP + IFN group (37 versus 25%) (50).

Two other prospective randomized studies are comparing CT alone to CT + IFN as induction treatment of MM. One of these studies, conducted by the cooperative acute leukemia group B (CALGB), is comparing conventional MP treatment to MP + IFN. The other study of the ECOG is comparing VMBCP polychemotherapy to VMBCP + IFN. However, no data from these studies are thus far available.

III. SALVAGE TREATMENT OF RELAPSING, REFRACTORY, OR RESISTANT MM PATIENTS

A. Chemotherapeutic Modalities as Salvage Treatment

Successful treatment with previous discontinued regimens has been reported in 50–80% of patients relapsing while off therapy. On the contrary, the response rate of MM patients refractory or resistant to first-line chemotherapies is very poor. Those patients who first respond to treatment and then relapse despite continuing treatment (refractory patients) have a poorer prognosis, with an average response rate of 25% to alternative regimens. Moreover, patients primarily resistant (resistant patients) to any of the first-line treatments have the poorest prognosis and are less likely to respond to alternative chemotherapies than refractory or relapsing patients. At present good results in resistant and refractory MM patients have been obtained employing high dose of dexamethasone alone or in combination with continuous infusion of vincristine and adriamycin (51,52). Similar results, associated with minor toxicity, have been obtained with intermediate doses of intravenous melphalan (53).

B. IFN as Salvage Therapy

The first observation of a transient response obtained in a patient with MM refractory to melphalan was reported in 1979 by Indestrom et al. (54) using the human leukocyte IFN-α. Since then, several other studies in which IFN has

TABLE 2 Results of Salvage Treatment with IFN Alone in MM

Number of patients			
Evaluable	Responders	% Responses	Reference
1	1	100	54
7	2	29	34
2	0	0	55[a]
5	1	20	56[a]
9	2	22	35
16	0	0	57[a]
8	7	87.5	58
19	7	37	59
20	2	10	60
18	2	11	61
13	2	15	39
13	0	0	62[b]

[a]Studies with IFN-β.
[b]Study with IFN-γ.

been used as salvage treatment in MM have been published. These studies are reported in Table 2.

The majority of these studies employed IFN-α as treatment; however, in a few studies the human fibroblastoid IFN-β as well as IFN-γ have been utilized.

The overall response rate observed in studies utilizing IFN-α as salvage therapy was about 20%; the three studies in which nonrecombinant IFN-β underwent clinical testing showed a response in only 1 of 23 evaluable patients with refractory myeloma (55–57).

This negative result observed with IFN-β may at least partially depend on the use of an intravenous route of administration. As a consequence, inadequate exposure to the biologic agent because of its short plasma half-life may result when IFN-β is administered by this route.

To date there are only a few published reports in which IFN-γ was used as salvage therapy (62). The overall results with IFN-γ are similar to those observed using IFN-β. As far as IFN-α is concerned, the observed response rate of 20% in refractory or resistant myeloma patients is noteworthy and makes IFN-α one of the most effective second-line treatments for MM.

Moreover, data from these studies indicate that for some refractory patients it was possible to achieve responses lasting more than 3 years (59). Furthermore, an improvement in the levels of normal immunoglobulins has been noted in some patients (38,59). Finally, a few patients presented a progressive healing with recalcification of lytic bone lesions.

C. Effect of Previous IFN Therapy on the Outcome of Relapsing, Resistant, or Refractory Patients

An important observation made using IFN as salvage treatment was that following IFN therapy in some MM patients independently of the response to IFN, there was a restoration of sensibility to the chemotherapy, thus prolonging the duration of survival of these patients. We recently confirmed this observation.

In particular we observed that patients receiving maintenance treatment with IFN who once relapsed and were then retreated had a better survival duration than patients not receiving IFN as maintenance therapy (63).

IV. MAINTENANCE TREATMENT IN MM

A. Chemotherapy as Maintenance Treatment

Because induction treatment does not eradicate the disease it seems appropriate in responding patients to provide maintenance treatment hoping to delay relapse. However, responding patients treated with maintenance therapy have not shown a prolonged duration of survival compared to patients not on maintenance therapy (30,64,65). An explanation of this behavior in responding MM patients is that these patients are in a "plateau phase" in which plasma cells are in a resting state resembling monoclonal gammopathy of undetermined significance (MGUS). It is therefore possible that in this state plasma cells are less vulnerable to the available chemotherapeutic agents. At present, no standardized maintenance chemotherapies exist for responding myeloma patients during this plateau phase.

B. IFN as Maintenance Treatment of Responding Myeloma Patients

The biologic knowledge that myeloma patients responding to induction chemotherapy are in a plateau phase, associated with the evidence that IFN inhibits the in vitro colony formation and labeling index of myeloma cells (66–68), as well as reduces the self-renewal capacity of myeloma forming cells (69), suggested that in MM this biologic agent might be better used as an agent for maintaining rather than for inducing a response (70).

Therefore, from April 1985 to May 1988, a total of 101 responding MM patients with symptomatic MM responding to standard induction chemotherapy were randomized to receive recombinant IFN-α_{2b} as maintenance therapy or no treatment in an attempt toward improving survival and response duration. As of December 1989, the overall median response duration from the time of randomization was 26 months for patients receiving IFN and 14 months for untreated patients ($P = 0.0002$). Moreover, the overall median survival duration from time of randomization was 39 months for the untreated control group and 52 months for the group receiving maintenance treatment (P = 0.0526). However, the survival duration for objective responders with MM to induction chemotherapy (reduction < 50% of the monoclonal component) is significantly longer for the IFN maintenance group (P = 0.0352). These results indicate that maintenance treatment with IFN significantly prolongs the response and duration of survival in MM patients responding to conventional induction chemotherapy (70).

Other studies dealing with the use of IFN (mainly recombinant IFN-α) as maintenance therapy are ongoing in different parts of the world.

Preliminary data from a Swedish study confirm that the use of IFN as maintenance treatment during the plateau phase of MM can significantly prolong the duration of response (71). Moreover, in the study of Ludwig et al. comparing VMCP to VMCP + IFN as induction treatment, patients in response or with stable disease after induction are randomized to receive or not to receive IFN as maintenance treatment. Thus far, in this study 62.5% of the IFN maintenance patients are still in response versus only 10% of the control group (50), confirming the results of our study.

Finally, two well-designed prospective randomized studies (one of the SWOG cooperative group and the other of the NCI of Canada) on the use of IFN as maintenance therapy are still open to randomization; therefore, no data are thus far available.

V. CONCLUDING REMARKS

A. The Present

Since its first use in the treatment of MM, IFN has proved to be the new single therapeutic agent of the last decade useful in the treatment of MM. It is our opinion that the best indications for the use of this biologic response modifier (BRM) in MM treatment are (1) as a response inducer, combined with standard chemotherapies, in previously untreated as well as in refractory MM patients; and (2) as maintenance treatment after obtaining a response or stabilization of the disease.

B. The Future

Thus far the majority of studies using IFN in MM patients have utilized IFN-α. IFN-β and IFN-γ have not been sufficiently explored in the clincial setting. In the future the use of IFN-α as well as IFN-β and IFN-γ in the treatment of MM will increase. Moreover, IFN will be used more frequently in association with other BMRs.

REFERENCES

1. Osgood EE. The survival time of patients with plasmocytomic myeloma. Cancer Chemother Rep 1960; 9:1–10.
2. Bergsagel DE, Rider WD. Plasma cell neoplasms. In: De Vita VT, Hellmann S. Rosenberg SA, eds. Cancer: principles and practice of oncology, 2nd ed. Philadelphia: J. B. Lippincott, 1985; 1753–95.
3. Buzaid AC, Durie GM. Management of refractory myeloma: a review. J Clin Oncol 1988; 6:889–905.
4. Durie BGM, Salmon SE. A clinical staging system for multiple myeloma. Cancer 1975; 36:842–54.
5. Merlini G, Waldenstrom JA, Jayakar SD. A new improved clinical staging system for multiple myeloma based on analysis of 123 treated patients. Blood 1980; 55:1011–9.
6. Medical Research Council Working Party on Leukemia in Adults. Prognostic features in the third MRC myelomatosis trial. Br J Cancer 1980; 42:831–40.
7. Bataille R, Durie BGM, Grenier J. Serum β_2-microglobulin and survival duration in multiple myeloma: a simple reliable marker for staging. Br J Haematol 1983; 55:439–47.
8. Boccadoro M, Durie BGM, Frutiger Y, et al. Lack of correlation between plasma cell thymidine labelling index and serum β_2-microglobulin in monoclonal gammopathies. Acta Haematol 1987; 78:239–42.
9. Cavo M, Galieni P, Zuffa E, Baccarani M, Gobbi M, Tura S. Prognostic variables and clinical staging in multiple myeloma. Blood 1989; 74:1774–80.
10. Cimino G, Avvisati G, Amardori S, et al. High serum IL-2 levels are predictive of prolonged survival in multiple myeloma. Br J Haematol 1990; 75:373–7.
11. Selby PJ, McElwain TJ, Nandi AC, et al. Multiple myeloma treated with high-dose intravenous melphalan. Br J Haematol 1987; 66:55–62.
12. Slavin M, Selby PJ, Clark PI, et al. Intensive treatment for multiple myeloma and criteria for complete remission. Lancet 1989; 2:879–81.
13. Barlogie B, Hall R, Zander A, et al. High dose melphalan with autologous bone marrow transplantation for multiple myeloma. Blood 1986; 67:1298–301.
14. Barlogie B, Alexanian R, Dicke KA. High-dose chemoradiotherapy and autologous bone marrow transplantation for resistant multiple myeloma. Blood 1987; 70:869–72.
15. Gahrton G, Tura S, Flesh M, et al. Bone marrow transplantation in multiple myeloma: report from the European Cooperative Group for bone marrow transplantation. Blood 1987; 69:1262–4.
16. Anderson K, Barut B, Takvorian T, et al. Monoclonal antibody purged autologous bone marrow transplantation for multiple myeloma (abstract 753). Blood 1989; 74 (Suppl. 1): 202a.
17. Reece DE, Barnett MJ, Connors JM, et al. Intensive therapy with busulfan, cyclophosphamide and melphalan and 4-hydroperoxycyclophosphamide purged autologous bone marrow transplantation for multiple myeloma (abstract 754). Blood 1989; 74 (Suppl. 1): 202a.

18. Marit G, Boiron JM, Reiffers J. Autologous blood stem cell transplantation in high risk multiple myeloma (abstract 751). Blood 1989; 74 (Suppl. 1): 201a.
19. Bergsagel DE. Use a gentle approach for refractory myeloma patients. J Clin Oncol 1988; 6:757–8.
20. Bergsagel DE, Phil D, Bailey AJ, et al. The chemotherapy of plasma-cell myeloma and the incidence of acute leukemia. New Engl J Med 1979; 301:743–8.
21. Alexanian R, Dreier R. Chemotherapy for multiple myeloma. Cancer 1984; 53:583–8.
22. Hansen OP, Toffner Clausen NA, Drivsholm A, Laursen B. Phase III study of intermittent 5-drug regimen (VBMCP) versus intermittent 3-drug regimen (VMP) versus intermittent melphalan and prednisone (MP) in myelomatosis. Scand J Haematol 1985; 35:518–24.
23. Cooper MR, McIntyre OR, Propert KJ, et al. Single sequential and multiple alkylating agent therapy for multiple myeloma: a CALGR study. J Clin Oncol 1986; 4:1331–9.
24. Palva IP, Ahrenberg P, Ala-Harja K, et al. Treatment of multiple myeloma with an intensive 5-drug combination or intermittent melphalan and prednisone: a randomized multicentre trial. Eur J Haematol 1987; 38:50–4.
25. Pavlovsky S, Corrado C, Santarelli MT, et al. An update of two randomized trials in previously untreated multiple myeloma comparing melphalan and prednisone versus three-and-five drug combinations: an Argentine group for the treatment of acute leukemia study. J Clin Oncol 1988; 6:769–75.
26. Osterborg A, Ahre A, Bjorkholm M, et al. Alternating combination chemotherapy (VMCP/VBAP) is not superior to melphalan/prednisone in the treatment of multiple myeloma patients stage III. A randomized study from MGCS. Eur J Haematol 1989; 43:54–62.
27. Alexanian R, Bonnet J, Gehan E, et al. Combination chemotherapy for multiple myeloma. Cancer 1972; 30:382–9.
28. Cavagnaro F, Lein JM, Pavlovsky S, et al. Comparison of two combination chemotherapy regimens for multiple myeloma: methyl-CCNU, cyclophosphamide and prednisone versus melphalan and prednisone. Cancer Treat Rep 1980; 64:73–9.
29. Ahre A, Bjorkholm M, Mellstedt H. Intermittent high-dose melphalan/prednisone vs continuous low-dose melphalan treatment in multiple myeloma. Eur J Cancer Clin Oncol 1983; 19:499–506.
30. Belch A, Shelley W, Bergsagel DE, et al. A randomized trial of maintenance versus non maintenance melphalan and prednisone in responding multiple myeloma patients. Br J Cancer 1988; 57:94–9.
31. Rivers SL, Patno ME. Cyclophosphamide vs melphalan in the treatment of plasma cell meyloma. JAMA 1969; 207:1328–34.
32. Mellstedt H, Ahre E, Bjorkholm G, Holm G, Johanson B, Stander H. Interferon therapy in myelomatosis. Lancet 1979; 1:245–7.
33. Osserman ET, Sherman WF, Alexanian R, Gutterman JU, Humphrey RL. Preliminary results of the American Cancer Society-sponsored trial of human leukocyte interferon in multiple myeloma (abstract). Proc Am Assoc Cancer Res 1980; 21:161.

34. Gutterman JU, Blumenschein GR, Alexanian R, et al. Leucocyte interferon induced tumor regression in human metastatic breast cancer, multiple myeloma and malignant lymphoma. Ann Intern Med 1980; 93:399–406.
35. Alexanian R, Gutterman JU, Levy H. Interferon treatment in multiple myeloma. Clin Hematol 1982; 2:211–20.
36. Ahre A, Bjorkholm M, Mellstedt H, et al. Human leukocyte interferon and intermittent high-dose melphalan-prednisolone administration in the treatment of multiple myeloma: a randomized clinical trial from the Myeloma Group of Central Sweden. Cancer Treat Rep 1984; 68:1331–8.
37. Ludwig H, Cortelezzi A, Scheithauer W, et al. Recombinant interferon alpha-2c versus polychemotherapy (VMCP) for treatment of multiple myeloma: a prospective randomized trial. Eur J Cancer Clin Oncol 1986; 22:1111–6.
38. Quesada JR, Alexanian R, Hawkins M, et al. Treatment of multiple myeloma with recombinant alfa-interferon. Blood 1986; 67:275–8.
39. Cox EB, Laszlo J, Krown S, Mintzer D, Sarna G. Phase II study of human lymphoblastoid interferon in patients with multiple myeloma. J Biol Resp Mod 1988; 7:318–25.
40. Ahre A, Bjorkholm M, Osterborg A, et al. High doses of natural alpha interferon (alpha-IFN) in the treatment of multiple myeloma. A pilot study from the Myeloma Group of Central Sweden (MGCS). Eur J Haematol 1988; 41:123–30.
41. Aapro MS, Alberts DS, Salmon SE. Interaction of human leukocyte interferon with *Vinca* alkaloids and other chemotherapeutic agents against human tumors in clonogenic assay. Cancer Chemother Pharmacol 1983; 10:161–6.
42. Kataoka T, Fusiko OH, Sakura Y. Enhancement of antiproliferative activity of vincristine and Adriamycin by interferon. Gann 1984; 75:548–56.
43. Balkwill FR, Monshowitz S, Seilman S. Positive interactions between interferon and chemotherapy due to direct tumor action rather than effects on host drug-metabolizing enzymes. Cancer Res 1984; 44:5249–55.
44. Balkwill FR, Moodey EM. Positive interactions between human interferon and cyclophosphamide or adriamycin in a human tumor model system. Cancer Res 1985; 44:906–8.
45. Cooper MR, Fefer A, Thomson J, et al. Alpha-2 interferon, melphalan/prednisone in previously untreated patients with multiple myeloma. A phase I-II trial. Cancer Treat Rep 1986; 70:473–6.
46. Kyle RA, Oken MM, Greipp PR, Kay NE, Tsiatis A. VBMCP/r-IFN alpha 2 induction therapy in multiple myeloma (abstract). V Hannover Interferon Workshop, IFN Therapy in B Cell Malignancies. Hannover, Germany, 1990; 46.
47. Alexanian R, Barlogie B, Gutterman J. Alpha interferon combinaton therapy for multiple myeloma (abstract). V Hannover Interferon Workshop, IFN Therapy in B Cell Malignancies. Hannover, Germany, 1990; 43.
48. Scheithauer W, Cortelezzi A, Fritz E, et al. Combined alpha-2c interferon/VMCP polychemotherapy versus VMCP polychemotherapy as induction therapy in multiple myeloma. A prospective randomized trial. J Biol Respir Modif 1989; 8:109–15.
49. Mellstedt H. MP versus MP/IFN alpha induction therapy: a randomized trial in multiple myeloma (abstract). V Hannover Interferon Workshop, IFN Therapy in B Cell Malignancies. Hannover, Germany, 1990; 44.

50. Ludwig H, Gisslinger H, Cohen AM, et al. VMCP versus VMCP/IFN alpha induction therapy: a randomized trial in multiple myeloma (abstract). V Hannover Interferon Workshop IFN Therapy in B Cell Malignancies. Hannover, Germany, 1990; 45.
51. Barlogie B, Smith L, Alexanian R. Effective treatment of advanced multiple myeloma refractory to alkylating agents. N Engl J Med 1984; 310:1353–6.
52. Alexanian R, Barlogie B, Dixon D. High dose glucocorticoid treatment for resistant multiple myeloma. Ann Intern Med 1986; 105:8–11.
53. Petrucci MT, Avvisati G, Tribalto M, Cantonetti M, Giovangrossi P, Mandelli F. Intermediate-dose (25 mg/m^2) intravenous melphalan for patients with multiple myeloma in relapse or refractory to standard treatment. Eur J Haematol 1989; 42:233–237.
54. Indestrom K, Canthel K, Killander D, Nilsson K, Strander H, Willems J. Interferon therapy in multiple myeloma. Acta Med Scand 1979; 205:149–54.
55. Billau A, Bloemmen J, Bogaerts M, et al. Interferon therapy in multiple myeloma: failure of human fibroblast interferon administration to affect the course of light chain disease. Eur J Cancer Clin Oncol 1981; 17:875–82.
56. Ezaki K, Ogawa M, Okabe K, et al. Clinical and immunological studies of human fibroblastoid interferon. Cancer Chemoter Pharmacol 1981; 8:145–58.
57. Misset JL, Mathé J, Gastiaburu A, et al. Treatment of lymphoid neoplasis with interferon. I. Human fibroblastic beta-interferon in malignant gammapathies. Phase II trial. Anticancer Res 1982; 2:63–6.
58. Medenica R, Slack N. Clinical results of leucocyte interferon-induced tumor regression in resistant human metastatic cancer resistant to chemotherapy and/or radiotherapy-pulse therapy schedule. Cancer Drug Deliv 1985; 2:53–76.
59. Costanzi JJ, Cooper R, Scarffe JH, et al. Phase II study of recombinant alfa-2 interferon in resistant multiple myeloma. J Clin Oncol 1985; 3:654–9.
60. Oken MM, Kyle RA, Kay NE, et al. A phase II trial of interferon alpha-2 (rIFN alpha-2) in the treatment of resistant multiple myeloma (MM) (abstract). Proc Am Soc Clin Oncol 1985; 4:215.
61. Wagstaff JK, Loynos P, Scarffe JH. Phase II study of rDNA human alpha-2-interferon in multiple myeloma. Cancer Treat Rep 1985; 69:495–8.
62. Quesada JR, Alexanain R, Kurzrock R, Barlogie B, Saks S, Gutterman JU. Recombinant interferon gamma in hairy cell leukemia, multiple myeloma and Waldenstrom macroglobulinemia. Am J Hematol 1988; 29:1–4.
63. Avvisati G, Petrucci MT, Giovangrossi P, et al. Second induction treatment in relapsing multiple myeloma patients receiving or not maintenance treatment with alpha-b interferon (Intron A) (abstract). International Conference on Multiple Myeloma, Bologna, Italy, 1989; 127.
64. Alexanian R, Gehan E, Haut A, et al. Unmaintained remissions in multiple myeloma. Blood 1978; 51:1005–11.
65. Southwest Oncology Group Study. Remission maintenance therapy for multiple myeloma. Arch Intern Med 1975; 135:147–52.
66. Salmon SE, Durie BGM, Young Y, et al. Effects of cloned leucocyte interferons in the human tumor stem cell assay. J Clin Oncol 1983; 1:217–25.

67. Browning G. The in vitro effect of leucocyte alpha-interferon on human myeloma cell in a semisolid agar culture system. Scand J Haematol 1985; 55:178–85.
68. Brenning G, Ahre A, Nillson K. Correlation between in vitro and in vivo sensitivity to human leukocyte interferon in patients with multiple myeloma. Scand J Haematol 1985; 35:543–9.
69. Bergsagel DE, Haas RH, Messner HA. Interferon alpha-2b in the treatment of chronic granulocytic leukemia. Semin Oncol 1936; 13 (Suppl. 2):27–34.
70. Mandelli F, Avvisati G, Amadori S, et al. Maintenance treatment with alpha-2b recombinant interferon significantly improves response and survival duration in multiple myeloma patients responding to conventional induction chemotherapy. Results of an Italian randomized study. New Engl J Med 1990; 322:1430–4.
71. Westin J, Cortelezzi A, Hjorth M, Rodgers J, Turesson I, Zador G. Interferon-alpha-2b therapy during the plateau phase of multiple myeloma (abstract). V Hannover Interferon Workshop, IFN Therapy in B Cell Malignancies. Hannover, Germany, 1990; 50.

6

Induction Therapy with Interferon in Multiple Myeloma and Possible Mechanisms of Action

Anders Österborg and Håkan Mellstedt for the Myeloma Group of Central Sweden

Karolinska Hospital, Stockholm, Sweden

I. INTRODUCTION

Multiple myeloma is a lymphoid malignancy of B cell origin involving not only plasma cells but also clonal B lymphocytes at various stages of maturation (for references see Ref. 1). The main evidence for a differentiating B cell compartment in multiple myeloma is based on the identification of idiotypic (id) immunoglobulin (Ig) structures on the surface of B lymphocytes and in the cytoplasm of lymphoid cells as well as of plasma cells, identical to those of the serum M component (1), and on the identification of identical clonal immunoglobulin (heavy and light chains) gene rearrangements in bone marrow plasma cells and in peripheral blood B lymphocytes (2). The earliest involved B lymphocyte has been proposed to be an early B cell or a pre-B cell (1,3). Also, a pluripotent stem cell origin has been suggested, based on the finding of myelomonocytic antigens on myeloma cells (4). An aberrant expression of such antigens due to malignant transformation cannot be excluded, however.

Regulatory cell subsets seem to be involved in the disease process. Large numbers of natural killer (NK) cells and a high NK cell activity have been found in patients with a small tumor burden (stages I and II) and in the response/plateau phase, and patients with advanced (stage III) and progressive disease had low NK cell functions (5). Normally, NK cells are cytotoxic for B lymphoid cells at restricted stages of differentiation and may also suppress B cell differentiation (6). In analogy, NK cells may also have a role in the regulation of multiple myeloma. Furthermore, T lymphocytes with receptors for the idiotype have been cloned (7). Such cells may be part of a regulatory network. Moreover, anti-idiotypic antibodies against the M component have been described, further indicating the possibility of immune network regulation in monoclonal gammopathies (8).

II. CYTOKINES IN MULTIPLE MYELOMA

During the last few years increasing knowledge has been generated on the diversified effects of cytokines. These polypeptide molecules produced by a variety of hematopoietic, lymphopoietic, and endothelial cells act in an unspecific manner. A regulatory effect on normal B cells at various stages of differentiation has been demonstrated for some of these cytokines as IL-2, IL-3, IL-4, IL-5, and IL-6 (9–13). A regulatory function on neoplastic B cells in multiple myeloma may also be anticipated.

Major interest has been focused on interleukin-6 (IL-6). Normally, IL-6 is a growth factor for terminal differentiation of B cells to antibody-producing plasma cells (13) but it is also a potent growth factor for multiple myeloma cells in vitro (14). The role of IL-6 with regard to the pathophysiology of multiple myeloma is not clear, but various mechanisms may be operating. Multiple myeloma cells seem to produce IL-6 because IL-6 mRNA can be detected in plasma cells and supernatants from freshly isolated myeloma cells stimulated the proliferation of an IL-6-dependent myeloma cell line (14). However, the level of IL-6 mRNA seems to be very low (15). Myeloma cells also express the receptor for IL-6 (IL-6R) (14). Because myeloma cells may be dependent on IL-6 for growth and proliferation and IL-6 and IL-6R are produced by the same cell, an autocrine loop may be operating. However, in many cases no IL-6 mRNA can be detected, either in fresh biopsy materials or in myeloma cell lines (16). In such cases bone marrow stromal cells, monocytes, and feeder cells were found to produce large amounts of IL-6. This is in good agreement with the experience that for in vitro growth most myeloma cells are dependent on feeder cells that produce IL-6 (16). These findings may indicate a paracrine loop. IL-6 also seems to be the single most important soluble factor responsible for myeloma cell growth. Thus, both an autocrine and a paracrine mechanisms are probably operating.

Myeloma cells from patients with a large tumor burden (stage III) showed a relatively low proliferative response to IL-6; cells from patients with a small tumor burden (stage I) and from those in the response phase had a high proliferative response (17). This observation is very interesting compared to results obtained in vitro. The 4-year-old myeloma cell line U-266/84 showed an exclusive growth dependence for IL-6 but the same cell line cultured for 18 years

(U-266/70) showed neither feeder cell nor IL-6 dependence for in vitro growth. A similar phenomenon has also been observed for other myeloma cell lines. Moreover, myeloma cell lines successfully grown in vitro gradually lost their feeder cell dependence (16). Myeloma cell lines established from ascitic or pleural fluid, that is, from patients with advanced disease, never require feeder cells.

Taken together, IL-6 may be both an autocrine and a paracrine growth factor for multiple myeloma. The IL-6 dependence seems to be restricted to early and less advanced tumors but in advanced disease the malignant cells have lost their IL-6 dependence. In the last case the uncontrolled growth may be supported by mutated *ras* oncogenes (18) acting in synergy with amplified or translocated *myc* oncogenes, which have shown a remarkable synergy with regard to tumor cell proliferation in mice (19).

Thus IL-6 is an important but not universal growth factor for multiple myeloma; some myelomas do not respond to IL-6, and IL-6 exerts its activity only on mature terminally differentiated B cells, but probably not on the less mature B lymphocyte compartment or on early B cells belonging to the myeloma tumor cell clone.

Other cytokines also may be involved in regulation of the tumor cell clone. IL-5 and IL-3 have been shown to induce the proliferation of cultured myeloma cells when used alone or in combination (20). The myeloma cells line RPMI-8226 has been found to produce IL-5, which acted as an autocrine growth factor (21).

Although a high activity of tumor necrosis factor (TNF) and IL-1β has been detected in the supernatants of cultured myeloma plasma cells, no growth- or differentiation-promoting effect has been ascribed to these cytokines (22,23). Both cytokines have an osteoclast-activating activity, so that a role in the pathogenesis of osteolytic lesions in myeloma might be anticipated. IL-1α, which by itself has no demonstrable effect on myeloma cell growth (20), has been found to indirectly promote the growth of myeloma plasma cells by stimulating the production of IL-6 (24).

IL-2 and IL-4, both of which have regulatory functions on normal B cells, have not been shown to stimulate the growth of cultured myeloma plasma cells (20). IL-2, however, was found to inhibit the growth of a murine myeloma cell line (25). In the normal situation, IL-4 predominantly stimulates B cells at an early stage of differentiation after antigenic presentation. It might be speculated that IL-4 exerts a regulatory effect on the differentiating myeloma B lymphocyte compartment, possibly by supporting the maturation of clonal B lymphocytes.

III. MECHANISMS OF ACTION OF INTERFERON

Interferon (IFN) is a biologic therapeutic agent with an antitumoral activity in experimental systems and in humans (26–29). The exact mechanisms for interferon's antitumoral activities are still unknown, and several functions may be operating. A summary of possible IFN activities in myeloma is shown in Table 1.

A direct cytotoxic effect of IFN on cultured myeloma plasma cells has been observed (30,31). A dose-dependent growth inhibitory effect of interferon has also been described in several experimental systems, including myeloma (32,33). In the clinical situation it is controversial whether such a relationship exists (34), although there are clinical observations that may indicate that such a correlation may exist (35).

An enhanced cytotoxic effect of interferon-α might be obtained when combined with chemotherapeutic agents. In an in vitro colony formation assay, an additive cytotoxic effect was seen when IFN was combined with prednisone. IFN in combination with melphalan resulted in a synergistic growth inhibitory effect. When all three agents were added together, an even greater cytotoxic activity was noted (36). This study also showed a dose-dependent effect of IFN-α.

IFN may also have an impact on the pharmacokinetics of melphalan. A decrease in the area under the curve (AUC) of melphalan was observed when IFN was given to patients (37). This effect may be ascribed to IFN itself or to the elevated body temperature induced by IFN. The clinical significance of the finding is not yet established but may indicate an increased cellular uptake of melphalan with a concomitant increase in the cytotoxic effect of melphalan.

IFN has also been shown to inhibit the growth-promoting effect of various growth factors. Cell lines dependent on epidermal growth factor (EGF) or platelet-derived growth factor (PDGF) for proliferation in vitro were arrested after addition of IFN, probably by interfering with the binding of growth factors to the cells (38). In hairy cell leukemia IFN has been found to inhibit the growth-promoting effect of low molecular B cell growth factor ($BCGF_{low}$) (39).

TABLE 1 Possible Mechanisms of Action of IFN-α In Vivo in the Treatment of Multiple Myeloma

Function	Reference
Direct cytotoxic effect	30, 31
Synergistic cytotoxic effect with alkylating agents and prednisone	36
Change in the pharmacokinetics of melphalan	37
Inhibition of growth-promoting effect of various growth factors (IL-6)	38
Downregulation of oncogene expression	40
Increase in NK cell functions	44
Increase in the tumor cell surface antigens and augmentation of immunogenicity	48
Expansion of specific T cells	49

A similar inhibitory effect of IFN on IL-6-induced growth stimulation may be operating. This assumption fits well with some clinical observations. A high responsiveness of myeloma cells to IL-6 from patients with stage I disease was noted compared to stage III myeloma (17). Patients with a small tumor burden showed a significantly higher therapeutic response to IFN than patients with advanced disease (see subsequent discussion).

Another IFN-mediated effect may be downregulation of oncogene expression. IFN has been shown to downregulate various oncogenes in experimental systems (40). Amplification of the c-*myc* and *bcl*-1 oncogenes and *ras* mutation has been described in myeloma (41,42), as well as various chromosomal translocations (43). Thus, IFN may also inhibit myeloma tumor cell progression by downregulation of oncogenes.

In vitro and in vivo natural killer cell activity is enhanced by IFN. Large numbers of NK cells and an increased NK cell function have been described in myeloma patients with a small tumor burden and in patients responding to therapy; patients with advanced disease had low NK activity (16). Thus, patients with a reduced tumor mass seem to have an intact NK cell system that may be functionally augmented after IFN administration (44) and thereby exert antitumoral effects.

In a mouse myeloma system, idiotype-reactive T cells with specific regulatory functions on the expanding myeloma clone have been described (45). In humans, idiotype-reactive T cells (7) and clonal rearrangements of $TCR_{v\beta}$ (46) have been found in patients with smoldering myeloma. IFN can enhance a specific T cell response (47), and thus IFN-stimulated expansion of specific T cells may also be a mechanism of action, as well as increased immunogenicity of the tumor cells by increased expression of tumor-associated antigens and major histocompatibility complex (MHC) antigens (48).

In summary, various direct or indirect IFN-mediated effects may be operating to explain the antitumoral effects in multiple myeloma. Based on experimental results and clinical observations, IFN should be combined with an alkylating agent and prednisone for induction therapy when the tumor cell compartment is large and the proliferating capacity comparatively high (at diagnosis) to utilize the direct cytotoxic effect and to obtain a reduction of the tumor load within a short time. In the response or plateau phase IFN may be used alone to await the effects on various immune functions. Moreover, in the response or plateau phase the proliferative capacity is low and the direct cytotoxic effect of IFN alone is more pronounced on cells in G_0.

IV. INDUCTION THERAPY WITH INTERFERON AS A SINGLE AGENT

Intermittent high-dose melphalan + prednisone (MP) treatment (49) is regarded by many clinicians as the primary standard therapy for patients with multiple myeloma. For previously untreated patients with small or intermediate tumor loads, combination chemotherapy has not been shown to improve the response rate or to prolong survival. Even for patients with large tumor loads there is no convincing evidence that combination chemotherapy consistently improves the response rate or extends survival (50,51). Since the overall prognosis for myeloma patients is rather poor, there is a need for better therapeutic modalities.

The first report of IFN-α in the treatment of multiple myeloma was published in 1979 (52). In a subsequent study the Myeloma Group of Central Sweden (MGCS) studied the therapeutic effect of natural IFN-α in previously untreated patients with multiple myeloma. In a randomized trial a dose of 3×10^6 U of IFN-α daily was compared to MP. The response rate of IgG myelomas was low (5%); in IgA and Bence-Jones (BJ) myelomas the response frequency (26%) was not statistically significant different from that of MP-treated patients (53). The IFN-α dose was well tolerated. The overall survival did not differ significantly between the two treatment groups.

To test a possible dose-response relationship in vivo, 50 patients with IgA and BJ myelomas entered an MGCS pilot study using high doses of natural IFN-α (35). This study clearly showed that the highest dose tested, 30×10^6 U of IFN-α daily, caused unacceptable adverse reactions, predominantly a flulike syndrome. The maximal tolerable dose that could be given with only minor side effects to most patients was 10×10^6 U daily for 7 consecutive days repeated every third week. The overall response rate was 36%. The highest response frequencies were seen in those treatment groups who received the highest IFN-α doses, which, however, were associated with unacceptable toxicity. The response duration was usually of considerable length, exceeding 1 year in 11 of 18 responding patients. The median survival was more than 3 years, which is very comparable to the results of conventional chemotherapy regimens.

Several reports have confirmed the clinical effect of IFN-α as a single agent in the treatment of multiple myeloma. In chemotherapy-resistant patients, the overall response rate was 17% (95% confidence levels between 12 and 22%) (54). Some patients achieved complete and partial responses of long duration. In previously untreated patients a response was obtained in 14–50% of the patients (51,52), the overall response rate being 34% (Table 2).

In two studies a correlation was found between the response rate and the IFN dose (35,55). This may indicate the existence of a dose-response relationship for IFN in multiple myeloma, although this finding has not been confirmed by others.

A particularly good effect in IgA myeloma has been noted in three studies (35,56,57). The reason for this difference, which was not found in other studies, remains largely unclear (see later).

Only scanty information is available about the clinical effect of other types of IFN, that is, IFN-γ and IFN-β, in multiple myeloma. Some antitumoral effects

TABLE 2 Response Rates in Newly Diagnosed Multiple Myeloma Patients Treated with IFN–α Alone

	Response rate (%)		
Number of patients	Mean	95% Confidence limits	Reference
14	14	0–44	Ludwig et al. (56)
14	50	22–78	Quesada et al (55)
50	36	22–50	MGCS (35)
192	34	27–41	All published studies

of IFN-β have been reported, but IFN-γ seems to have no or only a marginal effect on multiple myeloma (58).

V. INDUCTION THERAPY WITH INTERFERON AND CHEMOTHERAPY

Based on the findings already mentioned and on the in vitro synergism of IFN-α and melphalan + prednisone (36), the MGCS started in April 1986 a randomized clinical trial with the aim to analyze whether the addition of IFN-α to MP could improve the therapeutic outcome in previously untreated patients with multiple myeloma.

The maximal tolerable dose of IFN for induction therapy was used, taking advantage of a possible dose-response relationship and synergism with MP to achieve a maximal reduction in the myeloma tumor cell mass. At clinical response, which is associated with stable disease and a low proportion of proliferating cells (59), the IFN schedule was changed to a low-dose regimen in an attempt to inhibit the self-renewal capacity of myeloma clonal cells (60) and interfere with various immune functions (discussed earlier).

Natural IFN-α was prepared from human leukocytes and enriched to a specific activity of approximately 5×10^6 U/mg protein. INF-α (Finnferon) was obtained from the Finnish Red Cross Blood Transfusion Service (Helsinki).

The criteria for response were (1) a decrease in serum M component concentration by $> 50\%$ of the pretreatment value; and (2) a decrease in urinary light-chain excretion to < 0.2 g per 24 h. In addition, patients were classified as responders only if the hemoglobin level was > 90 g/L, serum albumin level > 30 g/L, and serum calcium level ≥ 2.6 mmol/L. Progression or relapse was attained when one or more of the following criteria were fulfilled: (1) an increase in the serum M component concentration with at least 25% of the pretreatment or response value, respectively; (2) a 100% increase in Bence-Jones protein 24 h urinary excretion of pretreatment or response value, respectively; (3) serum calcium ≥ 3 mmol/L; and (4) progression of osteolytic lesions.

The patients were randomized to either intermittent melphalan (0.25 mg/kg/day) and prednisone (2 mg/kg/day) for 4 days repeated every sixth week (MP) or to intermittent MP every sixth week plus 7×10^6 U/m^2/day of IFN-α for 5 consecutive days repeated every third week. When the patients obtained a response, MP was continued but the IFN dose was reduced to 3×10^6 U/day, 3 days a week continuously (MP + IFN). Treatment was continued to progression or relapse. At progression or relapse all patients received the same combination chemotherapy regimen.

The pretreatment characteristics of the patients in this MGCS study are shown in Table 3 and the response frequencies in Table 4. A statistically significant higher response rate was noted in the MP + IFN group compared to patients receiving standard MP therapy. In clinical stage II the response rate was significantly higher in the MP + IFN group than in the MP group; in stage III the difference between the two groups was not statistically significant. Patients with IgA myelomas had a significantly higher response rate in the MP + IFN group compared to the MP group; in IgG and BJ myelomas the response frequencies were numerically higher in the MP + IFN group, although the differences were statistically not significant.

During the induction period, 64% of the patients had no reduction in the IFN dose (Table 5). In 11 patients (12%) IFN-α had to be withdrawn because

TABLE 3 Pretreatment Patients Characteristics

	MP group	MP + IFN group
Total	111	109
Clinical Stage		
II	50	51
III	61	58
Serum Creatinine		
<170 mmol/L	80	84
≥170 mmol/L	31	25
M component		
IgG	56	62
IgA	26	24
Bence-Jones	23	21
Nonsecretory	5	2
IgD	1	—
Number of patients evaluable for response by September 1989	91	94

TABLE 4 Response Frequency (%) in Relation to Treatment Schedule

	MP group (n = 91)[a]	MP + IFN group (n = 94)[a]	*p* Value
Total	48	66	0.02
Clinical stage			
II	48 (20/42)	76 (34/45)	0.01
III	49 (24/49)	57 (28/49)	NS[b]
M component			
IgG	56 (25/45)	62 (31/50)	NS
IgA	52 (11/21)	91 (20/22)	0.01
Bence-Jones	26 (5/19)	50 (10/20)	NS

[a]Number of evaluable patients, September 1989.
[b]Not significant.

TABLE 5 Frequency (%) of Patients Requiring a Reduction in the IFN Dosage During the Induction Treatment Period

IFN reduction %	Frequency of patients %
0	64
25	15
50	8
75	1
100	12[a]

[a]Eleven patients.

of side effects. The reasons for withdrawals were one myocardial infarction, one congestive heart failure, one coma with hemiparesis, two flulike syndrome, one mental confusion, one allergic reaction, one thrombocytopenia, and three compliance problems. Various dose reductions were incorporated in 26% of the patients.

The hematologic side effects are shown in Table 6. There were no major differences between the two groups. Nonhematologic toxicities during the induction phase in the MP + IFN group were flulike syndrome (58%), myocardial infarction (1%), congestive heart failure (1%), allergic edema (1%), diarrhea (3%), and central nervous system (CNS)-related symptoms (4%).

Of 62 responders in the MP + IFN group 43 were evaluable for toxicity during the maintenance phase: 14% had a flulike syndrome and 37% hematologic toxicity grade III. In 8 of the responders IFN-α was discontinued after a median time of 3 months (range 1–9 months). The reasons for withdrawal were two flu-

TABLE 6 Hematologic Toxicity During the Induction Phase in Relation to Treatment Schedule

Treatment group	Number of patients with toxicity[a] (%)		
	Grade I	Grade II	Grade III
MP (n = 91)	27 (30)	15 (16)	24 (26)
MP + IFN (n = 89)	16 (18)	21 (24)	33 (37)

[a]I, leukopenia 2–3 × 10^9 L^{-1} and/or thrombocytopenia 100–150 × 10^9 L^{-1}.
II, leukopenia 1.5– < 2.0 × 10^9 L^{-1} and/or thrombocytopenia 50–< 100 × 10^9 L^{-1}.
III, leukopenia < 1.5 × 10^9 L^{-1} and/or thrombocytopenia < 50 × 10^9 L^{-1}.

like syndromes, one thrombocytopenia, two compliance problems, one nausea, one myelodysplastic syndrome, and one patient refused further IFN therapy.

There was no difference in response duration time and total survival between the two treatment groups. The median survival time has not yet been reached. However, looking at patients with a small tumor burden (stage II), there was a tendency for a longer response duration time as well as for survival of patients receiving MP + IFN therapy. Similar results were obtained for patients ≤ 65 years of age (the median age for all our myeloma patients). Considering IgA myelomas, there was a clear tendency to increased survival, duration of response, and survival from response in the MP + IFN group compared to the MP group. The number of patients in each group is still small, however.

This study clearly shows that MP + IFN therapy is an effective treatment for patients with multiple myeloma and superior to standard MP treatment with regard to response induction. The best therapeutic effect of MP + IFN was seen in patients with a small tumor mass (stage II) compared to patients with a large tumor burden (stage III). This effect may fit a difference in IL-6 dependence and a growth inhibitory effect of IFN by interaction with the binding of the growth factor to the tumor cell surface. Moreover, the very high response rate in IgA myelomas may partly also be explained by an interaction with IL-6. IL-6 has been shown to induce a high rate of IgA secretion in IgA-comitted B cells (61), and thus if one effect of IFN is to inhibit the growth stimulatory effect of IL-6, then IgA myelomas may be a particularly favorable target for IFN.

The observation time is still too short to reach conclusions about the survival effects, but at present there seems to be a survival advantage in the MP + IFN group for stage II patients, patients ≤ 65 years, and those with IgA myelomas.

The results of other studies on chemotherapy plus IFN-α for induction therapy are summarized in Table 7. A high response rate for chemotherapy plus IFN-α was found in the studies by Cooper et al. (62) and Montuoro et al. (63).

Oken et al. (64) showed in a nonrandomized study that 80% of untreated patients responded to vincristine BCNU melphalan cyclophosphamide prednisone (VBMCP) plus IFN-α and that 26% achieved a complete remission, that is, disappearance of the M protein and normalization of the bone marrow. Complete remission in multiple myeloma is a rare event. Using a combination of vincristine melphalan cyclophosphamide prednisone (VMCP) plus IFN compared to VMCP alone, Preis et al. (65) also showed superiority of the IFN-containing regimen for response induction, 57 versus 41%. In a relatively small study by Corrado et al. (66), however, a lower response rate was found for the IFN-α regimen, although 7% showed a complete response in the MP + IFN group.

Another approach has been used by the Italian Multiple Myeloma Study Group. After induction chemotherapy, responding patients were randomized to low-dose IFN (3×10^6 U/m^2 three times a week) continuously or to no maintenance therapy (67). A significant prolongation of duration of response and survival time was found for patients receiving IFN therapy. This therapeutic strategy is discussed in another chapter.

There is now substantial evidence showing the superiority of chemotherapy plus IFN-α for response induction in myeloma compared to chemotherapy alone. Whether this kind of therapy also prolongs survival cannot yet firmly be established and awaits further follow-up. However, the results of the Italian Multiple Myeloma Study Group using IFN as maintenance therapy and the tendency to a better survival for patients with a small tumor burden (stage II), patients ≤ 65 years of age, and IgA myelomas receiving MP plus IFN in the MGCS trial may support the assumption that IFN may also have an impact on survival.

TABLE 7 Response Frequencies (%) of α-IFN and Chemotherapy for Induction Treatment of Previously Untreated Multiple Myeloma Patients

Treatment schedule	Response rate (%) Mean	95% Confidence limits	Reference
MP + IFN-α (n = 26)	69	50–88	Cooper et al. (62)
MP (n = 21)	71	50–92	Montuoro et al. (63)
MP + IFN-α (n = 16)	81	60–100	
MP (n = 24)	54	33–75	Corrado et al. (66)
MP + IFN-α (n = 29)	41 (CR 7%)[a]	22–60	
VBMCP + IFN-α (n = 54)	80% (CR 26%)	69–91	Oken et al. (64)
VMCP (n = 27)	41	22–60	Preis et al. (65)
VMCP + IFN-α (n = 21)	57	34–80	

[a]Complete remission.

ACKNOWLEDGEMENTS

This study was supported by grants from the Swedish Cancer Society, the Cancer Society in Stockholm, and the Elina Andersson Foundation. For valuable scientific discussion we thank Professor Kenneth Nilsson. For excellent secretarial help we thank Ms. Marie Karlsson. Members of the Myeloma Group of Central Sweden (MGCS) and participating hospitals: B. Johansson, H. Mellstedt (Chairman), A. Österborg (Secretary), H. Strander, and E. Svedmyr, Department of Oncology (Radiumhemmet), Karolinska Hospital; M. Björkholm, G. Grimfors, and E. Ösby, Department of Medicine, Karolinska Hospital; R. Hast and E. Kimby, Department of Medicine, Danderyds Hospital; H. Gyllenhammar, R. Lerner, and A.-M. Udén, Department of Medicine, South Hospital; G. Gahrton, G. Juliusson, and C. Paul, Department of Medicine, Huddinge Hospital, Stockholm; G. Brenning, A. Killander, B. Simonsson, and B. Svedmyr, Department of Medicine, Academic Hospital, Uppsala; and Björeman, M. Järnmark, A.-M. Stalfelt, and B. Wadman, Department of Medicine, Örebro Hospital, Örebro, Sweden.

REFERENCES

1. Mellstedt H, Holm, G, Björkholm M. Multiple myeloma, Waldenström's macroglobulinemia and benign monoclonal gammopathy. Characteristics of the B cell clone, immunoregulatory cell populations and clinical implications. Adv Cancer Res 1984; 41:257–89.
2. Berenson J, Wong R, Kim K, Brown N, Lichtenstein A. Evidence for peripheral blood B lymphocyte but not T lymphocyte involvement in multiple myeloma. Blood 1987; 70:1550–3.
3. Kubagawa H, Vogler LB, Capra JD, Conrad ME, Lawton AR, Cooper, MD. Studies on the clonal origin of multiple myeloma. Use of individually specific (idiotype) antibodies to trace the oncogenic event to its earliest point of expression in B-cell differentiation. J Exp Med 1979; 150:792–807.
4. Epstein J, He XY, Xiao H, Barlogie B. Multi-lineage involvement in multiple myeloma (MM). Proc Annu Meet Am Soc Clin Oncol 1989; 8:256.
5. Österborg A, Björkholm M, Nilsson B, Holm G, Mellstedt H. Natural killer cell activity in monoclonal gammopathies: relation to disease activity. Eur J Haematol 1990; 45:153–157.
6. Targan S, Brieva J, Neuman W, Stevens R. Is the NK lytic process involved in the mechanism of NK suppression of antibody-producing cells? J Immunol 1985; 134:666–9.
7. Österborg A, Masucci M, Bergenbrant S. Generation of T cell clones binding $F(ab')_2$ fragments of the idiotypic immunoglobulin in patients with monoclonal gammopathy. Cancer Immunol Immunother 1992. In press.
8. Andersson M, Holm G, Lefvert A-K, Mellstedt H. Anti-idiotypic B cell lines from a patient with monoclonal gammopathy of undetermined significance. Scand J Immunol 1990; 30:489–2.

9. Mingari M, Gerosa CF, Carra G, et al. Human interleukin-2 promotes proliferation of activated B cells via surface receptors similar to those of activated T cells. Nature 1984; 312:641.
10. Palacios R, Henson G, Steinmetz M, Kearn JP. Interleukin-3 supports growth of of mouse pre-B cell clones in vitro. Nature 1984; 309:126–31.
11. Defrance T, Vanbervliet B, Aubry JP. B cell growth-promoting activity of recombinant human interleukin 4. J Immunol 1987; 139:1135–41.
12. Azuma C, Tanabe T, Konishi M, Cloning of cDNA for human T-cell replacing factor (interleukin 5) and comparison with the murine homologue. Nucleic Acids Res 1986; 14:9149–58.
13. Muraguchi A, Hirano T, Tang B, et al. The essential role of B cell stimulatory factor 2 (BSF-2/IL-6) for the terminal differentiation of B cells. J Exp Med 1988; 167:332–44.
14. Kawano M, Hirano T, Matsuda T, et al. Autocrine generation and requirement of BSF-2/IL-6 for human multiple myelomas. Nature 1988; 332:83–5.
15. Mushinski JF. B-CLL, multiple myelomas, benign monoclonal gammopathies. In: Melchers F, Potter M, eds. Mechanisms of B cell neoplasia. Basel: Roche, 1989; 262–5.
16. Nilsson K. B-CLL, multiple myelomas, benign monoclonal gammopathies. In: Melchers F, Potter M, eds. Mechanisms of B cell neoplasia. Basel: Roche, 1989; 229–35.
17. Asaoku H, Kawano M, Iwato K, et al. Decrease in BSF-2/IL-6 response in advanced cases of multiple myeloma. Blood 1988; 2:429–32.
18. Dalla-Favera R. Endemic Burkitt's, sporadic Burkitt's and AIDS lymphomas. In: Melchers F, Potter M, eds. Mechanisms of B cell neoplasia. Basel: Roche, 1989; 135–45.
19. Adams J. B-CLL, multiple myelomas, benign monoclonal gammopathies. In: Melchers F, Potter M, eds. Mechanisms of B cell neoplasia. Basel: Roche 1989; 236–42.
20. Anderson KC, Jones RM, Morimoto C, Leavitt P, Barut BA. Response patterns of purified myeloma cells to hematopoietic growth factors. Blood 1989; 73:1915–24.
21. Klein B, Jourdan M, Vazquez A, Dugas B, Bataille R. Production of growth factors by human myeloma cells. Cancer Res 1987; 47:4856–60.
22. Bataille R, Klein B, Jourdan M, Rossi JF, Durie BGM. Spontaneous secretion of tumor necrosis factor-β by human myeloma cell lines. Cancer 1989; 63:877–80.
23. Yamamoto I, Kawano M, Sone T, et al. Production of interleukin 1β, a potent bone resorbing cytokine, by cultured human myeloma cells. Cancer Res 1989; 49:4242–6.
24. Kawano M, Tanaka H, Ishikawa H, et al. Interleukin-1 accelerates autocrine growth of myeloma cells through interleukin-6 in human myeloma. Blood 1989; 73:2145–8.
25. Maekawa R, Matsumoto M, Kitagawa T, Harada M, Sato, K. Effect of recombinant interleukin 2 (R-IL 2) on in vivo growth of murine myeloma X5563. Cancer Immunol Immunother 1986; 23:25–30.
26. Taylor JL, Sabran JL, Grossberg SE. The cellular effects of interferon. In: Came PE, Carter WA, eds. Interferon and their applications. New York: Springer-Verlag, 1984; 169–205.

27. Weck PK, Came PE. Comparative biologic activities of human interferon. In: Came PE, Carter WA, eds. Interferon and their applications. New York: Springer-Verlag, 1984; 339–57.
28. Salmon SE, Ozer H. Alpha interferon therapy in oncology: clinical update. Semin Oncol 1986; 13:1–2.
29. Strander H. Interferon treatment of human neoplastia. Adv Cancer Res 1986; 46:1–256.
30. Aapro MS, Alberts DS, Salmon SE. Interactions of human leukocyte interferon with vinca alkaloids and other chemotherapeutic agents against human tumors in clonogenic assay. Cancer Chemother Pharmacol 1983; 10:161–6.
31. Einhorn S, Fernberg JO, Grandér D, Lewensohn R. Interferon exerts a cytotoxic effect on primary human myeloma cells. Eur J Cancer Clin Oncol 1988; 24:1505–10.
32. Adams A, Strander H, Cantwell K. Sensitivity of the Epstein-Barr virus transformed human lymphoid cell lines to interferon. J Gen Virol 1975; 28:207–17.
33. Einhorn S, Strander H. Interferon therapy for neoplastic diseases in man: in vitro and in vivo studies. Adv Exp Med Biol 1978; 110:159–74.
34. Case DC, Someborn HL, Paul SD, et al. Phase II study of rDNA alpha-2 interferon (Intron A) in patients with multiple myeloma utilizing an escalating induction phase. Cancer Treat Rep 1986; 70:1251–4.
35. Åhre A, Björkholm M, Österborg A, et al. High doses of natural α-interferon (α-IFN) in the treatment of multiple myeloma. A pilot study from the Myeloma Group of Central Sweden (MGCS). Eur J Haematol 1988; 41:123–30.
36. Cooper MR, Welander CE. Interferon in the treatment of multiple myeloma. Semin Oncol 1986; 13:334–40.
37. Ehrsson H, Eksborg S, Wallin I, Österborg A, Mellstedt H. Oral melphalan pharmacokinetics—influence of interferon induced fever. Clin Pharmacother 1990; 47:86–90.
38. Friedman RM. Growth factors, oncogenes, and interferon. J Exp Pathol 1986; 2:223–8.
39. Paganelli KA, Evans SS, Han T, Ozer H. B cell growth factor-induced proliferation of hairy cell lymphocytes and inhibition by type 1 interferon in vitro. Blood 1986; 67:937–42.
40. Clemens M. Interferons and oncogenes. Nature 1985; 313:531–2.
41. Pegoraro L, Malavesi F, Bellone G, et al. The human myeloma cell line LP-1: a versatile model in which to study early plasma-cell differentiation and c-*myc* activation. Blood 1989; 73:1020–7.
42. Krolewski JJ, Dalla-Favera R. Oncogenes and their relevance in the pathogenesis of hematologic malignancies. In: Luzzatto L, Mauer AM, eds. Education book. Milan, XXII International Congress of Hematology, August 28–September 3, 1988; 20–8.
43. Gazdar AF, Oie HK, Kirsch IR, Hollis GF. Establishment and characterization of a human plasma cell myeloma culture having a rearranged cellular *myc* proto-oncogene. Blood 1986; 67:1542–9.
44. Einhorn S, Åhre A, Blomgren H, Johansson B, Mellstedt H, Strander H. Interferon and natural killer activity in multiple myeloma. Lack of correlation between interferon induced enhancement of natural killer activity and clinical response to human interferon-α. Int J Cancer 1982; 30:167–72.

45. Flood PM, Phillips C, Taupier MA, Schreiber H. Regulation of myeloma growth in vitro by idiotype-specific T lymphocytes. J Immunol 1980; 124:424–30.
46. Tao W, Mellstedt H, Jondal M. Presence of clonal T cell populations in B-CLL and smouldering myeloma. J Exp Med 1990; 171:659–6.
47. Lindahl P, Leary P, Gresser I. Enhancement by interferon of the specific cytotoxicity of sensitized lymphocytes. Proc Natl Acad Sci USA 1972; 69:1721–5.
48. Lindahl P, Gresser I, Leary P, Tovey M. Interferon treatment of mice: enhanced expression of histocompatibility antigens on lymphoid cells. Proc Natl Acad Sci USA 1976; 73:1284–7.
49. Alexanian R, Haut A, Khan AU, et al. Treatment for multiple myeloma. Combination chemotherapy with different melphalan dose regimens. JAMA 1969; 208:1680–5.
50. Sporn JR, McIntyre OR. Chemotherapy of previously untreated multiple myeloma patients: an analysis of recent treatment results. Semin Oncol 1986; 13:318–25.
51. Österborg A, Åhre A, Björkholm M, et al. Alternating combination chemotherapy (VMCP/VBAP) is not superior to melphalan/prednisone in the treatment of multiple myeloma patients stage III—a randomized study from MGCS. Eur J Hematol 1989; 43:54–62.
52. Mellstedt H, Åhre A, Björkholm M, Holm G, Johansson B, Strander H. Interferon therapy in myelomatosis. Lancet 1979; 1:245–7.
53. Åhre A, Björkholm M, Mellstedt H, et al. Human leukocyte interferon and intermittent high dose melphalan/prednisolone administration in the treatment of multiple myeloma: a randomized clinical trial. Cancer Treat Rep 1984; 68:1331–8.
54. Goldstein D, Laszlo J. Interferon therapy in Cancer—from imaginon to interferon. Cancer Res 1986; 46:4315–29.
55. Quesada JR, Alexanian R, Hawkins M, et al. Treatment of multiple myeloma with recombinant α-interferon. Blood 1986; 67:275–8.
56. Ludwig H, Cortelezzi A, Scheithauer W, et al. Recombinant interferon alpha-2C versus polychemotherapy (VMCP) for treatment of multiple myeloma: a prospective randomized trial. Eur J Cancer Clin Oncol, 1986; 22:1111–6.
57. Ohno R, Kimura K. Treatment of multiple myeloma with recombinant interferon alpha-2a. Cancer 1986; 57:1685–8.
58. Ohno R. Interferons in the treatment of multiple myeloma. Int J Cancer (Suppl) 1987; 1:14–20.
59. Durie BGM, Russel DH, Salmon SE. Reappraisal of plateau phase in myeloma. Lancet 1980; 2:65–7.
60. Taetle R, Buick RN, McCulloc EA. Effect of interferon on colony-formation in culture by blast cell progenitors in acute myeloblastic leukemia. Blood 1980; 56:549–52.
61. Beagley KW, Eldridge JH, Lee F, et al. Interleukins and IgA synthesis. Human and murine interleukin-6 induce high rate IgA secretion in IgA-committed B cells. J Exp Med 1989; 169:2133–48.
62. Cooper MR, Fefer A, Thompson J, et al. Alpha-2-interferon/melphalan/prednisone in previously untreated patients with multiple myeloma: a phase I-II trial, Cancer Treat Rep 1986; 70:473–9.
63. Montuoro A, De Rosa L, De Blasio A, et al. Alpha-2-interferon/melphalan/prednisone versus melphalan/prednisone in previously untreated patients with mul-

tiple myeloma: preliminary results (Abstract) XXII International Congress of Hematology, August 28–September 3, Milan, 1988.
64. Oken MM, Kyle RA, Greipp PR, Kay NE, Tsiatis A, O'Connell MJ. Complete remission (CR) induction with VBMCP + interferon (rIFN-alpha-2b) in multiple myeloma: 3-year follow-up. Abstract: I International Symposium on Cytokines in Hematopoesis, Oncology and AIDS, June 14–17, Hannover, Germany, 1989.
65. Preis P, Sheithauer W, Fritz E, et al. VMCP chemotherapy with or without Interferon-alpha-2 in newly diagnosed patients with multiple myeloma. Onkologie 1989; 12:27–9.
66. Corrado C, Pavlovsky S, Saslasky J, Lein J, Palau V, Santarelli MT. Randomized trial comparing melphalan-prednisone with or without recombinant alpha 2 interferon (r-alpha-2-IFN) in multiple myeloma. Proc Am Soc Clin Oncol 1989; 8:258.
67. Mandelli F, Amadori S, Avvisati G, et al. Recombinant interferon alpha-2b as maintenance therapy in responding multiple myeloma patients: preliminary report of the Italian multiple myeloma study group (IMMSG) (Abstract). XXII International Congress of Hematology, August 28–September 3, Milan, Italy, 1988.

7

Interferons in the Treatment of Lymphomas

Linda M. Bavisotto

University of Washington, Seattle, Washington

Ernest C. Borden

Medical College of Wisconsin, Milwaukee, Wisconsin

I. INTRODUCTION

Preclinical and early clinical investigation with natural human interferons as antineoplastic agents indicated significant responsiveness in the lymphoid malignancies, including lymphomas (1–5). Since 1981, the availability of recombinant preparations of single-species human leukocyte interferon-α has facilitated confirmation of the antitumor efficacy seen with earlier crude preparations of mixed leukocyte interferons in the lymphomas. Significant single-agent responses have been achieved with interferon-α, most notably in the indolent lymphomas of both B and T cell origin, first in heavily pretreated advanced stages resistant to conventional therapy and more recently, as initial systemic therapy. Although interferon-β and -γ have been less extensively studied to date, several preliminary reports suggest activity in the lymphomas.

Accumulated experience defining the activity of interferon-α across the spectrum of other B cell lymphoid neoplasms (hairy cell leukemia, multiple myeloma, and acute and chronic lymphocytic leukemia), reviewed in other chapters, reflects a wide-ranging variation in degree of responsiveness between these disorders. The indolent lymphomas, in addition to historical responsiveness, present several features that have made them particularly appropriate for phase I/II clinical trials using interferons: these are malignancies that tend to disseminate early; unlike the more aggressive lymphomas, stage III and IV remain incurable with the best available combinations of conventional agents, and the natural history of these disorders (with median survival of 6–10 years) permits the protracted observation of patients with reasonable performance status over time. The possibility that immune defects associated with lymphomas might be amenable to interferon biotherapy was also anticipated (6–8,180). A number of reviews have chronicled the early therapeutic utility of the interferons for non-Hodgkin's lymphomas and cutaneous T cell lymphomas (9–16,187,193,196). Although substantially fewer in number, significant responses have also been documented in some instances in the diffuse lymphomas, in peripheral T cell lymphomas and other variant T cell lymphomas, in Hodgkin's disease, in acute lymphocytic leukemia, and in chronic lymphocytic leukemia with single-agent and combination therapy using interferons.

It is the aim of this chapter to provide an updated overview of the growing experience with interferons in the treatment of the malignant lymphomas of both B cell and T cell origin. The first section briefly highlights selected preclinical and clinical correlate studies that formed the rationale for subsequent introduction into lymphoma clinical trials. The focus of the second section is to summarize the safety and efficacy trials to date in the lymphomas, to examine critically the subtypes of disease with most efficacy, and to briefly survey current study design strategies and future directions. The final section seeks to place in perspective the questions challenging investigative oncologists caring for patients with lymphomas, taking into account currently unsettled questions relating to optimal management of the indolent lymphomas.

II. PRECLINICAL STUDIES

Despite extensive preclinical testing, much remains to be learned about the mechanism of action and differences in activity between interferons α, β, and γ and their potential for integration with chemotherapeutic agents, other biologic agents, or other modalities. Both antiproliferative and immunomodulatory effects may contribute to the antitumor mechanism of the interferons, and in different cell types the relative contribution of these effects may differ. The impetus for efforts to establish the explicit nature of the interferon antitumor effect in a given tumor has been to provide a rational guide to the design of biotherapeutic trials favoring either a cytotoxic or a biologic response modifier model (17,18, 192). In the latter, unlike the former, the optimal biologic dose may not be equal to the maximum tolerated dose (MTD), and responses may not be as prompt as expected with cytotoxic chemotherapy. Because it has not been simple to draw consistent conclusions from the preclinical setting, phase I/II trials with the interferons have necessarily been largely empiric in terms of dose, sequence, and duration. In the case of the lymphoid malignancies, several productive lines of preclinical investigation deserve mention.

A. Deficiency of Interferon Production in Lymphoid Malignancies

First, and perhaps most compelling, production of endogenous interferon has been found to be deficient in patients with non-Hodgkin's lymphoma, chronic lymphocytic leukemia (both interferon-α and -γ), acute lymphocytic leukemia, hairy cell leukemia (interferon-α), and advanced Hodgkin's disease (19–27). In some of the patients studied, production of interferon normalized with remission of the disease (22). Ho and co-workers (27) examined 13 patients with low-grade non-Hodgkin's lymphoma, 15 patients with high-grade non-Hodgkin's lymphoma, 20 patients with chronic lymphocytic leukemia, and 21 normal control subjects for induction of interferon in peripheral blood leukocytes by phytohemagglutinin (PHA), conconcavalin A (ConA), pokeweed mitogen (PWM), *Corynebacterium parvum* (*C. parvum*), Newcastle disease virus (NDV), herpes simplex virus (HSV), and interleukin-2 (IL-2). In all three patient groups, stimulation of interferon production in response to NDV was significantly lower than that measured in normal controls. In all non-Hodgkin's lymphoma patients, a blunted responsiveness to *C. parvum* was also observed. By contrast, PWM, HSV, ConA, and IL-2 produced little difference in interferon production between patients and controls. Since NDV and *C. parvum* induce mainly interferon-α and the mitogens PHA and ConA mainly stimulate interferon-γ production, the authors suggest that a selective deficiency in the interferon-α response occurs in patients with non-Hodgkin's lymphoma, an observation that may carry implications for the choice of subtypes of interferon in the treatment of non-Hodgkin's lymphoma.

A molecular basis for such a deficiency in interferon production in a subset of patients may lie in the loss of bands p21–22 from one or both of the chromosome 9 homologs as a consequence of the deletion of the short arm [del(9p)], unbalanced translocation, or monosomy 9 frequently observed in the malignant cells of patients with lymphoid neoplasms, including acute lymphoblastic leukemia and non-Hodgkin's lymphoma (28). The interferon-α gene cluster and interferon β_1 gene localize to this region. Homozygous or hemizygous deletions of the interferon genes were detected by Southern blotting in 7 of 15 cell lines established from patients with acute lymphocytic leukemia (ALL) (28). Complete deficiency of methyl thioadenosine phosphorylase (MTAP), an enzyme involved in purine metabolism and gene product of a closely linked gene mapping to 9pter-q12, accompanied the interferon gene deletions in these cell lines. To confirm that the deletions did not arise de novo during subcultivation of these cell lines, primary uncultured leukemic cells of 62 patients with ALL were examined (29), showing that 18 (overall 29%) had such deletions. About half these deletions were detectable cytogenetically as structural rearrangements of the short arm of chromosome 9, and half were submicroscopic deletions revealed only by Southern blotting. Homozygous deletions of the interferon-α cluster occurred in

4 (7%); 1 of these also had a homozygous deletion and 3 of these, hemizygous deletions, respectively, of the interferon-β_1 gene. Overall, 14 (23%) had hemizygous deletions of both interferon-α and interferon-β_1 genes. The minimal region of overlap of all these deletion patterns proved to be 9p22. These authors reasoned that in view of the frequency of structural rearrangements of 9p22 in ALL, the chromosomal and molecular deletions are likely to be related to loss of a tumor suppressor gene(s) on chromosome 9p, which may be an interferon gene itself or a closely linked gene. Thus, the interferon-α and -β_1 genes could behave as tumor suppressor genes in normal individuals, and their acquired deletion or inactivation could be associated with the initiation or progression of these lymphoid neoplasms. A significant incidence of 9p abnormalities has also been associated with melanoma and glioblastoma. In the setting of diseases in which such an interferon deficiency state is found, the long-term therapeutic administration of continuous low-dose interferon (which might be viewed as "replacement therapy") may have clinical utility. Indeed, more than a decade ago speculation existed that the interferon response may play a defensive part against the development of tumors, as it is produced by lymphocytes in response to encounter with foreign antigens or tumor cells (3). Since production of interferon is regulated by interaction with immunocompetent cells, and interferon itself causes activation of cellular defense elements, defects in the interferon system may be involved in the progression of lymphoid neoplasms as well as in some of their attendant complications, particularly frequency of infections (27).

The follicular non-Hodgkin's lymphomas are characterized, in approximately 85–90% of the cases, by a specific cytogenetic abnormality, the t(14;18) (q32;q21) translocation, providing a marker chromosome for these indolent lymphomas (30–33). In this translocation, the *bcl*-2 protooncogene translocates to chromosome 14 near the immunoglobulin heavy-chain genes in a manner analogous to the Burkitt's lymphoma t(8;14) translocation in which the *myc* protooncogene translocates to 14q32. Rearrangement of *bcl*-2 in patients undergoing treatment for follicular non-Hodgkin's lymphomas can be monitored using Southern blotting and, more recently, polymerase chain reaction (PCR) techniques (34–36). Recently, the establishment and characterization of a human lymphoma cell line (WSU-NHL) that carries the t(14;18) translocation from a patient with nodular histiocytic (follicular large cell) lymphoma has been reported (37). Those authors noted that interferon-γ at 500 U/ml inhibits growth and differentiation of this cell line. Whether cytogenetic reversions of this marker chromosome for follicular NHL occur in interferon-treated patients, as in the suppression of the Philadelphia chromosome in approximately 40% of patients with chronic myelogenous leukemia (CML) treated in the chronic phase with interferon-α, must be determined.

B. Direct Antiproliferative Effects of Interferon in Lymphoid Cell Lines

The direct (non-host mediated) antiproliferative activity of interferon may be due to cytotoxic or cytostatic effects, induced maturation and terminal differentiation of committed cells, or a combination of these. Recently, differentiation-inducing effects of interferon-α have been implicated in hairy cell leukemia, as indicated by surface marker changes to a more mature phenotype (38) and also in blast cells from acute myelogenous leukemia (AML) and CML in blast crisis, in which the presence of Auer rods in interferon-γ or tumor necrosis factor α (TNF-α)-induced macrophages show that these cytokines can induce differentiation of a leukemic clone in uncultured cells (188).

Interferons can be viewed in the context of a homeostatic network of counteracting growth inhibitors secreted in response to growth factors, normally limiting cell proliferation after growth stimuli (39). Antagonism between interferons and known physiologic growth factors (e.g., epidermal growth factor and fibroblast growth factor) suggests that interferons may be physiologic growth regulators. The antiproliferative effect of interferons in the Burkitt's lymphoma-derived Daudi cell line may be due to the induction of cellular differentiation and loss of responsiveness to autocrine growth factors (40). This clonal cell line, transformed at a late stage of B cell maturation, is blocked in its ability to differentiate to plasma cells and continues to proliferate. The block to differentiation can be overcome by such agents as interferon or the phorbol ester tetradecanoyl phorbol acetate (TPA), both of which suppress overexpression of c-*myc* (40). Interferons have positively or negatively affected the expression of a number of oncogenes implicated in cell cycle progression, potentially correlating with a cytostatic effect (39,41). In malignant cells from patients with hairy cell leukemia, interferon has induced both in vivo and in vitro a state of functional unresponsiveness to B cell growth factor (BCGF; IL-5), to which these cells may respond in an autocrine fashion (42).

It is possible to demonstrate direct growth inhibition by interferon-α in clonogenic assays using human tumor cell lines in vitro and in xenografts of human tumors in athymic nude mice in vivo, both assay systems that remove host immune function as a variable. Although not linear, a dose-response effect can be seen in sensitive tumors, both for interferon dose and for tumor burden (43). Furthermore, only sporadic correlations have been shown between augmentation of measurable host defense parameters (such as normalization of natural killer, NK, activity) and antitumor efficacy. Other lines of evidence, however, implicate the importance of host response factors in the antiproliferative response. A murine lymphoma with resistance to interferon in vitro has exhibited sensitivity in vivo (44). Several human clinical trials have indeed observed a consistent correlation between antitumor effect and increases in NK activity (see Ref. 45). Increased tumor growth and transplantability were observed when athymic nude mice carrying various human tumor xenografts in the absence of exogenous interferon were injected with an antiserum to murine interferon, supporting a role for endogenous interferons in the normal host effector immune response (46). Like other cytokines, interferons induce a formidable array of pleiotropic responses, including biochemical-metabolic changes, broad alterations in RNA and protein synthetic profiles, and surface membrane changes, which may contribute to antiproliferative and immunomodulatory properties and perhaps to the antitumor effectiveness (47). Yet another type of indirect antitumor mechanism may be operative in the inhibition of angiogenesis by interferons (48) or in the microvascular injury implicated in the pathogenesis of interferon-induced necrosis of subcutaneous tumors in mice (49).

Studies of lymphoid cell lines have shown mixed responses to interferons (190, 194). A potent growth inhibitory effect of interferon-α_{2b} was seen in a number of normal and malignant human cell lines, including Burkitt's lymphoma-derived Daudi, T cell lymphocytic leukemia-derived RPMI-8402, and B cell lymphocytic leukemia-derived BALM-2. Not all lymphoid cell lines showed decreased proliferation, however (50). Interferon-β_1 inhibited T cell proliferation while augmenting cytolytic activity (51,52). Growth inhibition in the presence of interferon-β_2 (interleukin-6) has been shown in Daudi (Burkitt's lymphoma-derived B cell), U-937 (diffuse histiocytic lymphoma-derived monocytic), and Molt-4 (T cell lymphoma-derived) cell lines (53). The antiproliferative effects could be blocked by antibodies directed to the N terminus of the interleukin-6 synthetic peptide. Like the classic type I interferon-β_1, IL-6 is produced in fibroblasts and induces 2′,5′-oligo-adenylate synthetase, but is localized on chromosome 7 rather than 9 and has distinctive effects as a B cell differentiation factor.

C. Potential Immunomodulatory Activity of Interferon in the Lymphomas

Immunomodulation by interferons occurs within a complex network of cytokine interactions that has yet to be fully delineated. Pleiotropic immunomodulatory effects of interferons have been observed (47,54–56). Several abnormalities characterize untreated patients with non-Hodgkin's lymphomas, including depressed antibody-mediated cellular cytotoxicity (ADCC), a defective proliferative response of lymphocytes to allogeneic cells and mitogens, and depressed natural killer cell activity (6,7). Natural interferon-α, and in some cases interferon-β and -γ, have induced proliferation and blast transformation of B cells from human lymph nodes taken from either B and T cell lymphoma patients or normal volunteers with enlarged, nonmalignant lymph nodes (57). Cytotoxic chemotherapy was found to enhance both ADCC and NK activity in non-Hodgkin's lymphoma patients over depressed pretreatment values, apparently by affecting postbinding events, causing an increase in the active killing potential of the NK cells. An augmentation of NK activity in vitro by exogenous interferon-α treatment of patient lymphocytes after chemotherapy was comparable to the augmentation seen in normal control subjects, suggesting a therapeutic role for interferon in combination with cytotoxic therapy (58). Time and dose dependence as well as assay methodology may be critical to measurement of in vivo augmentation of NK cell activity by interferons, however. By 1 week after initiation of interferon therapy, NK cell function in lymphoma patients was markedly depressed; upon discontinuation of interferon, NK cell activity quickly returned to pretreatment values (59). Furthermore, higher doses of interferon may result in less augmentation of NK cell or monocyte tumoricidal activity (60–62). Several groups have investigated the influence of interferon on NK activity in vivo in mice (63,64). Voiculescu et al. found significant augmentation of NK activity when interferon-β treatment was combined with indomethacin. In vitro, the cytotoxic supernatant activity of tumor target-stimulated IL-2-activated killer cells (LAK) has been found to be neutralized by polyclonal antibodies specific to interferon-γ and tumor necrosis factor α (65). Interferons differentially regulated expression of the HLA-B7 and HLA-A3 class I genes in the Jurkat T cell line, a low constitutive expressor of HLA class I antigens, but not in the JJK Epstein-Barr virus (EBV)-transformed human B lymphocyte line, a high constitutive expressor (66). Interferon-α inhibited the normal expression of heavy-chain μ messenger RNA in Daudi cells (67); this inhibition was not due to increased degradation, as it was in the case of the decline in c-*myc* expression following interferon treatment, or to an alteration in transcriptional rate. In co-culture experiments with fractionated B cells and highly purified NK cells, a subset of large activated B cells was found to stimulate production of interferon-γ by NK cells (68). This group found that, in turn, the interferon-γ inhibited polyclonally induced B cell proliferation; small resting B cells did not stimulate or respond to NK cells (68).

D. Interferon Antiviral Activity and the Lymphomas

Secretion of interferons may play a major role in natural host defense against viral infections, including those viruses capable of inducing tumor formation (190). Perhaps more than any other malignancy, lymphomas have been associated with tumor-inducing viruses, providing further rationale for assessment of interferons in these disorders. The human lymphotropic retroviruses HTLV-I, HTLV-II, and HIV-1 (HTLV-III) have been associated with adult T cell leukemia and lymphoma, T cell hairy cell leukemia variants, and the acquired immunodeficiency syndrome (AIDS), respectively (69–71). Serum antibodies to

HTLV-I have been found in a majority of patients with T cell lymphoma of the Caribbean, diffuse peripheral T cell lymphoma, and adult T cell leukemia of Japan, but in the United States less than 5% of patients with cutaneous T cell lymphoma (CTCL) are positive by sero-epidemiology. Another T lymphotropic retrovirus, HTLV-V, has been associated with cutaneous T cell lymphomas, particularly mycosis fungoides (72). A newly isolated herpesvirus (73), human B lymphotropic virus (HBLV), has been associated with lymphoproliferative disorders, including angioimmunoblastic lymphadenopathy, cutaneous T cell lymphoma, immunoblastic lymphoma, and acute lymphoblastic leukemia in HIV-seronegative patients (74). HBLV was also isolated from two HIV-seropositive patients in their sample, one with an AIDS-related lymphoma and another with dermatopathic lymphadenopathy. The well-characterized herpesvirus Epstein-Barr virus has been associated not only with Burkitt's lymphoma but also with nasopharyngeal carcinomas that may respond to interferon (75), thymic carcinomas (76), and lymphoproliferative disorders in patients who are immunosuppressed (77,78). Primates vaccinated against EBV membrane antigen were found to be completely protected against challenge with a 100% lymphoma-producing inoculum (79). Many clinical trials with interferons in the lymphomas have excluded patients in whom viral etiology was documented, with the exception of specific trials in the AIDS-associated malignancies (80,81). In vitro, suppression of HIV-1 (HTLV-III) replication by interferon-α has been documented (82). Other recently demonstrated antiviral effects of interferons in lymphoid cells are of interest. Decreased EBV-induced transformation and increased 2,5-oligo-A synthetase and RNAse L activity in peripheral blood leukocytes from patients treated with interferon-α_{2b} has been reported (83). B cell lines established from HTLV-I- or EBV-infected patients spontaneously produce an acid-labile interferon-α (84), suggesting polyclonal B cell activation. HTLV-I-infected T cells did not secrete interferon. An inverse relationship was found between constitutive interferon-γ production and HTLV-I expression in cultured T lymphocytes (85). These workers suggested that a greater number of HTLV-I-seropositive patients with cutaneous T cell lymphoma may be identified by maintenance of T cell cultures in antibodies to interferon-γ. Several workers have observed lupus inclusions or cylindrical confronting cisternae which are tubular or particulate structures that have been noted in lymphocytes and other cells of patients with AIDS and in lymphoblastoid Daudi cells treated with interferon-α (86,87). In the latter cells these inclusions were de novo synthesized complexes of ribonucleoprotein and membrane (88). A similar type of reticulotubular inclusion in the BALB/c S49 mouse lymphoma cell line was regulated by interferon-α treatment both in vitro and in vivo. Immunoelectron microscopy using antibodies to murine mammary tumor virus (MMTV) showed these inclusion structures to be correlated with stages of MMTV morphogenesis (89).

E. Correlation with Receptor Binding Studies

Interferons initiate their activity via binding to specific receptors for type I (α and β) or type II (γ) interferon. Differences between cell lines with regard to growth inhibition may relate to differences in receptor number or affinity. In some cases receptor number and internalization upon binding have correlated with antiproliferative effects, in other cases not (for review see Ref 90). Interferon-α receptors on human lymphoblastoid cells were related to antitumor response in patients with lymphoproliferative disease (91,92). Recently, this group characterized the human type I interferon receptor by ligand blotting (93). A correlation by Scatchard analysis in several children with refractory ALL showed 50% modulation of interferon-α receptors 24 h after initiation of treatment with interferon-α; such modulation did not occur in a patient who failed to respond to interferon-α in vivo (94). Binding, internalization, and degradation of interferon-α in human Burkitt's lymphoma-derived Daudi cells (95), of interferon-γ by human Raji cells (96), and of interferon-γ by human diffuse histiocytic lymphoma U-937 cells (97) have been correlated with antiproliferative effects. Lymphoid and leukemic cells lines that showed growth inhibition upon interferon treatment bound more interferon-γ than resistant cell lines, and interferon-α_2 bound all cell lines irrespective of the antiproliferative susceptibility of the cells (98).

F. Synergistic Effects of Interferon in Combination with Other Agents

Different mechanisms of action and nonoverlapping toxicities suggest the potential for clinical benefit from combining interferons with other cancer treatment modalities. The synergism attainable from such combinations may be highly dose, sequence, and schedule dependent (17,99). In several animal models, prolongation of survival and reduction in tumor size have been at least additive and, in most instances, synergistic. The effectiveness of interferon combined with cytotoxic therapy has been demonstrated in the treatment of murine leukemias (100–102). The design of in vivo trials must take into consideration several additional aspects of potential interaction. Interferon-α inhibits hepatic P_{450} microsomal enzymes, which may affect the clearance of a coadministered agent and compromise the ability to deliver some conventional cytotoxic drugs; interferon-α may arrest cells in G_0 of the cell cycle, affecting the choice and scheduling of drugs; and cytotoxic drugs themselves can be immunomodulatory (16,99).

In vitro observations have indicated some beneficial combinations that may be exploitable in clinical trials (179,185). The human tumor clonogenic assay (HTCA) designed by Hamburger and Salmon has been employed to screen for synergy between interferons and conventional cytotoxic drugs (103,104). In some cases, the HTCA has indicated growth inhibition only at high doses of interferon, with lower doses actually enhancing clonal proliferation (105). A potential theoretical advantage of combining interferon with conventional cytotoxic therapy is the possibility that the antiproliferative effects of interferon on cells from many normal tissues spare organs with rapid cell turnover (gastrointestinal tract or bone marrow) from the toxicity of chemotherapeutic drugs selective for cycling cells (106). Combinations utilizing different cytokines are also being actively investigated. A rationale for combining interferon-γ with other biologic agents lies in observations that interferon-γ may activate macrophages, has shown a stronger antiproliferative effect than interferon-α for many cell types, and has shown synergy when combined with other interferons (107). In a variety of cultured cell types, treatment schedules combining type I and type II interferons, acting on different receptors, has produced synergistic antiproliferative effects, even in cells with relative resistance to one interferon type (108).

In lymphoid cells, additive or synergistic effects of interferon combination treatments are of interest. Combination treatment with tumor necrosis factor-α and interferon-γ inhibited the development of thymic lymphomas induced by whole-body split-dose radiation in C57BL/Ka mice compared to untreated control mice (109). The protection was similar to that obtained by grafting normal bone marrow after irradiation. Combined treatment with interferon-γ and tumor necrosis factor-α upregulated the expression of HLA class I determinants in HLA class I-deficient Burkitt's lymphoma cell lines (110). Concomitant addition of glucocorticoids and interferon-α_{2a} to some lymphoid cell lines produced synergistic antiproliferative effects (111). Enhancement of interferon-induced 2,5-oligo-adenylate synthetase activity by retinoic acid in human histiocytic lymphoma U-937 cells and WISH cells has been studied: the potentiation was dose and time dependent but did not appear to coincide with the antiproliferative or differentiation-inducing effects of interferon in these cells (112). The combination of tumor necrosis factor-α and interferon-α or -γ enhanced antiproliferative effects on several lymphoid and leukemic cell lines (113). Regulation of Fc receptor for IgE (CD23) and class II major histocompatibility complex (MHC) antigen expression in Burkitt's lymphoma cell lines by human IL-4 and interferon-γ has been demonstrated (114), as has expression of an Fc receptor on U-937 cells by interferon-γ (97).

III. IN VIVO ANIMAL STUDIES

Interferons are highly species specific, and only limited murine interferon has been available. Thus, animal modeling of the activity and toxicity of human interferons has been limited largely to studies of human tumor xenografts in athymic nude mice. In an AKR murine lymphoid leukemia model (115–117) administration of murine brain-derived interferon reduced the high incidence of spontaneous lymphoma development and, when administered only after lymphoma was diagnosed, induced tumor regression. Another useful murine model has investigated potential in vivo mechanisms for the synergistic antitumor effect seen with combination interferon + antiidiotype monoclonal antibody therapy. This model compared responses in normal C3H/HeN and their respective Fc-γ receptor-defective counterpart C3H/HeJ mice injected intraperitoneally with cells from a syngeneic murine B cell lymphoma cell line, C3H 38C13 (118). The C3H 38C13 cell line, derived from a dimeth[a]anthracene-induced lymphoma in a C3H/eB mouse depleted of T cells, expresses IgM κ and a unique idiotype to which a panel of syngeneic monoclonal antibodies has been produced. Antiidiotype therapy alone (leading to cure in 80% of mice previously injected with the murine B cell lymphoma-derived 38C13 tumor cells) resulted in the selection of idiotype-negative tumors, similar to those arising in human B cell lymphomas treated by this group with antiidiotype monoclonal antibodies (119). Human hybrid interferon-α A/D administered alone in high concentrations has direct antitumor effects in vivo in these mice; lower concentrations of interferon alone showed virtually no direct antitumor effect. Coadministration of monoclonal antiidiotype antibody and low-dose interferon-α A/D resulted in a synergistic increase in survival in C3H/HeN mice challenged with a lethal tumor dose (118). By contrast, the lipopolysaccharide (LPS)-hyporesponsive and Fc-γ receptor-defective C3H/HeJ mice responded less well to antiidiotype treatment alone. The diminished responsiveness to antiidiotype treatment in the latter mice was fully corrected by simultaneous administration of interferon. Fluorescence-activated cell sorting (FACS) analysis did not detect increased idiotype expression in response to interferon in these mice, making it unlikely that the interferon effect was due to enhancement of idiotype as a tumor target (as has been described for tumor-associated antigens in other tumor types). In the same cells, enhancement of H_2 expression by interferon treatment was readily detected. Antiidiotype monoclonal antibodies cleaved into F(ab′)2 fragments were not active. Taken together, these results suggested that the antiidiotype antibodies probably functioned through increased Fc-γ receptor-bearing effector cells resulting from interferon co-administration.

In further support of this conclusion, a stable subclone of the C3H 38C13 murine B cell lymphoma cell line used in these studies (SIR-1 variant) was selected in soft agar for normal expression of the parental tumor idiotype but total resistance to the most commonly measured effects of interferons, including antiviral and antiproliferative properties, 2′,5′oligo-adenylate synthetase induction, H_2 expression augmentation, and transient induction with subsequent repression of c-*myc*. Surprisingly, antitumor effects were seen in vivo following interferon-α treatment of C3H mice inoculated with these variant cultured lymphoma tumor cells, despite the demonstrated in vitro resistance of these lymphoma cells to all the previously mentioned effects of interferon (44). Combination treatment routinely protected 100% of the mice. Tumor cells reisolated from spleen, liver, and peritoneal washings of these mice retained complete resistance to the antiproliferative effects of human interferon-α A/D at 104 U/ml, indicating that there was not a phenotypic switch of the SIR-1 cells in vivo. These and other such studies suggest that the antitumor effects of interferon in vivo may result from an altered host response that more readily recognizes tumor cells and thereby eliminates them (44,120).

IV. CLINICAL RESULTS

The non-Hodgkin's lymphomas are a heterogeneous group, encompassing disorders of B or T cell origin with widely divergent natural histories. The International Working Formulation (199) has provided a pathologically and prognostically useful classification into two major groupings: low-grade (indolent) versus high-grade (aggressive) lymphomas. The indolent follicular non-Hodgkin's lymphomas (follicular NHL) and the cutaneous T cell lymphomas (CTCL), including mycosis fungoides and Sézary syndrome, have median survivals of 6 and 8–10 years, respectively (14). Studies that document a high frequency of malignant microscopic but clinically inapparent dissemination to extracutaneous sites in the blood, lymph nodes, and viscera of patients with CTCL at the time of diagnosis (121) suggest that the natural history of CTCL is indolent and similar to that in patients with low-grade NHL of B cell origin. Complete responses are readily induced with conventional chemotherapeutic agents in early stages of indolent NHL of both B and T cell origin, but remissions are short-lived and the course despite therapy is one of continuing relapse and preterminal transformation to diffuse aggressive lymphomas (12,122). Thus, whether early therapeutic intervention in patients with low-grade "favorable" histologic subtypes and advanced disease (stage III–IV NHL) offers superior palliation or survival compared to deferral of treatment until patients are symptomatic or threatened by their lymphoma is actively debated. Therefore, effective new treatments, such as biologic agents, could have significant clinical impact.

Evaluation of treatment strategies must take into account the spontaneous regression of NHL reported by the Stanford group (9,123,124). Of 44 patients with favorable histology NHL initially observed without therapy at Stanford University, 7 experienced spontaneous regression of measurable tumor during their disease course. Advocates of an early aggressive multimodality approach, on the other hand, have emphasized that attainment of complete response (CR) status may correlate with survival advantage. In practice, these two divergent approaches have been reflected by the experience at Stanford (124–126) and at the National Cancer Institute (127).

A. Single-Agent Interferon Treatment of the Non-Hodgkin's Lymphomas of B Cell Origin

The earliest phase I clinical trials utilized natural interferons crudely purified from supernatants of virus-stimulated leukocyte buffy coats or lymphoblastoid cells, which represented a mixture of interferon-α subspecies. Both the scarcity and low purity (typically $< 1\%$) of natural interferon preparations limited these trials (18). Nonetheless, responses were consistently seen in the lymphoid malignancies. Among the first clinical cases were anecdotal reports of decreased adenopathy, pulmonary infiltrate, and symptoms in a single patient with Hodgkin's lymphoma (1) and two patients with ALL treated with interferon in whom substantial decreases in peripheral and marrow leukemic blasts were observed by 2–3 weeks (2).

A consistent finding since the earliest trials has been a much higher response rate in the low-grade (nodular follicular, classifications A–C in the International Working Formulation, "favorable" histology) lymphomas than that in the high-grade (IWF classifications D–J, "unfavorable" histology) non-Hodgkin's lymphomas (Tables 1 and 2). In initial observations on the effect of partially purified natural human leukocyte interferon in non-Hodgkin's lymphoma, none of 3 patients with heavily pretreated advanced high-grade NHL (DHL) responded, but all three patients with low-grade favorable histology NHL did (1 CR and 2 partial response PR) (3). In a follow-up report (Louie et al., 1981) these observations were expanded to 11 patients, of whom 7 with favorable histology non-Hodgkin's were evaluable: 1 complete response, 2 partial responses, and 2 minor responses were seen. Of 5 responders 3 were previously untreated; unmaintained remission durations ranged from 6 to 12 months. Notably, a second PR was obtained in one patient upon retreatment with interferon after becoming refractory to a course of chemotherapy in the interval between interferon treatments. Leukopenia was the dose-limiting toxicity in this trial. The long time to response (3 months) in some responders suggested that interferon worked by more than a simple direct antiproliferative effect. These results were confirmed in a group of 6 low-grade NHL patients in whom 2 CR and 1 PR occurred; minor responses were seen in 2 of 4 patients with CLL and 1 patient with DHL (128). In a follow-up report using higher doses, a 3 month administration, and three times weekly schedule, no CRs were seen, and the 2 PRs occurred at the highest doses (129). The results of the American Cancer Society Lymphoma Trial (1979–1982) using partially purified leukocyte interferon were reported in 1985 (130). No CR, 3 PR, and 3 minor responses were seen in 18 evaluable patients with low-grade NHL treated for only 1 month at doses ranging from 3 to 9 × 106 U IM (intramuscular) daily. The 3.5 month time to maximum response suggested the value of a longer treatment period. Median response duration was

TABLE 1 Interferon-α Efficacy in the Low-Grade non-Hodgkin Lymphomas[a]

Group	Schedule and route	Response					Time to progression
		N	CR	PR	MR	RR(%)	
Stanford							
Merigan et al. (3)	2.5–5 × 10^6 U IM twice a day for 1 month	3	1	2	—	3 (100)	Not stated
Louie et al. (173)	5 × 10^6 U IM twice a day for 1 month	7	1	3	3	4 (57)	1.5–18$^+$ months
M. D. Anderson							
Gutterman et al. (128)	3–9 × 10^6 U IM daily for 1–3 months	6	2	1	—	3 (50)	Not stated
Quesada and Gutterman (129)	9–86 × 10^6 U IM daily for 3 months	3	0	2	—	2 (66)	Not stated
Southeastern Cancer Group (5)	5 × 10^6 U IM three times a week for 2 months, escalating if stable disease	25	2	4	—	6 (24)	Not stated
Phase I MTD studies[b] (174)	50 × 10^6U/m^2 IM three times a week for 3 months	25	2	14	—	16 (64)	Not stated
Multigroup phase I[b] (132)	3–50 × 10^6 U IM daily for 56 days, in escalating dose	17	2	4	2	6 (35)	
ACS lymphoma trial (130)	1, 3, or 9 × 10^6 U IM daily for 1 month	18	0	3	3	3 (17)	Median 6 months
NCI BRMP[b] (133)	50 × 10^6 IM three times a week for 3 months	24	4	9		13 (54)	Median 8 months

ECOG pilot study[b] (45)	12×10^6 U/m^2 IM three times a week for 2 months; maintenance for responders	16	1	6		7 (44)	Median 26^+ weeks (7–84^+)
University of Maryland[b] (135)	10×10^6 U SC three times a week for 6 months, or 2 months beyond	15	3	7	—	10 (67)	Median 7 months
Ozer et al.[b] (175–177)	2–30 $\times 10^6$ U/m^2 IV or SC daily	10	0	4		4 (40)	Not stated
Oslo, Edinburgh[b]	100×10^6 U/m^2 IV day D1; 2×10^6 U/m^2 SC three times a week from day 8, repeat cycle monthly	9	0	2		2 (22)	2, 6^+ months
Manchester, Paris[b] (138)	2×10^6 U/m^2 SC three times a week until disease progression or one year	34	2	15		17 (50)	Median 11 months
Van der Molen et al.[b] (139)							
low dose	3×10^6 U SC daily	19	0	5		5 (26)	Median 3 months
High dose	50×10^6 U/m^2 IM twice a week	20	2	5		7 (35)	Median 5 months

[a]"Low-grade" lymphomas include those in the International Working Formulation (IWF) classified A, B, or C. For Tables 1–4, *N* indicates the number of patients evaluable for response among those enrolled. CR (complete response) was defined as disappearance of all clinically measurable disease, with pathologic confirmation in most cases, including disappearance of marrow lymphoma by sequential bone marrow biopsy, lasting at least 1 month. PR (partial response) represented a reduction of 50% or greater in product in the biperpendicular diameters of measurable indicator lesions, without evidence of progression elsewhere, lasting at least 1 month. Minimal responses (MR) were recorded for measurable responses not attaining 50% regression. RR is the overall objective response rate = CR + PR.
[b]Indicates trial using recombinant IFN-α.

TABLE 2 Interferon-α Efficacy in the High-Grade non-Hodgkin Lymphomas[a]

Group	Schedule and route	Responses					Time to progression
		N	CR	PR	MR	RR(%)	
Stanford (3)	2.5–5.0 × 10^6 U IM twice a day for 1 month	3	0	0	0	0	
M. D. Anderson (128)	3–9 × 10^6 U IM daily for >1 month	1	0	0	0	0	
Southeastern Cancer Center (5)	5 × 10^6 U/m^2 IM three times a week for eight weeks, escalating if stable disease	7	0	2	—	2 (29)	Not stated
ACS lymphoma trial (130)	9 × 10^6 U IM daily for 1 month	11	0	0	2	0	Minimum responses, 1, 2$^+$ months
Ozer et al.[b] (175–177)	2–3 × 10^6 U/m^2 IM three times a week for >3 months	11	0	1	—	1 (9)	
Sherwin et al.[b] (174)	50 × 10^6 U/m^2 IM three times a week for >3 months	6	0	2	—	2 (33)	
NCI BRMP[b] (133)	50 × 10^6 U/m^2 IM three times a week for 3 months	6 7	1 0	1 1	— —	2 (33) 1 (14)	Intermediate grade, high grade; median 8 months
Wagstaff et al.[b] (138)							
Edinburgh	20 × 10^6 U/m^2 SC three times a week	10	0	3	—	3 (30)	2, 2, 6$^+$ months
Manchester	250 × 10^6 U/m^2 IV continuous infusion monthly						
Leavitt et al.[b] (136)	50 × 10^6 U/m^2 IV continuous infusion daily × 5 days every 3 weeks, escalated	25	0	4	—	4 (16)	3–12 months

[a]"High-grade" lymphoma includes those in the International Working Formulation (IWF) classified D–J. N, CR, PR, MR, and RR are defined as in Table 1.
[b]Indicates trial using recombinant IFN-α.

6 months. Serum levels of interferon drawn 3–4 h posttreatment varied widely among individuals receiving the same batch and dose level. An unusual toxicity in this study was the development 30 months subsequent to a 1 month course of interferon (at the 3×10^6 dose) of an Auer rod-positive acute nonlymphocytic leukemia in one previously untreated patient with low-grade NHL (131).

With the advent of recombinant DNA technology, interferon-α was among the earliest proteins to be cloned and expressed, making available since 1981 large quantities of uniform, well-characterized single-species material to facilitate phase II trials in larger numbers of patients and for longer treatment intervals (reviewed by Spiegel, Ref. 18). Stanford University, M. D. Anderson Cancer Center, and the University of Wisconsin collaborated in an escalating multidose phase I study (132), using $3\text{–}50 \times 10^6$ U of interferon-α_2 for 56 days, yielding 2 CR and 4 PR in 17 evaluable patients with low-grade NHL. No responses occurred at doses below 9×10^6 U. In a study by the Biological Response Modifiers Program at the NCI (133) of heavily pretreated patients with advanced (stage III–IV) NHL treated at 50×10^6 U/m^2 IM three times per week (134) with interferon-α_{2a}, 13 of 24 evaluable patients with low-grade NHL responded. Of these, 4 were complete responders, for an overall response rate of 54% and with an average response duration of 8 months. Complete responders cleared both bulky disease and previously involved bone marrow, dispelling the idea that interferon may be active only as an adjuvant in the minimal disease setting. Second responses upon reinstitution of interferon-α after evidence of disease progression were seen in 2 of 6 retreated patients (197). The response rates were equivalent between chemoresistant and nonresistant patients; both CRs occurred in chemoresistant patients. Most patients relapsed within 2–7 months after discontinuation of interferon, usually in sites of previous disease, suggesting the possible value of maintenance therapy. All patients required dose reductions to 50%, and some to 10%, for considerable toxicity. Of 6 patients with intermediate and 10 patients with high-grade lymphoma treated in this trial, only 13 patients were evaluable. In 1, a CR (a patient with diffuse poorly differentiated lymphocytic lymphoma) was achieved and in another a PR for an overall response rate of 15%.

The University of Maryland Cancer Center coordinated a multiinstitutional phase II trial from 1982 to 1984 in which 45% of patients with low-grade NHL receiving interferon-α_{2b} at 10×10^6 U subcutaneous, (SC) three times per week for 6 months (or for 2 months after best response) had CR or PR with a medium duration of 7 months. Responses were seen only in the nodular histologies (135,136); no responses were seen in 7 patients with CLL, Waldenström's macroglobulinemia, or diffuse well-differentiated lymphocytic lymphoma. Median time to response was 2.4 months, and for many patients undergoing prolonged treatment, responses slowly improved. A more intensive regimen was employed for patients with heavily pretreated high-grade non-Hodgkin's lymphomas.

Patients with high-grade lymphomas were treated with 50×10^6 U/m^2 intravenous (IV) continuous infusion daily for 5 days, repeated every 3 weeks, and escalated by 25% each cycle if no dose-limiting toxicity was encountered. The overall response rate in heavily pretreated patients was 16%. Toxicities were more substantial than in the low-grade lymphomas, likely due in part to more compromised marrow reserve or residual toxicity from prior chemoradiotherapy; only 29 were evaluable of 40 enrolled because of early cessation of treatment from interferon toxicity or progressive disease. A partial response was attained by 4 patients with diffuse undifferentiated lymphoma with T cell markers, diffuse large cell lymphoma, and diffuse poorly differentiated lymphocytic lymphoma.

An Eastern Cooperative Oncology Group (ECOG) pilot study investigated the efficacy of interferon-α administered in moderate dose as initial systemic therapy of favorable histology NHL and CLL (45). Interferon-α_{2a} at 12×10^6 U/m^2 IM was administered three times weekly for 2 months, followed by maintenance for 16 weeks at the same dose for responders or for those with stable disease at an escalated dose of 25×10^6 U/m^2 IM three times weekly for an additional 4 weeks. Of 16 previously untreated patients with low-grade NHL, 1 complete and 6 partial responders were seen for an overall response rate of 44%. Median time to progression from initiation of therapy in responders was 26+ weeks (range 7–84). The onset of objective response was frequently delayed until 2 months or more after initiation of treatment. In 15 patients with stable disease after the 8 week induction, dose escalation failed to achieve any objective responses. In every patient studied, a decline in the T3 and T4 subsets and in NK functional activity was seen within 6 h of initial interferon-α dose, with rebound in 48 h. The NK cell activity of patients with objective responses was 25–28% (significantly) higher at 2 and 4 weeks of therapy than those in patients with progressive disease. Of 4 patients with CLL, no complete and only 1 partial response was seen; a 50% reduction in peripheral lymphocytosis was observed on induction, but these counts increased 2 weeks into the maintenance treatment. Although this trial confirmed activity in low-grade NHL, since only partial responses were seen in this trial, the authors conclude that conventional chemotherapy has a better response rate and duration than single-agent interferon as initial therapy for low-grade NHL.

The Southeastern Cancer Study Group used high- and low-dose lymphoblastoid interferon-α (Wellferon) in patients with lymphoma refractory to conventional therapy (5). Initial treatment was 5×10^6 U/m^2 three times weekly for 8 weeks, with those failing to respond proceeding to 30×10^6 U/m^2 for 10 additional days. Of 25 patients with low-grade NHL, 6 responded at the lower dose, 2 CR and 4 PR. Of 7 patients with high-grade NHL, 2 experienced partial responses.

The European experience has been summarized in a report of four phase II trials (137,138,200,201) that enrolled patients from 1982 through January

1985. Indications for previously untreated patients to enter the study were bulky disease > 5 cm, systemic symptoms, or life-threatening organ involvement. In the low-grade non-Hodgkin's lymphomas, two schedules were employed, either 2×10^6 U/m^2 SC three times per week until disease progression or 1 year (Manchester and Paris), or 100×10^6 U/m^2 on day 1, then 2×10^6 U/m^2 SC three times per week from day 8, with cycles repeated at monthly intervals (Oslo and Edinburgh). In the first, 29 patients were treated, with 11 responders (1 CR and 10 PR, duration 1–10+ months). This regimen could be managed entirely on an outpatient basis, with the majority of patients self-administering their subcutaneous injections. Toxicities were mild, with no patient having to stop or delay treatment from myelosuppression or toxicity; no patient developed abnormal liver function tests. In the second, 2 of 9 patients had a partial response (2–6+ months). Toxicity was more severe with the second regimen. Several patients with a prior history of cardiovascular disease experienced cardiac symptoms in this study. The authors observed that this was less likely a direct interferon toxicity than a reflection of underlying cardiovascular disease exacerbated by the "stress" induced by interferon treatment. In the high-grade lymphomas, 3 of 10 patients had a partial response, with a median duration of 4 months.

The relationship of interferon-α dose to tumor response remains an open question. The early results of a prospective randomized trial designed to explore this issue in low-grade NHL were recently reported (139). Previously treated patients with favorable histology NHL were randomized to receive either low-dose (3×10^6 U SC daily) or high-dose (50×10^6 U/m^2 IM twice weekly) interferon-α. Of 19 patients evaluable at the lower dosage, no CR and 5 PR were seen (26% overall response rate). At the higher dosage, in 20 patients there were 2 CR and 5 PR (35% overall response rate). The complete remissions lasted 12 and 24$^+$ months. Median durations of response were 3 months in the low-dose and 5 months in the high-dose regimen. Median times to attain maximal response were 3 and 4 months, respectively. Most high-dose patients required dose reduction before maximum response would be expected. Of 8 patients with stable or progressive disease on the low-dose regimen crossed over to the high-dose regimen, no further responses occurred. These authors concluded that interferon-α was minimally effective as single-agent treatment of relapsed indolent NHL at its maximum tolerated dose, but that sustained treatment at higher doses is associated with a higher response rate.

Interferon-β has also been administered in low doses to patients with favorable histology NHL and CLL (140). Minimal responses were noted in two patients, and eight patients progressed.

Occasional correlations between production of antibodies to interferon and loss of clinical response in the lymphomas has been noted (136,141). In the NCI and ECOG studies, no correlation was found (45,142). Development of antibodies has not been accompanied by any acute adverse clinical symptoms (186,195).

B. Single-Agent Interferon Treatment of the Non-Hodgkin's Lymphomas of T Cell Origin

Clinical trials to date have reproducibly shown significant and durable antitumor responses to interferon-α in the cutaneous T cell lymphomas (Table 3, and earlier reviewed in refs. 181,182,183). Recent reports in smaller numbers of patients with more aggressive T cell lymphomas, including adult T cell leukemia and lymphoma and peripheral T cell lymphoma, have also demonstrated activity of interferons.

The indolent cutaneous T cell lymphomas, mycosis fungoides (MF) and Sézary syndrome (SS), are clonal malignancies of the helper T cell phenotype with initial skin manifestations. Mycosis fungoides typically demonstrates an apparent orderly progression from patch to plaque to tumor stage to generalized erythroderma with malignant lymphadenopathy preceding other extracutaneous spread, but a high frequency of microscopic early dissemination has been documented (121). In Sézary syndrome, leukemic involvement and erythrodermic skin disease are earlier findings. In those cases associated with HTLV-I seropositivity, extracutaneous disease is widespread at the time of diagnosis and immunodeficiency and hypercalcemia are prominent (143). Conventional treatments concentrating on the skin, including topical mechlorethamine, whole-body electron beam x-ray therapy, and psoralen + ultraviolet A (UV-A; PUVA), or combination chemotherapy, have yielded variable complete response rates (reviewed by Jones, Ref. 107, and Kuzel et al., Ref. 144) accompanied by universal relapse.

In a phase II trial, 20 patients with heavily pretreated advanced refractory CTCL received high-dose interferon-α_{2a} (145). None were HTLV-I seropositive; none had peripheral T cell lymphoma. Most patients were stage T3 or T4 (according to Bunn and Lamberg, Ref. 146), and 15 had visceral extracutaneous disease. As first reported in 1984, no CR and 9 PR were observed, giving a response rate of 45%. An updated report on this cohort (142,191) indicated that 2 of the 9 patients in whom partial responses were attained converted to pathologic CRs. No correlation between response and any monitored changes in immune function or development of antibodies to interferon was apparent. Response frequency was equal between cutaneous and extracutaneous sites, with all partial responses occurring within 4 weeks of initiating interferon-α_{2a} therapy. Extracutaneous as well as cutaneous disease regression occurred in 8 of 9 patients.

In a subsequent trial at the same institution, the efficacy and toxicity of an intermittent schedule of high-dose interferon-α was assessed in 24 patients with advanced, refractory CTCL (147). Patients received 10×10^6 U/m^2 IM on day 1 and 50×10^6 U/m^2 on days 2–5 repeated every 3 weeks for 4 cycles, thereby withholding interferon-α treatment 16 days during each 3 week cycle. After four cycles, those with a partial response or stable disease were given additional treatment at twice the initial starting dose. An overall response rate of 29%

TABLE 3 Interferon-α Efficacy in the T Cell Lymphomas[a]

Group	Schedule and route	Responses N	CR	PR	MR	RR (%)	Time to progression
NCI-BRMP[b] (145)	50 × 10^6 U/m^2 IM three times a week	20	2	7	5	9 (45)	Median 5.5 months ($3–36^+$)
Wolff et al.[b] (153)	2 × 10^6 U three times a week intralesionally	9					
Tura et al.[b] (178)	3–18 × 10^6 U IM daily for 3 months; maintain responders	15	3	8	—	11 (73)	Not stated
Vonderheid et al.[b] (154)	1 × 10^6 U/site intralesionally;	6		(see text, p. 95)			Not stated
	5 × 10^6 U IM three times a week × 4 weeks	5	0	0	—	0	
Hagberg et al.[b] (149)	2–4 × 10^6 U/m^2 three times a week	4	1	1	1	2 (50)	20^+ months CR
Thestrup-Pedersen et al.[b] (164)	3–36 × 10^6 U IM daily for 3 months; 18 × 10^6 U IM three times a week × 3–6 months for responders	11	1	6	—	7 (64)	23, 4^+ months
Olsen et al.[b] (148)	3 or 36 × 10^6 U IM daily × 10 weeks; maintain responders	22	6	8	—	14 (64)	4–27.4 months for complete responders
Covalli et al.[b] (151,152)	3–18 × 10^6 SC daily escalating × 12 weeks maintain responders	22	8	9	—	17 (77)	1.5^+ years CR 1.2 years PR
Kohn et al.[b] (147)	10 × 10^6 U/m^2 IM day 1, 50 × 10^6 U/m^2 IM days 2–5, repeat every 3 weeks	24	1	6	—	7 (29)	Median 8 months (4–19)

[a]N, CR, PR, MR, and RR are defined as in Table 1.
[b]Indicates trial using recombinant IFN-α.

(1 CR and 6 PR) occurred. No further response was observed in 8 patients who received dose escalations after the first four cycles. Dose reduction was required in 8 of 22 patients. All patients experienced a drop in ECOG performance status of one level. None of 4 patients with visceral infiltration of mycosis fungoides or Sézary syndrome responded in this trial. Compared to the earlier NCI-BRMP trial of continuous high-dose interferon-α in advanced, refractory CTCL, this trial achieved a similar mean weighted dose rate intensity (65.5×10^6 U/m^2/week over the first four cycles compared to 73.2×10^6 U/m^2/week in the previous trial) but with a lower response rate (29 versus 45% in previous trial, not a statistically significant difference).

Between 1984 and 1986, 22 patients with both early and advanced stages of CTCL but no clinical evidence of visceral disease were treated with either low-dose (3×10^6 U) or high-dose (36×10^6 U) interferon-α IM daily for 10 weeks, with further maintenance for responders (148). At the end of the induction period, 3 CR, 10 PR, and 1 MR were observed. With further therapy, 3 of the patients in whom partial responses had been attained converted to pathologically proven CR status, giving an overall CR response rate of 27%. Mean time to CR was 21 weeks (7–47), and mean time to PR was 8 weeks (2–10). Mean response duration was 14 weeks (2–52). All 6 patients who attained CR remained in remission with the interferon therapy continued generally for 1 year following attainment of CR. One patient relapsed when interferon was discontinued but achieved a second CR upon reinduction with interferon-α. The response rate was higher in the high-dose (11 of 14) than in the low-dose arm (3 of 8) at the end of induction, but only 1 high-dose patient was able to tolerate the 10 week induction without dose reduction. The maximal tolerated dose was 18×10^6 U IM daily. Relapses in objective responders were noted when dose reduction to less than 18×10^6 U daily was made before a patient attained CR. Of particular interest in this trial was the observation that progressive disease in previous responders was correlated with a rise in leukecyte count above 4000/mm^{-3}, due to interferon-α_{2a} dose reduction, tachyphylaxis, or absence of neutropenic effect. Neutralizing antibodies to interferon-α_{2a} developed in 6 of 10 patients studied. No correlation was found to disease response; in fact, 2 of the complete responses developed after discovery of an interferon-neutralizing antibody titer.

Low-dose therapy was explored in four patients with advanced stage CTCL in Sweden (149). The initial dose of 2×10^6 U IM three times per week was doubled after 1 month if no response was obtained; one CR, one PR, and one MR resulted. The time to CR was 4 months, with a response duration of 20^+ months. One patient in whom recurring lesions were seen on dose reduction had disease regression again with dose reescalation.

Japanese workers reported the outcome of 10 evaluable patients with CTCL treated with natural human lymphoblastoid interferon-α. A 33% response rate was noted (8 PR) (150).

In Rome and Milan, 23 patients with newly diagnosed and previously untreated mycosis fungoides received daily subcutaneous interferon-α (151,152). None had known visceral disease or lymphadenopathy. The schedule provided for rapid dose escalation from 3 to 18 × 10^6 U SC daily for a 12 week induction course, followed in responders by maintenance at the individual's maximum tolerated dose three times weekly for an additional 6 months. In 1987, 5 CR and 6 PR were seen in 12 evaluable patients (overall response rate 92%), with a median of 5 months to respond from treatment initiation. All CRs in this trial were pathologically restaged. In their expanded report in 1989, a total of 23 patients were similarly treated, with 8 CR (36%) and 9 PR (39%); 5 patients had resistant disease. Dose modifications were due to liver toxicity (10 cases), fatigue (6 cases), or hematologic toxicity (4 cases). A clear correlation of response rate to stage of disease was reported, with 100, 83, and 57% of stage I, II, and IV patients responding, respectively. Of patients with preexisting antibodies to interferon-α, 2 of 2 failed to respond; 1 of 14 antibody-negative patients failed to respond. The elevated pretreatment CD4/CD8 ratio in all these patients tended to normalize upon treatment, particularly in those attaining CR. None of the patients in CR status had relapsed after 1.5 years of follow-up; 5 of 9 partial responders progressed within 1.2–2 years.

Intralesional interferon-α therapy of CTCL has been reported by several groups. A randomized double-blind trial of 12 patients with plaque-stage mycosis fungoides administered intralesional interferon-α to 9 patients and vehicle only to 3 patients (153). In each patient, two additional plaques were evaluated: one untreated, and one treated topically with either placebo ointment or betamethasone ointment. Of 9 interferon-injected lesions, 3 showed total clearing; all interferon-injected lesions showed improvement. Of 18 noninjected lesions 13 also improved in all patients who received intralesional interferon, suggesting a systemic effect not seen in the vehicle-injected patients. The design of another two-part randomized double-blind trial of intralesional versus systemic intramuscular interferon-α in plaque-phase mycosis fungoides allowed individual patients to serve as their own controls (154). In each of 6 previously untreated patients with mycosis fungoides, 2 representative plaques were injected with 1 × 10^6 U interferon-α and 2 plaques were injected with placebo three times weekly for 4 weeks. By 8 weeks, 10 of 12 interferon-injected plaques had completely cleared histopathologically and 2 of 12 showed improvement, in contrast to only 1 of 12 placebo-injected plaques with complete clearing and 2 of 12 improved. The authors assert that the different response rates between intralesional and systemic therapy may result from different intralesional interferon concentrations attainable by these routes.

Two published reports have explored the efficacy of interferon-β or interferon-γ in T cell lymphomas. In 16 patients with refractory heavily pretreated cutaneous T cell lymphoma of various stages given interferon-γ at

0.25 mg/m^2/day IM for the first week and then 0.5 mg/m^2 IM daily, the objective response rate was 31%, with an additional 38% exhibiting lesser degrees of response (0 CR, 5 PR, and 6 MR; median response duration 10 months, range 3–32$^+$ months) (155). In addition to cutaneous responses, regression of palpable lymphadenopathy and peripheral blood involvement resulted. None of 3 patients with stage IVB disease had responses in the visceral sites, but 2 had brief cutaneous responses. Otherwise, responses did not correlate with disease stage or type of previous treatment. An additional benefit in the majority of patients, even in those without a documented antitumor response, was resolution or improvement of chronic pruritus.

Five patients had received previous treatment with interferon-α_{2a}; of two previous interferon-α_{2a} responders, one responded to interferon-γ with a PR (duration 4 months), and another attained a minor response with interferon-γ. Of the three interferon-α_{2a} nonresponders, two subsequently had minor responses and one had no response to interferon-γ. No antibodies to interferon-γ were detectable by radio-immunoprecipitation in this trial. One patient experienced a treatment-related nephrotic syndrome that abated with discontinuation and reappeared upon reinstitution of interferon-γ.

A Japanese trial treated 11 patients with adult T cell leukemia, all HTLV-I seropositive, with either interferon-β or interferon-γ (156). All patients received interferon-β as a 36 $\times$ 10^6 U IV 1 h infusion daily for 5 days with 9 days off treatment followed by the same dose three times per week for 4 weeks or longer. Of 6 treated patients 3 attained PR (durations 1, 1.5, and 12 months). In 5 patients receiving interferon-γ in escalating doses from 1 to 8 $\times$ 10^6 IM or IV daily until relapse, 1 CR and 2 PR were observed (durations 4, 4, and 2 months). One of these patients was treated with interferon-β initially and then with interferon-γ on relapse. All patients died of infection or hypercalcemia. These short response durations must be compared to the 3–6 month median survival in this aggressive disease despite intensive supportive as well as conventional antileukemic treatment. Endemic in southern Japan, neighboring Taiwan, and parts of the Caribbean, the clinical course of HTLV-I associated adult T cell leukemia and lymphoma in the United States has been described (143).

Peripheral T cell lymphoma (PTCL) has been recognized as a subset of diffuse aggressive non-Hodgkin's lymphomas incurable with conventional chemotherapy. In four patients with stage IV PTCL (all HTLV-I seronegative and without cutaneous disease) treated with interferon-α at varying doses according to individual tolerance, CR occurred in three, one of which lasted 10$^+$ months at a dose of 10 $\times$ 10^6 U/m^2 SC three times per week, one of which lasted 9$^+$ months at the same dose, and one of which lasted 6.5 months at 3 $\times$ 10^6 U/m^2 SC three times weekly (157). Another T cell malignancy, lethal midline granuloma, was found to be responsive to interferon-α_{2a} in three patients (158). Further studies are indicated to determine whether other lymphomatous or prelymphomatous variants of T cell origin (198), including angioimmunoblastic lymphadenopathy, Lennert's (epithelioid) lymphoma, and perhaps chronic lymphomatoid granulomatosis, may be responsive to the interferons. One patient with angioimmunoblastic lymphadenopathy treated with interferon-β has attained a complete response.

C. Combination Therapies of Non-Hodgkin's Lymphoma of B or T Cell Origin Including Interferon

With the expectation of nonoverlapping toxicities and preclinical studies suggesting a potential synergistic antitumor effect, a reasonable initial approach to combination therapy has been to combine interferon with the conventional regimens for the lymphomas (17,185).

Three separate trials have explored the use of interferon in combination with chlorambucil in NHL. In Great Britain, 23 patients with recurrent low-grade NHL (including 1 peripheral T cell lymphoma) received 10 mg oral chlorambucil daily, concurrent with interferon-α, 2×10^6 U/m^2 SC three times per week. Of 23 patients, 14 responded (1 CR and 13 PR). Of these, 8 were patients with follicular NHL (1 CR and 7 PR). In 4 patients, combination treatment resulted in a greater response than previously observed with chlorambucil alone (159). In Italy, a response rate of 70% (8 of 11), including 2 complete responders, was attained in follicular NHL treated with chlorambucil and low-dose interferon-α_{2b} (160). When patients with diffuse intermediate- and high-grade NHL are included, the overall response rate in these heavily pretreated patients was 64% (14 of 22). Response durations varied from 2 to 9^+ months. No hematologic CRs were achieved in patients with bone marrow involvement. This study prompted an ongoing trial by the Italian Cooperative Lymphoma Group comparing chlorambucil alone versus concurrent chlorambucil + interferon-α in the initial treatment of stage III–IV follicular NHL to determine whether continuous interferon treatment increases the frequency or prolongs the duration of complete response. A phase II study of intermittent interferon-α and high-dose chlorambucil in NHL resistant to conventional therapy has been reported from the Michigan State University Cancer Treatment Consortium (161). Of 13 patients with advanced refractory NHL treated with chlorambucil, 16 mg/m^2 on day 5, with interferon α, 6×10^6 U IM, on days 1–5 and 8, repeated monthly, 5 CR and 1 PR (overall 46%) occurred. Responses were quite durable, with a median of 456^+ days, and occurred primarily in the low- and intermediate-grade lymphomas.

Combination therapy with oral cyclophosphamide and subcutaneous interferon-α_{2b} has also been explored (162) in favorable histology B cell NHL. A multigroup CALGB and ECOG trial is now investigating cyclophosphamide induction with or without interferon-α, with subsequent randomization to interferon maintenance or observation. In a pilot study at the University of Wisconsin, interferon-α_{2a} (6×10^6 U/m^2 $\times$ 5 days) did not delay recovery from combination chemotherapy-induced leukopenia using the COPA regimen (cyclophosphamide, vincristine, prednisone, and doxorubicin) (189). This has served as the rationale for a larger ongoing ECOG phase III study randomizing low-grade NHL patients to either COPA alone every 28 days or combined I-COPA with interferon-α (6×10^6 U/m^2 × 5 days) interspersed on days 22–26 of each cycle. Recently in The Netherlands, interferon-2c was combined with ProMACE-cytaBOM induction chemotherapy in patients with intermediate- or high-grade NHL (163). Of seven evaluable patients, two CR (8 and 6 months) and one PR were achieved. The Lymphoma Group at the M. D. Anderson Cancer Center has incorporated interferon-α induction sequentially followed by a COPA-like combination cytotoxic therapy and, in responders, 2 years of interferon maintenance in the early aggressive treatment of stage IV follicular NHL patients (184). Examining the adjuvant role of interferon in the minimal disease setting, EORTC is conducting a randomized trial of maintenance interferon-α in complete responders to CVP combination chemotherapy on a continuous schedule of 3×10^6 U SC three times per week for 12 months. A SWOG study proposes to employ intensive chemotherapy and radiation in indolent NHL followed by randomization to maintenance with interferon-α versus observation.

Another potentially valuable combination has been that of antiidiotype monoclonal antibody treatment concurrent with interferon-α for B cell non-Hodgkin's lymphomas. A recent report has identified 1 CR and 7 PR in 16 patients treated with antiidiotype antibody alone, whereas in 12 patients treated with combination antiidiotype + interferon-α, 2 CR and 7 PR were achieved (119).

A trial comparing interferon-α alone to interferon-α + etretinate in patients with mycosis fungoides has been reported (164). Escalating doses of interferon-α, 3–36 × 10^6 U SC daily, were given for 3 months, followed by administration three times weekly at the same dose for another 12 months. When concurrent etretinate, 0.7 mg/kg, was added, a dose reduction of interferon-α to 18×10^6 U/dose was required. The maximum interferon-α dosage was attained in only 2 patients, and only 4 patients were able to complete 12 months of treatment. Of 7 patients, 1 CR and 6 PR were observed; the complete responder received combination treatment. Another of the partial responders in the group that received interferon-α alone had a clinical CR but histopathologically failed to clear a pleomorphic skin infiltrate.

Combination therapy with deoxycoformycin has been explored in two reported trials. In a phase I trial in patients with hairy cell leukemia, T cell ALL, T cell lymphoma, and B cell lymphomas, the maximum tolerated dose for interferon-α given concurrently with deoxycoformycin (the latter at a fixed dose of 4 mg/m^2) was 4×10^6 U IM three times per week (165). In a phase II trial in 18 patients with advanced mycosis fungoides or Sézary syndrome, deoxyco-

See page 103 for abbreviations.

formycin (4 mg/m^2 IV, days 1–3) or interferon-α_{2a} (10 $\times$ 10^6 U/m^2 IM, day 1, and 50 $\times$ 10^6 U/m^2 IM, days 2–5) was given in alternating 3 week cycles until disease progression or toxicity (166). Of 8 evaluable patients 5 achieved a partial response (RR 58%), with a median duration of 35 weeks. Interferon-α dose reductions were required in 5 patients. This combination may provide palliation in treatment-refractory patients.

Combination therapy using escalating doses of interferon-α_{2a} and phototherapy with psoralen + UV-A was tested in a phase I trial in pretreated CTCL patients (stages IB–IVB). Interferon doses were escalated in groups of three patients from 6 to 30 $\times$ 10^6 U IM three times per week. Of 15 patients, 12 achieved CR and 2 PR for an overall response rate of 93% (167). The median duration of response exceeded 13 months (range 3–15$^+$ months). All responders have been maintained on therapy. The maximal tolerated dose was 18 $\times$ 10^6 U IM three times per week.

D. Other Lymphoid Neoplasms

Despite that the initial case report of interferon activity in the lymphomas occurred in a patient with Hodgkin's disease, the high number of complete durable responses induced with conventional chemotherapy in this disease has precluded large studies of responsiveness to interferons. The experience in refractory heavily pretreated Hodgkin's disease in limited numbers of patients from the trials already discussed are summarized in Table 4. The largest experience is at the University of Maryland, where 4 of 13 patients had brief partial responses (136).

The largest trial of interferons in chronic lymphocytic leukemia was reported by the group at the NCI-BRMP (168). Patients with advanced-stage CLL received either high-dose (50 $\times$ 10^6 U/m^2 IM three times per week) or low-dose (5 $\times$ 10^6 U/m^2 IM three times per week) interferon-α_{2a}. No CR and 2 brief PR were seen in 18 evaluable patients (overall RR = 11%); 5 patients experienced accelerated disease on treatment. In the American Cancer Society Lymphoma Trial, 10 patients with DLWD/CLL had no response except for a transient decrease in lymphocytosis (130). In the University of Maryland Cancer Center trial, no responses were seen in 7 patients with DLWD/CLL treated with interferon-α, 10 $\times$ 10^6 U SC three times per week for 6 months (136). More recently, early-stage previously untreated B-CLL patients younger than 60 years of age were treated with interferon-α_2 at a dose of 5 $\times$ 10^6 U SC three times per week for 8–16 months. All 9 patients responded with a decrease in white blood cells (WBC) and total lymphocyte count, 1 had a substantial decrease in splenomegaly, and 5 of 7 analyzed attained a partial response defined as a 50% reduction in CD20$^+$ B cells (a relatively specific clonal marker); in no case was complete eradication of CD20$^+$ B cells attained, however (169). Of particular interest in this study was the observation that nonleukemic components of the immune system were also favorably affected by interferon-α treatment. Immu-

TABLE 4 Interferon-α Efficacy in Hodgkin's Lymphomas[a]

Group	Schedule and route	Responses					Time to progression
		N	CR	PR	MR	RR (%)	
ACS lymphoma trial (130)	9×10^6 U IM daily for 1 month	10	0	0	2	0	Minimal responses 1, 7 months
Ozer et al.[b] 1983 (175–177)		4	0	2	0	2 (25)	Not stated
Leavitt et al.[b] (136)		13	0	4	—	4 (31)	4 months (1–6)

[a]Definitions of N, CR, PR, MR, and RR are found in Table 1.
[b]Indicates trial using recombinant IFN-α.

noglobulin levels substantially improved (serum IgG increased by more than 3 g/L) in 3 of 7 patients; class II HLA antigen expression was enhanced on Leu-M3$^+$ monocytes in several patients, suggesting an in vivo activation by interferon-α_2, and the increased numbers of CD2$^+$ T lymphocytes decreased in 6 of 7 patients. These authors concluded that whether interferon-α treatment will result in long-term beneficial effects in early-stage CLL merits investigation in a larger study.

The group at St. Jude Children's Research Hospital has reported the results of a phase I/II study of interferon-α against advanced leukemia and lymphoma in children (170). Of 17 children with refractory acute lymphoblastic leukemia in relapse treated with interferon-α, 1 child had an 11 month complete response; 2 others showed disease stabilization. The maximum tolerated dosage appears to be higher than reported for adults, as no dose-limiting toxicities were encountered.

E. Common and Unusual Toxicities of Interferon in Lymphoma Trials

The common and well-characterized toxicities attributed to interferons (fever, myalgias, fatigue, and anorexia), occurring with all routes of administration, are dose dependent, and in the studies discussed here have been the chief dose-limiting adverse effects. Some of the lymphoma trials illustrate innovations in dosage schedule designed to take advantage of the tachyphylaxis that occurs to some of the acute adverse effects, including gradual dosage escalation and continuous rather than intermittent scheduling. Hematologic toxicity, including leukopenia and thrombocytopenia, has generally been reversible, predictable, and not dose limiting. Occasional hepatotoxicity (reflected by a reversible rise in transaminases), adverse central nervous system (CNS) effects (confusion and somnolence), and adverse effects in patients with underlying cardiovascular disease have been reported in the lymphoma trials as in most interferon studies. In the NCI trial, one patient with underlying coronary artery disease suffered a massive myocardial infarction and died shortly after receiving the first dose of interferon-α, leading to the recommendation that persons with significant underlying cardiovascular disease or persons in whom fever might be life threatening should not receive high-dose interferon. A few unusual reported toxicities deserve mention. Acute interstitial nephritis with nephrotic syndrome was reported in a patient treated with interferon-α for mycosis fungoides (171). An atypical tumor lysis syndrome was seen in a patient with T cell lymphoma treated with interferon-α (172). One case of acute nonlymphocytic leukemia developed after treatment with human leukocyte interferon of a previously untreated non-Hodgkin's lymphoma patient (131). In the NCI trial of interferon-α in CLL, 7 of 19 patients developed large perioral herpes simplex lesions requiring discontinuation of interferon-α in all and institution of acyclovir treatment in 2 patients. Reported toxicities have not been cumulative.

V. SUMMARY AND FUTURE DIRECTIONS

Interferon-α is effective in both untreated and heavily pretreated chemoresistant indolent non-Hodgkin's lymphomas, with an overall response rate approaching 50% in follicular NHL and even higher in the cutaneous T cell lymphomas. Half of these are complete responses. Given the available data, interferon-α may be the best single-agent therapy for the cutaneous T cell lymphomas. Intralesional interferon may serve additionally as adjunctive treatment in residual refractory lesions in these disorders. When compared to other drugs currently used for the treatment of lymphomas, the level of activity of interferons for lymphomas suggest their ultimate usefulness in clinical practice.

Several generalizations emerge from the diversity of data gathered in the lymphoma trials. A prolonged time to response is characteristic; partial responses may convert to durable complete responses with continued dosing. Relapse in previous sites of disease occurs frequently upon withdrawal of treatment, suggesting a role for maintenance therapy in these disorders. Continuous (three times weekly or daily) dosing appears to be better tolerated than intermittent dosing. Lower dose subcutaneous regimens are amenable to long-term outpatient use. The question of dose responsiveness, examined in several of these trials, remains unsettled, but the data suggest an increased response rate (at the expense of a higher incidence of toxicity) with higher doses, and several studies were designed to escalate toward an individualized maximum tolerated dose.

Many questions regarding interferons in lymphomas remain unanswered (Table 5). Whether interferon is best used as an induction or maintenance agent, or both, cannot yet be determined. Tolerated doses of interferons are generally lower when combined with other modalities, although toxicities have not been worse than with either agent alone. Combination trials have shown the feasibility and safety of the inclusion of interferon with other modalities concurrently or sequentially in the lymphomas, but the data are not yet mature enough to judge whether synergistic antitumor activity is attained. The role of host factors, such as immune status, remain unclear. In the follicular non-Hodgkin's lymphomas, studies tracking the marker cytogenetic abnormalities of 14q and bcl-2 will be of considerable interest (such a study was initiated by the Cancer and Leukemia

TABLE 5 Interferons and the Lymphomas: Unanswered Questions

How much interferon?
Which interferon?
Which histology and phenotype?
Induction or maintenance?
What combinations?

Group B in 1988). Further studies of the effectiveness of interferon-α, as well interferon-β and -γ, alone and in combination with conventional modalities, are indicated in larger numbers of patients with refractory high-grade B and T cell non-Hodgkin's lymphomas and refractory Hodgkin's disease.

For optimal therapeutic use in lymphomas, innovative preclinical study will continue to be essential. Interferons regulate gene expression, modulate the expression of proteins intracellularly and extracellularly, regulate cell proliferation, and increase immune effector cell function. In addition to their potential for use in combinations with cytotoxic drugs, interferons are part of the cytokine cascade and potentiate actions of other biologic agents. The design of optimal therapeutic strategies will require determining how these pleiotropic effects mediate antitumor activity. These results can then be rigorously tested in phase III trials in lymphomas, some of which are underway.

ABBREVIATIONS *Multiinstitutional groups*—CALGB: Cancer and Leukemia Group B; ECOG: Eastern Cooperative Oncology Group; EORTC: European Organization for Research in the Treatment of Cancer; SWOG: Southwest Oncology Group. *Combination chemotherapy regimens*—COPA: cyclophosphamide, vincristine, prednisone, and doxorubizin; CHOP-Bleo: same agents as COPA with inclusion of bleomycin; CVP: cyclophosphamide, vincristine, and prednisone; Pro MACE-cyta BOM: prednisone, methotrexate, doxorubizin, cyclophosphamide, etoposide, cytarabine, bleomycin, and vineristine.

REFERENCES

1. Blomgren H, Cantell K, Johansson B, Lagergren C, Ringborg U, Strander H. Interferon therapy in Hodgkin's disease: a case report. Acta Med Scand 1976; 199:527–32.
2. Hill NO, Loeb E, Pardue A, et al. Leukocyte interferon production and its effectiveness in acute lymphatic leukemia. J Clin Hematol Oncol 1978; 8:66.
3. Merigan TC, Sikora K, Breeden JH, Rosenberg SA. Preliminary observations on the effect of human leukocyte interferon in non-Hodgkin's lymphoma. N Engl J Med 1978; 299:1449–53.
4. Clark RH, Dimitrov NV, Axelson JA, Charamella LJ. Leukocyte interferon as a biological modifier in lymphoproliferative disease resistant to standard therapy (abstract). Blood 1983; 62(suppl 1):657.
5. Gams R, Gordon D, Guaspari A, Tuttle R. Phase II trial of human polyclonal lymphobalstoid interferon (Welferon) in the management of lymphoma. Proc Am Soc Clin Oncol 1984; 3:65.
6. Keegan P, Ozer H. Immunology of the lymphomas. In: Wiernik PH, Canellos GP, Kyle RA, Schiffer CA, eds. Neoplastic diseases of the blood, Vol. 2. New York: Churchhill Livingstone, 1985; 748.
7. Healy F, Rees RC, Hancock BW. An assessment of natural cell-mediated cytotoxicity in patients with malignant lymphoma. Eur J Cancer Clin Oncol 1985; 21:775.

8. Chandor SB. Autoimmune phenomena in lymphoid malignancies. Clin Lab Med 1988; 8:373–84.
9. Horning S. Lymphoma. In: Sikora K, ed. Interferon in cancer. New York: Plenum Press, 1983; 77.
10. Canellos GP. Interferon in the treatment of malignant lymphoma. Semin Oncol 1985; 12(suppl 5):25–9.
11. Rohatiner AZ, Lister TA. Clinical interferon studies in leukemia and lymphoma. Dev Oncol 1985; 32:591–600.
12. Urba WJ, Longo DL. Alpha interferon in the treatment of nodular lymphomas. Semin Oncol 1986; 13:40–7.
13. Foon KA, Roth MS, Bunn PA Jr. Alpha interferon treatment of low-grade B-cell non-Hodgkin's lymphoma, cutaneous T-cell lymphoma, and chronic lymphocytic leukemia. Semin Oncol 1986; 13(suppl 2):35–42.
14. Cavalli F. Alpha interferon in the treatment of malignant lymphoma. Br J Clin Pract 1988; 42(suppl 62):16–21.
15. Gutterman JU. The role of interferons in the treatment of hematologic malignancies. Semin in Hematol 1988; 25(suppl 3):3–8.
16. Cheson BD. Interferon in the treatment of B-cell malignancies. Biother Cancer 1989; 2:1–5.
17. Borden EC, Hawkins MJ. Biologic response modifiers as adjuncts to other therapeutic modalities. Semin Oncol 1986; 13:144–52.
18. Spiegel RJ. The alpha interferons: clinical overview. Semin Oncol 1987; 14(suppl 2):1–12.
19. McKenzie AMR. Variations in interferon production by lymphocytes from patients with chronic lymphatic leukemia. J Clin Pathol 1972; 25:768–71.
20. Virelizier JL. Are there pathologic defects of interferon secretion in man? Biomedicine 1980; 32:105–7.
21. Lazar A, Jackson R, Grossmayer B, Mizrahi A, Freeman AI, O'Malley JA. Interferon production and lymphocyte transformation in lymphocytes of leukemic patients. J Interferon Res 1981; 2:97–102.
22. Quesada JR. Interferons in cancer research: an update. Cancer Bull 1983; 35:30–9.
23. Lee SHS, Fernandez LA, Rozee KR. Further observation on interferon production by chronic lymphocytic leukemia cells. Eur J Cancer Clin Oncol 1984; 20:719–20.
24. Papendick U, Heimpel H. Deficient interferon-alpha production in hairy cell leukemia. Blut 1986; 52:185–190.
25. Mohammed GS, Taylor CE, Dickson AM, et al. Interferon responses of peripheral blood mononuclear cells from normal and leukemic children. Br J Haematol 1986; 64:789–98.
26. Hooks JJ, Detrick B. Interferon production during immunologically related diseases. In: Baron S, Dianzani F, Stanton JFG Fleishman WR, eds. The interferon system: a current review to 1987, Austin: University of Texas Press, 1987; 319–325.
27. Ho AD, Moritz T, Rensch K, Hunstein W, Kirchner H. Deficiency in interferon production of peripheral blood leukocytes from patients with non-Hodgkin lymphoma. J Interferon Res 1988; 8:405-13.

28. Diaz MO, Ziemin S, Le Beau MM, et al. Homozygous deletion of the alpha and beta-1 interferon genes in human leukemia and derived cell lines. Proc Natl Acad Sci USA 1988; 85:5259–63.
29. Diaz MO, Rubin CM, Harden A, et al. Deletions of interferon genes in acute lymphoblastic leukemia. N Engl J Med 1990; 322:77–82.
30. Tsujimoto Y, Finger LR, Yunis JJ, Nowell PC, Croce JM. Cloning of the chromosomal breakpoint of neoplastic B cells with the t(14;18) chromosome translocation. Science 1984; 226:1097.
31. Bakhshi A, Jensen JP, Goldman P, et al. Cloning the chromosomal breakpoint of the t(14;18) human lymphomas: clustering around JH on chromosome 14 and near a transcriptional control unit on 18. Cell 1985; 41:899–904.
32. Weiss LM, Warnke RA, Sklar J, Cleary ML. Molecular analyses of the t(14;18) chromosome translocation in malignant lymphomas. N Engl J Med 1987; 317:1185.
33. Yunis JJ. bcl-2 oncogene rearrangement in follicular and diffuse large-cell and mixed-cell lymphoma. In: Furth M, Greaves M, eds. Cancer cells. 7. Molecular diagnostics of human cancer, Cold Spring Harbor, NY: Cold Spring Harbor Laboratory Press, 1989; 37–40.
34. Lee MS, Chang KS, Cabanillas F, Freireich EJ, Trujillo JM, Stass SA. Detection of minimum residual cells carrying the t(14;18) by DNA sequence amplification. Science 1987; 237:175–8.
35. Stetler-Stevenson M, Raffeld M, Cohen P, Cossman J. Detection of occult follicular lymphoma by specific DNA amplification. Blood 1988; 72:1822–5.
36. Crescenzi M, Seto M, Herzig GP, Weiss PD, Griffith RC, Korsmeyer SJ. Thermostable DNA polymerase chain amplification of t(14;18) chromosome breakpoints and detection of minimum residual disease. Proc Natl Acad Sci USA 1988; 85:4869.
37. Mohamed AN, al-Katib A. Establishment and characterization of a human lymphoma cell line (WSU-NHL) with (14;18) translocation. Leuk Res 1988; 12:833–43.
38. Gressler VH, Weinkauff RE, Franklin WA, Golomb HM. Is there a direct differentiation-inducing effect of human recombinant interferon on hairy cell leukemia in vitro? Cancer 1989; 64:374–8.
39. Clemens MJ. Molecular mechanisms of interferon action. Br J Clin Prac (suppl) 1988; 62:5–12.
40. Exley R, Gordon J, Nathan P, Walker L, Clemens MJ. Antiproliferative effects of interferons on Daudi Burkitt lymphoma cells: induction of cell differentiation and loss of response to autocrine growth factors. Int J Cancer 1987; 40:53–7.
41. Einat M, Resnitzky D, Kimchi A. Close link between reduction of c-*myc* expression by interferon and G0/G1 arrest. Nature 1985; 313:597–600.
42. Genot E, Billard C, Sigaux F, et al. Proliferative response of hairy cells to B-cell growth factor (BCGF): in vivo inhibition by interferon-alpha and in vitro effects of interferons alpha, beta, and gamma. Leukemia 1987; 1:590–6.
43. Smyth JF. Guidelines for the use of INTRON A (interferon alfa-2b) in clinical oncology: lessons from the laboratory. Cancer Treat Rev 1988; 15(suppl A):3–6.
44. Reid TR, Race ER, Wolff BH, Friedman RM, Merigan TC, Basham TY. Enhanced in vivo therapeutic response to interferon in mice with an in vitro interferon-resistant B-cell lymphoma. Cancer Res 1989; 49:4163–9.

45. O'Connell MJ, Colgan JP, Oken MM, Ritts RE, Kay NE, Itri LM. Clinical trial of recombinant leukocyte A interferon as initial therapy for favorable histology non-Hodgkin's lymphomas and chronic lymphocytic leukemia: an Eastern Cooperative Oncology Group pilot study. J Clin Oncol 1986; 4:126–36.
46. Gresser I, Belardelli F, Maury C, Maunoury M-T, Tovey MG. Injection of mice with antibody to interferon enhances the growth of transplantable murine tumors. J Exp Med 1983; 158:2095–107.
47. Gresser I. On the mechanism of the antitumor effects of interferon. Tex Rep Biol Med 1977; 35:394–8.
48. Sidky YA, Borden EC. Inhibition of angiogenesis by interferons: effects on tumor- and lymphocyte-induced vascular responses. Cancer Res 1987; 47:5155–61.
49. Dvorak H, Gresser I. Microvascular injury in the pathogenesis of IFN-induced necrosis of subcutaneous tumors in mice. J Natl Cancer Inst 1989; 81:497–502.
50. Trotta PP. Summary of pre-clinical data. In: Kisner DL, Smyth JF, eds. Interferon alpha-2; pre-clinical and clinical evaluation. Boston: Martinus-Nijhoff, 1985; 13–27.
51. Zarling JM, Sosman J, Eskra L, Borden EC, Horoszewicz JS, Carter WA. Enhancement of T-cell cytotoxic responses by purified human fibroblast interferon. J Immunol 1978; 121:2002–4.
52. Borden EC, Hogan TF, Voelkel JC. The comparative antiproliferative activity in vitro of natural interferons alpha and beta for diploid and transformed human cells. Cancer Res 1982; 42:4948–53.
53. Chen L, Mory Y, Zilberstein A, Revel M. Growth inhibition of human breast carcinoma and leukemia/lymphoma cell lines by recombinant interferon beta-2. Proc Natl Acad Sci USA 1988; 85:8037–41.
54. Paulnock DM, Borden EC. Modulation of immune functions by interferons. In: Reif AE, Mitchell MS, eds. Immunity to cancer. Orlando, FL: Academic Press, 1985; 545–59.
55. Borden EC, Spear GT, Edwards BS, Paulnock DM, Hawkins MJ. Immunoregulatory effects of interferons in man. In: Dianzani F, Rossi G, eds. Proceedings of the International Symposium on the Interferon System, New York: Raven Press, 1985; 385–9.
56. Foon KA. Biologic response modifiers: the new immunotherapy. Cancer Res 1989; 49:1621–39.
57. Ostlund L, Biberfeld P, Robert KH, Christensson B, Einhorn S. Induction of proliferation and blast transformation by interferon in human malignant and nonmalignant lymph node B cells. Blood 1989; 73:2171–81.
58. Mehta BA, Satam MN, Advani SH, Nadkarni JJ. In vitro modulation of natural killer cell activity in non-Hodgkin's lymphoma patients after therapy. Cancer Immunol Immunother 1989; 28:148–52.
59. Spina DA, Fahey JL, Durkos-Smith D, Dorey F, Sarna G. Suppression of natural killer cell cytotoxicity in the peripheral blood of patients receiving interferon treatment. J Biol Response Mod 1983; 2:458–69.
60. Edwards BS, Merritt JA, Fulbrigge RC, Borden EC. Low doses of interferon alpha result in more effective clinical natural killer cell activation. J Clin Invest 1985; 75:1908–13.

61. Kleinerman ES, Kurzrock R, Wyatt D, Quesada JR, Gutterman JU, Fidler IJ. Activation or suppression of the tumoricidal properties of monocytes from cancer patients following treatment with human recombinant γ-interferon. Cancer Res 1986; 46:5401–5.
62. Maluish AE, Ortaldo JR, Conlon JC, et al. Depression of natural killer cell cytotoxicity after in vivo administration of recombinant leukocyte interferon. J Immunol 1983; 131:503–7.
63. Marini S, Guadagni F, Bonmassar E, Potenza P, Giuliani A. Influence of interferon on the functional expression of natural killer target structures of murine lymphoma cells. Cell Immunol 1986; 102:113–25.
64. Voiculescu CL, Rosu L, Rogoz S. Modulation of mouse spleen natural killer cell activity by beta-interferon, interleukin-1, and prostaglandins. Lymphology 1988; 21:144–51.
65. Chong AS, Scuderi P, Grimes WJ, Hersh EM. Tumor targets stimulate IL-2 activated killer cells to produce interferon-gamma and tumor necrosis factor-alpha. J Immunol 1989; 142:2133–9.
66. Hakem R, LeBouteiller P, Barad M. et al. IFN-mediated differential regulation of the expression of HLA-B7 and HLA-A3 class I genes. J Immunol 1989; 142:297–305.
67. Meurs E, Hovanessian AG. Alpha-interferon inhibits the expression of heavy-chain mu messenger RNA in Daudi cells. EMBO J 1988; 7:1688-96.
68. Michael A, Hackett JJ, Bennett M, Kumar V, Yuan D. Regulation of B lymphocytes by natural killer cells. Role of interferon-gamma. J Immunol 1989; 142:1095–101.
69. Poiesz BJ, Ruscetti FW, Reitz MS, Kalyanaraman VS, Gallo RC. Isolation of a new type-C retrovirus (HTLV) in primary uncultured cells of a patient with Sezary T-cell leukemia. Nature 1981; 294:268–71.
70. Kalyanaraman VS, Sarngadharan MG, Robert-Guroff M, et al. A new subtype of human T-cell leukemia/lymphoma virus (HTLV-II) associated with a T-cell variant of hairy cell leukemia. Science 1982; 218:571–5.
71. Fischinger PJ, Robey WG, Koprowski H, Gallo RC, Bolognesi DP. Current status and strategies for vaccines against diseases induced by human T-cell lymphotropic retroviruses (HTLV I, II, and III). Cancer Res 1985; 45:4694.
72. Manzari V, Gismondi A, Barillari G, et al. HTLV-V: a new human retrovirus isolated in a Tac-negative T-cell lymphoma/leukemia. Science 1987; 238:1581–3.
73. Josephs SF, Salahuddin SZ, Ablashi DV, Schachter F, Wong-Staal F, Gallo RC. Genomic analysis of the human B-lymphotropic virus (HBLV). Science 1986; 234:601–3.
74. Salahuddin SZ, Ablashi DV, Markham PD, et al. Isolation of a new virus, HBLV, in patients with lymphoproliferative disorders. Science 1986; 234:596–601.
75. Connors JM, Andiman WA, Howarth CB, et al. Treatment of nasopharyngeal carcinoma with human leukocyte interferon. J Clin Oncol 1985; 3:813–7.
76. Leyvraz S, Henle W, Chahinian AP, et al. Association of Epstein-Barr virus with thymic carcinoma. N Engl J Med 1985; 3129:1296–9.
77. Guillou PJ, Hegarty HH, Ransden CW, Giles GR. The response to interferon of natural killer (NK) and killer (K) cells from conventionally-immunosuppressed and cyclosporine-treated renal allograft recipients. Transplantation 1984; 38:130–6.

78. Schooley RT, Haynes BF, Payling-Wright CR, Grouse JE, Dolin R, Fauci AS. Mechanisms of Epstein-Barr virus induced human B-lymphocte activation. Cell Immunol 1980; 56:518–23.
79. Epstein MA, Morgan AJ, Finerty S, Randle BJ, Kirkwood JD. Protection of cottontop tamarinds against Epstein-Barr virus-induced malignant lymphoma by a prototype subunit vaccine. Nature 1985; 318:287–9.
80. Krown SE, Real FX, Cunningham-Rundles S, et al. Preliminary observations on the effect of recombinant leukocyte A interferon in homosexual men with Kaposi's sarcoma. N Engl J Med 1983; 301:1071–6.
81. Volberding P. Treatment of malignant disease in AIDS patients. AIDS 1988; 2(suppl 2):169–75.
82. Ho DD, Hartshorn KL, Rota TR, et al. Recombinant human interferon alpha-A suppresses HTLV-III replication in vitro. Lancet 1985; 1:602.
83. Fronko GE, Suhadolnik JR, Vonderheid EC, et al. Decreased Epstien-Barr virus-induced transformation, and elevated 2-5A synthetase and RNase L activity in peripheral blood mononuclear cells from patients treated with recombinant interferon alfa 2b. Biochem Biophys Res Commun 1988; 153:448–53.
84. Boumpas DT, Hooks JJ, Popovic M, Tsokos GC, Mann DL. Human T cell leukemia/lymphoma virus I and/or Epstein-Barr virus-infected cell lines spontaneously produce acid-labile alpha-interferon. J Clin Immunol 1985; 5:340–4.
85. Moore JL, Poiesz BJ, Zamkoff KW, et al. Inverse relationship between constitutive gamma-interferon production and human T-cell lymphoma/leukemia virus expression in cultured T lymphocytes. J Virol 1985; 53:440–6.
86. Rich SA. Human lupus inclusions and interferon. Science 1981; 213:772–5.
87. Bockus D, Remington F, Luu JY, Bean M, Hammar S. Induction of cylindrical confronting cisternae (AIDS inclusions) in Daudi lymphoblastoid cells by recombinant alpha-interferon. Hum Pathol 1988; 19:78–82.
88. Rich SA, Reilly AA. Evidence that the interferon-induced Daudi cell human lupus inclusions are de novo synthesized complexes of ribonucleoprotein and membrane. J Biol Chem 1989; 264:3529–37.
89. Hochman J, Mador N, Panet A. Tubular structures in S49 mouse lymphoma are regulated through in vivo host-cell interaction and in vitro interferon treatment. J Cell Biol 1985; 100:1351–6.
90. Taylor-Papadimitriou J, Rozengurt E. Interferons as regulators of cell growth and differentiation. In: Taylor-Papadimitriou J, ed. Interferons: their impact in biology and medicine. New York: Oxford University Press, 1985; 81–98.
91. Faltynek CR, Branca AA, McCandless S, Baglioni C. Characterization of an interferon receptor on human lymphoblastoid cells. Proc Natl Acad Sci USA 1983; 80:3269–73.
92. Faltynek CR, Princler GL, Rossio JL, et al. Relationship of the clinical response and binding of recombinant interferon alpha in patients with lymphoproliferative diseases. Blood 1986; 67:1077–82.
93. Schwabe M, Princler GL, Faltynek CR. Characterization of the human type I interferon receptor by ligand blotting. Eur J Immunol 1988; 18:2009–14.

94. Evans SS, Ozer H, Ochs J, Freeman AJ. Alpha-interferon receptor expression on lymphoblasts in children with acute lymphocytic leukemia during therapy (abstract). Proc Annu Meet Am Assoc Cancer Res 1987; 28:380.
95. Eid P, Bandu MT, Uze G, Mogensen KE. Interferon removes its own receptors as it blocks the division of Daudi cells. Eur J Biochem 1988; 171:675–82.
96. Filgueri L, Groscurth R, Aguet M. Binding and internalization of gold-labeled IFN-gamma by human Raji cells. J Immunol 1989; 142:3436–9.
97. Finbloom DA. Internalization and degradation of human recombinant interferon-gamma in the human histiocytic lymphoma cell line, U937: relationship to Fc receptor enhancement and antiproliferation. Clin Immunol Immunopathol 1988; 47:93–105.
98. Ishii Y, Tsukagoshi S. Specific binding of interferon-gamma and -alpha-2a to tumor cells and their antitumor activities. J Pharmacobiodyn 1988; 11:465–71.
99. Bonnem EM. Alpha-interferon: combinations with other antineoplastic modalities. Semin Oncol 1987; 14(2):48–60 (suppl. 2).
100. Mowshowitz SL, Chin-Bow ST, Smith GD. Interferon and cis-DDP: combination chemotherapy for P388 leukemia in CDF1 mice. J Interferon Res 1982; 2:587.
101. Slater WM, Wetzel MW, Cesario T. Combined interferon-antimetabolite therapy of murine L1210 leukemia. Cancer 1981; 48:5.
102. Chirigos MA, Pearson JW. Cure of murine leukaemia with drug and interferon treatment. J Natl Cancer Inst 1973; 51:1367.
103. Welander CE, Muss HB, Morgan TM, Trotta PP, Spiegel RJ. Synergy in vitro and in clinical trials. In: Kisner DL, Smyth JF, eds. Interferon alpha-2: preclinical and clinical evaluation. Boston: Martinus Nijhoff, 1985; 29–39.
104. Yamamoto S, Tanaka H, Kanamori T, Nobuhara M, Namba M. In vitro studies of potentiation of cytotoxic effects of anticancer drugs by interferon on a human neoplastic cell line (HeLa). Cancer Lett 1983; 20:131–8.
105. Ludwig CV, Durie BGM, Salmon SE, Moon TE. Tumor growth stimulation in vitro by interferons. Eur J Cancer Clin Oncol 1983; 19:1625–32.
106. Slapak C, Richman C. Interferon protects normal human granulocyte/macrophage progenitors (CFU-GM) from ara-C cytotoxicity in vitro. Proc Am Soc Clin Oncol 1986; 5:224.
107. Jones SE. Enigma of therapy for cutaneous T-cell lymphoma. J Natl Cancer Inst 1990; 82:169–70.
108. Schiller JH, Groveman DS, Schmid SM, Wilson JKV, Cummings KB, Borden EC. Synergistic antiproliferative effects of human alpha-54, beta-ser, and gamma-interferons on human cell lines of various histogenesis. Cancer Res 1986; 46:483–8.
109. Boniver, Jr, Humblet C, Desfresne MP. Human tumor necrosis factor and interferon-gamma inhibit the development of radiation-induced thymic lymphomas in C57BL/Ka mice. Leukemia 1989; 3:611–3.
110. Avila-Carino J, Torsteinsdottir S, Bejarano MT, Klein G, Klein E, Masucci MG. Combined treatment with interferon (IFN)-gamma and tumor necrosis factor

(TNF)-alpha up-regulates the expression of HLA class I determinants in Burkitt lymphoma lines. Cell Immunol, 1988; 117:303–11.

111. Elliot KRF, Princler GL, Urba WJ, Faltynek CR. Synergistic antiproliferative effects of glucocorticoids and interferon-alpha on some lymphoid cell lines. J Cell Physiol 1988; 123:85–92.

112. Ho CK, Wang SY, Ou BR, Shiao MS, Chen HY, Kuwata T. Enhancement of interferon-induced 2–5 oligoadenylate synthetase activity by retinoic acid in human histiocytic lymphoma U937 cells and WISH cells. Differentiation 1989; 40:70–5.

113. Shiiki S, Fuchimoto S, Orita K. Therapeutic potential of natural human tumor necrosis factor-alpha in combination with natural human interferon-alpha or -gamma on human cancer cells. Res Commun Chem Pathol Pharmacol 1988; 61:345–51.

114. Rousset F, Malefijt RW, Slierendregt B, et al. Regulation of Fc receptor for IgE (CD23) and class II MHC antigen expression on Burkitt's lymphoma cell lines by human IL-4 and IFN-gamma. J Immunol 1988; 140:2625–32.

115. Gresser I, Coppey J, Bourali C. Interferon and murine leukaemia. VI. Effect of interferon preparations on the lymphoid leukaemia of AKR mice. J Natl Cancer Inst 1969; 43:1086.

116. Gresser I, Maury C, Tovey M. Interferon and murine leukaemia. VII. Therapeutic effect of interferon preparations after the diagnosis of lymphoma in AKR mice. Int J Cancer 1976; 17:647.

117. Gresser I, Chantal M, Tovey M. Efficacy of combined interferon and cyclophosphamide therapy after the diagnosis of lymphoma in AKR mice. Eur J Cancer 1978; 14:97.

118. Basham TY, Race ER, Campbell MJ, Reid TR, Levy R, Merigan, TC. Synergistic antitumor activity with IFN and monoclonal antiidiotype for murine B cell lymphoma: mechanism of action. J Immunol 1988; 141:2855–60.

119. Brown SL, Miller RA, Horning SJ, et al. Treatment of B-cell lymphomas with antiidiotype antibodies alone and in combination with alpha interferon. Blood 1989; 73:651–61.

120. Bellardelli F, Gresser I, Maury C, Maunoury MT. Antitumor effects of interferon in mice injected with interferon-sensitive and interferon-resistant friend leukemia cells. Int J Cancer 1982; 30:813–20.

121. Bunn PA Jr, Huberman MS, Whang-Peng J, et al. Prospective staging evaluation of patients with cutaneous T-cell lymphomas: demonstration of a high-frequency of extracutaneous dissemination. Ann Intern Med 1980; 93:223–30.

122. Longo DL, Young RC, DeVita VT. What is so good about the "good prognosis" lymphomas? In: Williams CJ, Whitehouse JMA, eds. Recent advances in clinical oncology. Edinburgh: Churchill-Livingstone, 1982; 223–31.

123. Krikorian JG, Portlock CS, Cooney DP, Rosenberg SA. Spontaneous regression of non-Hodgkin's lymphoma: a report of nine cases. Cancer 1980; 46:2093–9.

124. Horning SJ, Rosenberg SA. The natural history of initially untreated low-grade non-Hodgkin's lymphomas. N Engl J Med 1984; 311:1471–5.

125. Portlock CS. Deferral of initial therapy for advanced indolent lymphomas. Cancer Treat Rep 1982; 66:417–9.

126. Portlock CS. "Good-risk" non-Hodgkin's lymphomas: approaches to management. Semin Hematol 1983; 20:25.
127. Young RC, Longo DL, Glatstein E, Ihde DC, Jaffe ES, DeVita VT. The treatment of indolent lymphomas: watchful waiting vs. aggressive combined modality treatment. Semin Hematol 1988; 25:11–6.
128. Gutterman JU, Seymour F, Quesada J, et al. Recombinant leukocyte A interferon: pharmacokinetics, single-dose tolerance and biological effects in cancer patients. Ann Intern Med 1982; 96:549–56.
129. Quesada JR, Gutterman JU. Clinical study of recombinant DNA-produced leukocyte interferon (clone A) in an intermittent schedule in cancer patients. J Natl Cancer Inst 1983; 70:1041–6.
130. Horning SJ, Merigan TC, Krown SE, et al. Human interferon alpha in malignant lymphoma and Hodgkin's disease: results of the American Cancer Society trial. Cancer 1985; 56:1305–10.
131. Warrell RP Jr, Krown SE, Koziner B, Andreef M, Kempin SJ. Acute nonlymphoid leukemia after treatment of nodular lymphoma with human leukocyte interferon. Ann Intern Med 1983; 98:482–3.
132. Quesada JR, Hawkins M, Horning S, et al. Collaborative phase I/II study of recombinant interferon (clone A) in metastatic breast cancer, malignant lymphoma, and multiple myeloma. Am J Med 1984; 77:427–32.
133. Foon KA, Sherwin SA, Abrams PG, et al. Treatment of advanced non-Hodgkin's lymphoma with recombinant leukocyte-A interferon. N Engl J Med 1984; 311:1148–52.
134. Sherwin SA, Knost JA, Fein S, et al. A multiple-dose phase I trial of recombinant leukocyte A interferon in cancer patients. JAMA 1982; 248:2461–6.
136. Leavitt RD, Kaplan S, Bonnem E, et al. High and low dose treatment for high and low grade non-Hodgkin's lymphoma. In: Kisner DL, Smyth JF, eds. Interferon alpha-2: pre-clinical and clinical evaluation. Boston: Martinus Nijhoff, 1985; 57–73.
137. Wagstaff J, Scarffe JH, Crowther D. Interferon in the treatment of multiple myeloma and the non-Hodgkin's lymphomas. Cancer Treat Rev 1985; 12(suppl B):39–44.
138. Wagstaff J, Loynds P, Crowther D. A phase II study of human rDNA alpha-2 interferon in patients with low grade non-Hodgkin's lymphoma. Cancer Chemother Pharmocol 1986; 18:54–58.
139. Van der Molen L, Duffey P, Urba W, et al. Low-dose vs high-dose recombinant interferon alpha-2a treatment in favorable histology non-Hodgkin's lymphoma (abstract). Proc Am Soc Clin Oncol 1989; 8:255.
140. Siegert W, Theml H, Fink U, et al. Treatment of non-Hodgkin's lymphoma of low-grade malignancy with human fibroblast interferon. Anticancer Res 1982; 2:193–8.
141. Itri LM, Campion M, Dennin RA, et al. Incidence and clinical significance of neutralizing antibodies in patients receiving recombinant interferon alpha-2b by intramuscular injection. Cancer 1987; 59:668–74.
142. Foon KA, Bunn PA. Alpha interferon treatment of cutaneous T cell lymphoma and chronic lymphocytic leukemia. Semin Oncol 1986; 13:35–9.
143. Bunn PA Jr, Schechter GP, Jaffe E, et al. Clinical course of retrovirus-associated adult T-cell lymphoma in the United States. Engl J Med 1983; 309:257–64.

144. Kuzel TM, Gilyon K, Springer E, et al. Interferon alfa-2a combined with phototherapy in the treatment of cutaneous T-cell lymphoma. J Natl Cancer Inst 1990; 82:203–7.
145. Bunn PA Jr, Foon KA, Ihde DC, et al. Recombinant leukocyte A interferon: an active agent in advanced cutaneous T-cell lymphomas. Ann Intern Med 1984; 101:484–7.
146. Bunn PA, Lamberg SI. Report of the committee on staging and classification of cutaneous T-cell lymphomas. Cancer Treat Rep 1979; 63:725–8.
147. Kohn EC, Steiss RG, Sausville EA, et al. Phase II trial of intermittent high-dose recombinant interferon-alfa 2a in mycosis fungoides and the Sezary syndrome. J Clin Oncol 1990; 8:155–60.
148. Olsen EA, Rosen ST, Vollmer RT, et al. Interferon alfa-2a in the treatment of cutaneous T-cell lymphoma. J Am Acad Dermatol 1989; 20:395–407.
149. Hagberg H, Juhlin L, Sheynius A, Tjernlund U. Low dosage alpha interferon treatment in patients with advanced cutaneous T-cell lymphoma. Eur J Haematol 1988; 40:31–4.
150. Ichimaru M, Kamihira S, Moriuchi Y, Kuraishi Y, Usui N, Toki H, Okabe K, Niho Y, Shibuya T, Umei T, et al. Clinical study of the effect of natural alpha-interferon (HLBI) in the treatment of adult T-cell leukemia. Gan To Kagaku Ryoho 1988 15:2975—2981.
151. Covelli A, Cavalieri R, Coppola G, et al. Recombinant leukocyte A interferon as initial therapy in mycosis fungoides (MF) and Sezary syndrome (SS). Proc Am Soc Clin Oncol 1987; 6:189.
152. Covelli A, Papa G, Vegna ML, et al. Recombinant alpha-2a interferon as initial therapy in mycosis fungoides: results of a 3-year follow-up (abstract). Proc Am Soc Clin Oncol 1989; 8:251.
153. Wolff JM, Zitelli JA, Rabin BS, Smiles KA, Abell E. Intralesional interferon in the treatment of early mycosis fungoides. J Am Acad Dermatol 1985; 13:604–12.
154. Vonderheid EC, Thompson R, Smiles KA, Lattanand A. Recombinant interferon alfa-2b in plaque-phase mycosis fungoides: intralesional and low-dose intramuscular therapy. Arch. Dermatol. 1987; 123:757–63.
155. Kaplan EH, Rosen ST, Norris D, Roenigk H Jr, Saks S, Bunn PA Jr. Phase II study of recombinant human interferon-gamma in cutaneous T-cell lymphoma (CTCL). J Natl Cancer Inst 1990; 82:208–12.
156. Tamura K, Makino S, Araki Y, Imamura T, Seita M. Recombinant interferon beta and gamma in the treatment of adult T-cell leukemia. Cancer 1987; 59:1059–62.
157. Schiff RD, Headley RN Jr, Self S, Garvin AJ, Stuart RK. Treatment of peripheral T-cell lymphoma (PTCL) with recombinant alpha-interferon (abstract). Proc Am Assoc Clin Oncol 1989; 8:267.
158. Rossi JF, Dubois A, Pignodel C, et al. Lethal midline granuloma: a particular T-cell lymphoma responding to interferon-alpha 2a (Roferon-A) treatment. Original report of 3 patients. Second International Congress on Neo-Adjuvant Chemotherapy, February 19–21, 1988, 1988; 76.
159. Rohatiner AZ, Richards MA, Barnett MJ, Stansfeld AG, Lister TA. Chlorambucil and interferon for low-grade non-Hodgkin's lymphoma. Br J Cancer 1987; 55:225–6.

160. Chisesi T, Capnist G, Vespignani M, Dini E. The role of interferon alfa-2b and chlorambucil in the treatment of non-Hodgkin's lymphoma. Cancer Treat Rev 1988; 15(suppl A):27–33.
161. Clark RH, Dimitrov NV, Axelson JA, Charamella LJ, Stott PB. A phase II trial of intermittent leukocyte interferon and high dose chlorambucil in the treatment of non-Hodgkin's lymphoma resistant to conventional therapy. Am J Clin Oncol 1989; 12:75–7.
162. Ozer H, Anderson JR, Peterson BA, et al. Combination trial of subcutaneous interferon alfa-2b and oral cyclophosphamide in favorable histology non-Hodgkin's lymphoma. Invest New Drugs 1987; 5:27–33.
163. Werter M, de Pauw B, Haanen C, Strijk S, Bogman M. Recombinant interferon alpha-2c in combination with cytostatic therapy in non-Hodgkin's lymphoma in high and intermediate grade malignancy (abstract). Proc Am Soc Clin Oncol 1988; 7:A935.
164. Thestrup-Pedersen K, Hammer R, Kaltoft K, Sogard H, Zachariae H. Treatment of mycosis fungoides with recombinant interferon alpha-2a alone and in combination with etretinate. Br J Dermatol 1988; 118:811–8.
165. Bernard S, Gill P, Gavigan M, et al. Deoxycoformycin and alpha-interferon in the treatment of hematologic malignancies: a phase I study (abstract). Proc Am Assoc Clin Oncol 1989; 8:264.
166. Foss F, Fischmann A, Schechter G, et al. Phase II trial of pentostatin and interferon-alfa-2a in advanced mycosis fungoides/Sezary syndrome (MF/SS) (abstract). Proc Am Assoc Clin Oncol 1989; 8:276.
167. Kuzel TM, Springer E, Roenigk HH Jr, Rosen ST. Mycosis fungoides: time to define the best therapy. J Natl Cancer Inst 1990; 82:183–5.
168. Foon KA, Bottino GC, Abrams PG, et al. Phase II trial of recombinant leukocyte A interferon in patients with advanced chronic lymphocytic leukemia. Am J Med 1985; 78:216–20.
169. Ziegler-Heitbrock HWL, Schlag R, Flieger D, Thiel E. Favorable response of early stage B-CLL patients to treatment with IFN-alpha 2. Blood 1989; 73:1426–30.
170. Ochs J, Abromowitch M, Rudnick S, Murphy SB. Phase I-II study of recombinant alpha-2 interferon against advanced leukemia and lymphoma in children. J Clin Oncol 1986; 4:883–7.
171. Averbuch SD, Austin HA III, Sherwin SA, Antonovych T, Bunn PA Jr, Longo DL. Acute interstitial nephritis with nephrotic syndrome following recombinant leukocyte A interferon therapy for mycosis fungoides. N Engl J Med 1984; 310:32-5.
172. Fer M, Bottino GC, Sherwin SA, et al. Atypical tumor lysis syndrome in a patient with T-cell lymphoma treated with recombinant leukocyte interferon. Am J Med 1984; 77:953–6.
173. Louie AC, Gallagher JG, Sikora K, Levy R, Rosenberg SA, Merigan TC. Follow-up observations on the effect of human leukocyte interferon in non-Hodgkin's lymphoma. Blood 1981; 56:712–8.
174. Sherwin S, Foon K, Bunn P, Longo DL, Oldham R. Recombinant leukocyte A interferon in the treatment of non-Hodgkin's lymphoma, chronic lymphocytic leukemia and mycosis fungoides (abstract). Blood 1983; 62(suppl 1):764.

175. Ozer H, Leavitt R, Ratanatharathorn V, et al. Experience in the use of DNA-alpha-2 interferon in the treatment of malignant lymphomas (abstract). Blood 1983; 62(suppl 1):761.
176. Ozer H, Ratanatharathorn V, Leavitt R, et al. A phase II trial of rDNA interferon in low-grade Non-Hodgkin's lymphoma. Proc Am Soc Clin Oncol 1983; 2:215.
177. Ozer H, Gavigan M, O'Malley J, et al. Immunomodulation by recombinant interferon-alpha 2 in a phase I trial in patients with lymphoproliferative malignancies. J Biol Resp Mod 1983; 2:499–515.
178. Tura S, Mazza P, Zinzani PL, et al. Alpha recombinant interferon in the treatment of mycosis fungoides (MF). Haematologica 1987; 72:337–40.
179. Balkiwill FR, Moodie EM. Positive interactions between human interferon and cyclophosphamide or adriamycin in a human tumour model system. Cancer Res 1984; 44:904–8.
180. Borden EC. Interferons: rationale for clinical trials in neoplastic diseases. Ann Int Med 1979; 91:472–9.
181. Bunn PA Jr, Foon KA. Therapeutic options in advanced cutaneous T-cell lymphomas: a role for interferon alpha-2a (Roferon A). Semin Oncol 1985; 12(suppl 5):18–24.
182. Bunn PA Jr, Ihde DC, Foon KA. The role of recombinant interferon alfa-2a in the therapy of cutaneous T-cell lymphomas. Cancer 1986; 57:1689–95.
183. Bunn PA Jr, Foon KA, Ihde DC, et al. Treatment of cutaneous T-cell lymphomas with biologic response modifiers: recombinant leukocyte A interferon and T101 monoclonal antibody. Dev Oncol 1985; 32:579–90.
184. Cabanillas FF. Management of patients with low-grade follicular lymphomas. Am J Clin Oncol 1989; 12:81–7.
185. Durie BGM, Clouse L, Braich T, Grimm M, Robertone AB. Interferon alfa-2b-cyclophosphamide combination studies: in vitro and phase I-II clinical results. Semin Oncol 1986; 13:84–8.
186. Figlin RA, Itri LM. Anti-interferon antibodies: a perspective. Semin Hematol 1988; 25(suppl 3):9–15.
187. Foon KA, Roth MS, Bunn PA Jr. Interferon therapy of non-Hodgkin's lymphoma. Cancer 1987; 59:601–4.
188. Geissler K, Tricot G, Leeimuis T, Walker E, Broxmeyer HE. Differentiation-inducing effect of recombinant human tumor necrosis factor-alpha and gamma-interferon in vitro on blast cells from patients with acute myeloid leukemia and myeloid blast crisis of chronic myelogenous leukemia. Cancer Res 1989; 49:3057–62.
189. Hawkins MJ, O'Connell MJ, Schiller JH, Davis TE, Sielaff KM, Aughey JL. Phase I evaluation of recombinant A interferon alpha (rIFN-alpha) in combination with COPA chemotherapy (I-COPA) (abstract). Proc Am Soc Clin Oncol 1985; 4:229.
190. Hilfenhaus J, Damm H, Johannsen R. Sensitivities of various lymphoblastoid cells to the antiviral and anticellular activity of human leukocyte interferon. Arch Virol 1977; 54:271–7.

191. Ihde DC, Steis R, Sausville EA, Veach SR, Eddy J, Bunn PA Jr. Phase II trial of intermittent high-dose recombinant interferon alpha 2-A in mycosis fungoides and Sezary syndrome (abstract). Proc Annu Meet Am Assoc Can Res 1987; 28:208.
192. Oldham RK. Interferon treatment of non-Hodgkin's lymphoma and myeloma: a model for biotherapy. Dev Med Virol 1988; 4:109–20.
193. Roth MS, Foon KA. Alpha interferon in the treatment of hematologic malignancies. Am J Med 1986; 81:871–82.
194. Sikora K, Basham T, Dilley J, Levy R, Merigan T. Inhibition of lymphoid hybrids by human interferon. Lancet 1980; 2:891.
195. Spiegel RJ, Spicehandler JR, Jacobs SL, Oden EM. Low incidence of serum neutralizing factors in patients receiving recombinant alfa-2b interferon (Intron-A). Am J Med 1986; 80:223–7.
196. Steiss RG, Foon KA, Longo DL. Current and future views of recombinant interferon alpha in the treatment of low-grade non-Hodgkin's lymphomas. Cancer 1987; 59:658–63.
197. Stevenson HC, Ochs JJ, Halverson L, Oldham RK, Sherwin SA, Foon KA. Recombinant alpha-interferon in the re-treatment of two patients with pulmonary lymphoma: dramatic responses with resolution of pulmonary complications. Am J Med 1984; 77:355–8.
198. Watanabe S, Sato Y, Shimoyama M, Minato K, Shimosato Y. Immunoblastic lymphadenopathy, angioimmunoblastic lymphadenopathy, and IBL-like T-cell lymphoma: a spectrum of T-cell neoplasia. Cancer 1986; 58:2224–32.
199. Non-Hodgkin's lymphoma pathologic classification project. National Cancer Institute-sponsored study of classifications of non-Hodgkin's lymphomas. Working formulation. Summary and description of a working formula for clinical usage. Cancer 1982; 49:2112–35.

II

IMMUNOTHERAPEUTIC APPROACHES TO HEMATOLOGIC MALIGNANCIES

8

Pathways and Signals to Activation of Human Leukemia-Directed NK and T Cell Subsets

Eva Lotzová and Cherylyn A. Savary

University of Texas, M. D. Anderson Cancer Center, Houston, Texas

I. INTRODUCTION

The first indication of the role of natural killer (NK) cells in defense against leukemia originated from experimental animal studies. These investigations demonstrated that murine strains exhibiting low NK cell activity or animals depleted of NK cells displayed high susceptibility to leukemias (1,2). Conversely, leukemia resistance in vivo could be induced after activation and/or adoptive transfer of NK cells (3,4).

Similarly, early studies in humans indicated an exquisite sensitivity of human leukemia-lymphoma targets to NK cell lysis and a high risk in individuals with NK cell defects of hematopoietic malignancies (5). Moreover, a low NK cell activity was detected in patients with leukemia and preleukemic disorders (5–9) and a high risk of leukemia relapse in patients unable to generate NK cell cytotoxic function (10). These indications were subsequently corroborated by the observations that NK cells were effective in the inhibition of the growth of human clonogenic leukemia (11) and after activation with interleukin-2 (IL-2), displayed lysis of human leukemic blasts (12).

The implication of NK cells in the control of human leukemia triggered our interest in this lymphocyte population and initiated studies aimed at the generation of highly oncolytic leukemia-directed NK cells. These investigations demonstrated that highly oncolytic NK cells can be generated from peripheral blood and bone marrow after activation with IL-2 in vivo or in vitro. In addition, these studies showed that T cells can also be signaled to mediate an antileukemia effect. In this chapter we discuss in vivo and in vitro pathways to activation of NK cells and T cells and their relevance to leukemia therapy.

II. INDUCTION OF ONCOLYTIC NK CELLS BY IL-2 IN VIVO

The clinically most direct approach to the generation of oncolytic effector cell populations is portrayed by an activation in vivo. We examined the efficacy of this approach using the potent NK cell stimulator, IL-2. Specifically, we analyzed the effect of repetitive cycles of continuous infusion of IL-2 on the growth and cytotoxic activity of NK cells and other lymphocyte subsets from patients with acute myelogenous leukemia (AML) in second remission. Patient treatment was composed of repeated cycles of 4 days of continuous IL-2 infusion with 10^6 U/m^2/day, followed by a 3 day treatment-free interval for 4 weeks. The patients treated > 4 weeks received the same IL-2 treatment, followed by a 10 day intermission.

A. Studies of Cell Surface Phenotype

As shown in Fig. 1, the repeated cycles of IL-2 treatment resulted in a substantial increase in both the percentage and the absolute numbers of CD56$^+$, CD3$^-$ NK cells in peripheral blood; a high percentage of these NK cells also expressed the CD8 cell surface molecule. The number of NK cells increased progressively with each IL-2 infusion and reached 80% of total lymphocytes at the end of the fourth cycle of IL-2. In contrast, the CD3$^+$, CD56$^+$ T cell subset, also mediating major histocompatibility complex-nonrestricted cytotoxicity, remained low during all cycles of IL-2 therapy; the percentage of CD56$^-$, CD3$^+$ T cells decreased sharply; however, a slight increase was observed in the absolute number of these cells after multiple IL-2 infusions. Similarly to peripheral blood, NK cell numbers were substantially potentiated (up to 60%) in bone marrow tissue. Some increase, although lower than that in peripheral blood, was observed in the CD56$^+$, CD8$^+$ subset, but CD56$^+$, CD3$^+$ T lymphocytes did not show any increase. The percentage of CD56$^-$, CD3$^+$ T cell subset decreased significantly, and only a slight increase was detected in absolute numbers of these lymphocytes. These data indicate that the treatment of AML patients in remission with multiple cycles of continuous IL-2 infusion was effective in the induction of high levels of NK cells in the peripheral blood and bone marrow compartments.

B. Analysis of the Cytotoxic Response

Analysis of the cytotoxic potential of peripheral blood lymphocytes after in vivo IL-2 treatment showed that the increase in NK cell numbers was accompanied

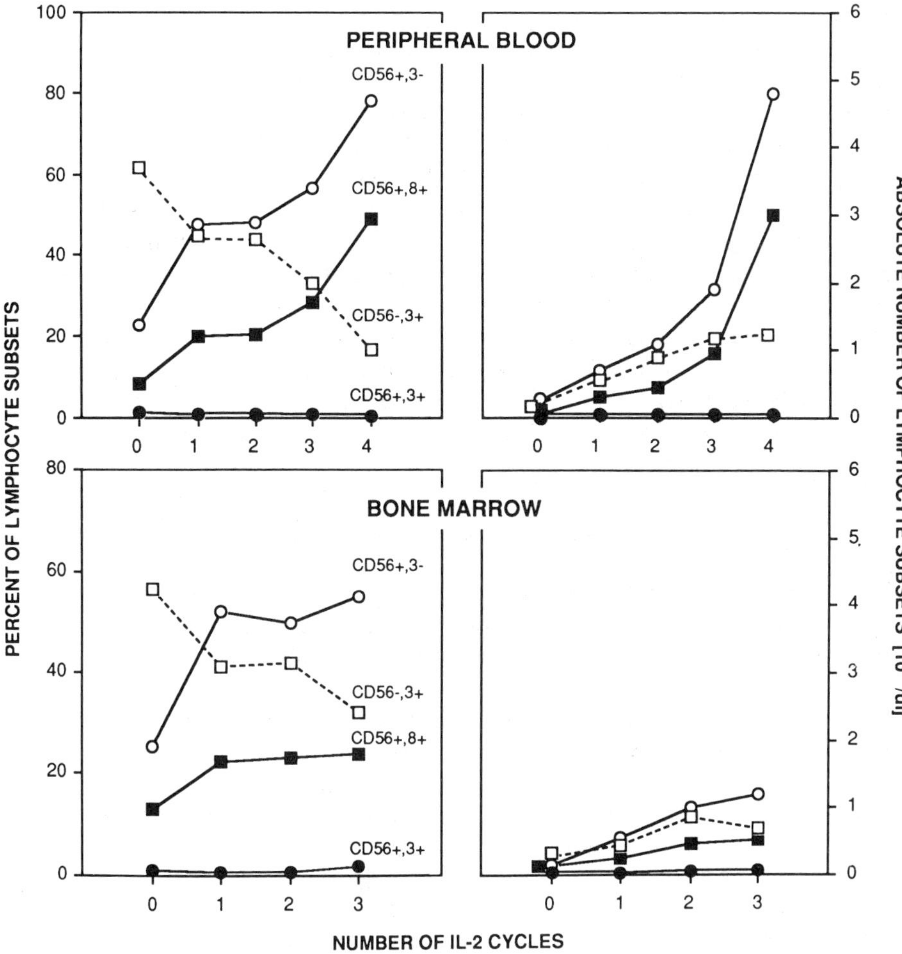

FIGURE 1 Effect of continuous IL-2 infusion on lymphocyte subsets in peripheral blood and bone marrow of AML patients. The percentage of each lymphocyte subset was determined by two-color flow cytometric analysis (gating on lymphocytes) using phycoerythrin- and fluorescein-conjugated monoclonal antibodies Leu-19, Leu-4, and Leu-2b recognizing CD56, CD3, and CD8 cell surface structures, respectively. Absolute numbers of individual subsets were calculated by multiplying the total number of lymphocytes (10^3/μl blood) by the percentage of lymphocytes displaying the particular phenotype. Analysis was made before (0) and 5–7 days after initiation of each IL-2 cycle.

by enhancement of lytic activity against NK-sensitive target K-562 cells as well as against the NK-resistant Daudi cell line in both peripheral blood and bone marrow (Fig. 2). The enhancement of lytic activity against K-562 was already manifested after the first or second IL-2 infusion; however, lytic activity was most pronounced after several IL-2 cycles. The peripheral blood cytotoxic activity against K-562 remained elevated for 5–6 days after the initiation of IL-2 treatment but declined thereafter; even after this decline, however, the cytotoxic levels were in general higher than those displayed before initiation of IL-2 treatment. The potentiation of cytotoxic activity against K-562 in bone marrow appeared to have a somewhat longer duration since increased cytotoxicity levels were still observed 10 days after initiation of IL-2 treatment. The cytotoxic response against the Daudi cell line was delayed in comparison to K-562; the high cytotoxicity was observed only after the third or fourth IL-2 infusion. Furthermore, cytotoxic activity against Daudi cells was always lower than that manifested against K-562 (Fig. 2).

C. Induction of Lytic Activity Against Fresh Leukemia

Despite the induction of high levels of cytotoxicity against the K-562 and Daudi cell lines, no or very low cytotoxicity was generated in peripheral blood against fresh AML blasts (Fig. 3). We considered the possibility that the IL-2 levels delivered by continuous IL-2 infusion might not be sufficiently high for induction of cytotoxic function against a highly resistant target, exemplified by AML blasts. Thus, in subsequent studies, we examined the effect of a short exposure (1 h) to a relatively high dose of IL-2 in vitro (100 U/ml in comparison to significantly lower levels administered by continuous infusion in vivo) on the induction of cytotoxicity against AML blasts. These studies, illustrated for three representative patients in Fig. 3, demonstrated that the in vitro IL-2 treatment resulted in the induction of high levels of an anti-AML-directed cytotoxic response. It is important to note that the in vivo priming with IL-2 was essential for induction of the in vitro cytotoxic response against AML, since lymphocytes unprimed in vivo with IL-2 did not respond to the in vitro IL-2 activation signal (Fig. 3).

These observations indicate that in vivo IL-2 treatment was effective in priming cytotoxic lymphocyte function but was not optimal for induction of oncolytic activity against highly resistant AML blasts. This is supported by the observation that lower activity was induced, and a longer time of in vivo activation was necessary, for manifestation of lytic activity against the resistant Daudi than against the highly sensitive K-562 target. Based on these data it is suggested that the treatment schedule resulting in higher IL-2 serum levels might be necessary for the induction of an optimal anti-leukemia effect. Perhaps a combination of continuous IL-2 infusion with periodic bolus injections may be effective in

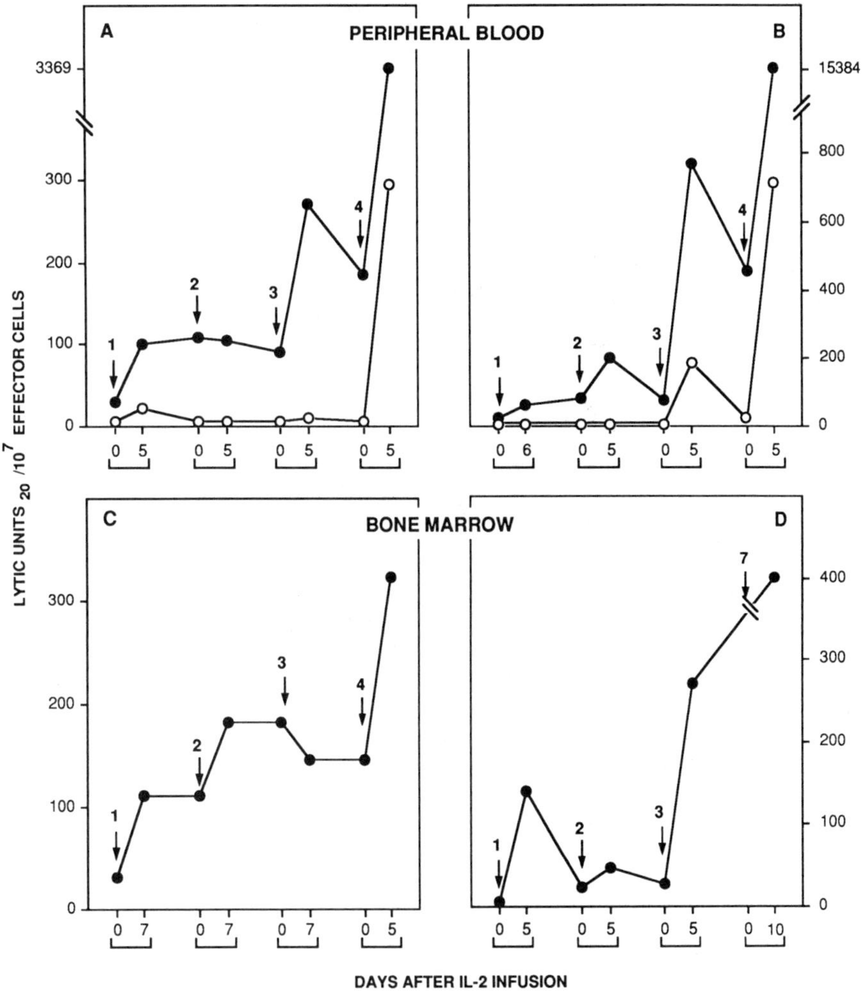

FIGURE 2 Effect of continuous IL-2 infusion on the cytotoxic response of AML patients. Peripheral blood (A and B) and bone marrow (C and D) of two representative AML patients were tested against K-562 (•) and Daudi (o) cell lines before (day 0) and after each IL-2 cycle in a 3 h ^{51}Cr release assay (12,14); arrows indicate the initiation of a 4 day IL-2 cycle. Data are expressed in lytic units calculated by linear regression analysis based on multiple effector-target ratios. One lytic unit represents the number of effector cells required for lysis of 20% of target cells. The hatched line indicates that cytotoxicity was not tested on day 0 of cycle 7 of IL-2.

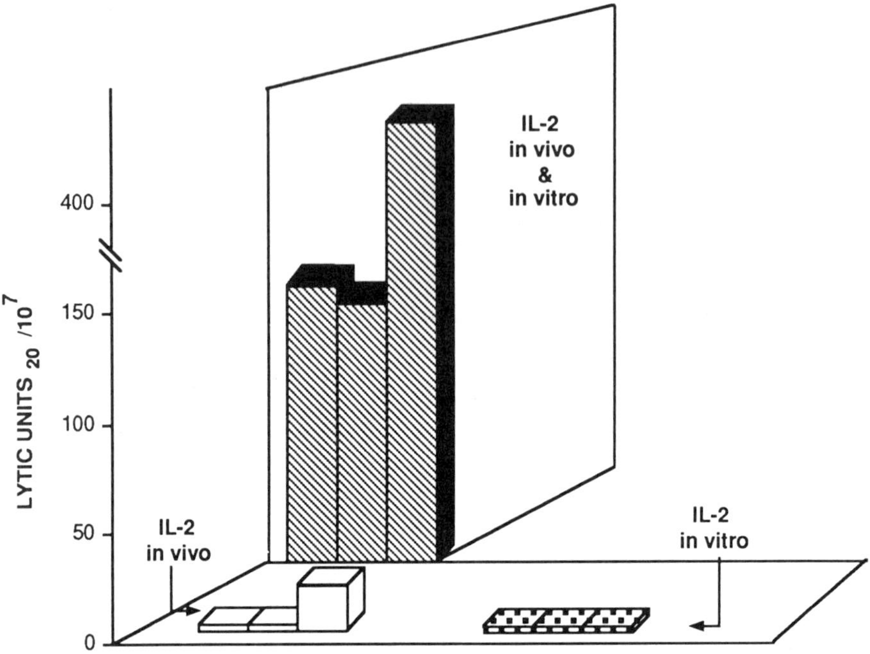

FIGURE 3 Activation of peripheral blood cytotoxic lymphocytes against AML blasts by combined in vivo and in vitro IL-2 treatment. Effector cells of three AML patients obtained after in vivo IL-2 infusion only (□) or activated additionally with 100 U/ml of IL-2 for 1 h in vitro (▧) were tested for cytotoxicity to allogeneic fresh AML blasts in a 4 h ^{51}Cr release assay; three normal donors were also tested after in vitro IL-2 activation (◘). Highly purified recombinant human IL-2 from *Escherichia coli* with a specific activity of 18×10^6 IU/mg (24,25) was provided by Cetus Corporation (Emeryville, CA).

achieving both an increase in NK cell numbers and optimal potentiation of the cytotoxic response.

D. Characterization of Oncolytic Cells Against Fresh Leukemia

To determine whether the oncolytic activity induced by combined in vivo and in vitro treatment with IL-2 was mediated by NK cells, we depleted either NK or T cells (both candidates for the cytotoxic function) from the peripheral blood and examined the efficacy of these depleted lymphocyte populations to lyse AML blasts and the Daudi cell line. These experiments showed that depletion of $CD56^+$ lymphocytes resulted in total removal and depletion of $CD16^+$ NK cells in partial (but significant) removal of cytotoxic function (Fig. 4). On the

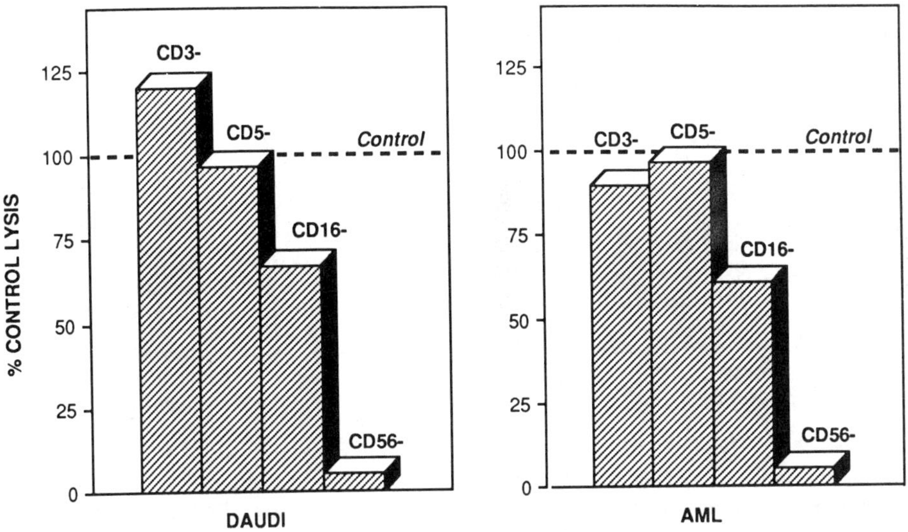

FIGURE 4 Characterization of in vivo and in vitro activated peripheral blood lymphocytes. Lymphocytes of a representative AML patient obtained after the fourth IL-2 infusion were activated in vitro with 100 U/ml of IL-2 for 1 h. These activated lymphocytes were then depleted of NK or T cells in a complement-dependent cytotoxicity assay using OKT3, NKH1, Leu-11b, and Leu-1 (anti-CD3 and anti-CD56, anti-CD16 and anti-CD5, respectively) monoclonal antibodies. Depleted populations were tested against Daudi and AML blasts in a 3 h ^{51}Cr release assay. As analyzed by a paired *t*-test, there was a significant decrease in cytotoxicity following removal of $CD56^+$ ($p < 0.005$ to $p < 0.02$) and $CD16^+$ ($p < 0.05$) lymphocytes.

contrary, the lymphocyte populations depleted of $CD3^+$ and $CD5^+$ T cells displayed cytotoxic levels equal to those in untreated controls. These observations clearly established the role of NK cells in the cytotoxic function generated after in vivo and in vitro IL-2 activation.

III. INDUCTION OF ONCOLYTIC LYMPHOCYTES BY IL-2 IN VITRO

A. Adherent IL-2-Activated Killer Cells

Adherent IL-2-activated lymphocytes (A-LAK) represent a population of killer cells that acquires the adherent properties shortly (24–48 h) after activation with IL-2 (13). This population can be further propagated in IL-2-supplemented cultures ex vivo. We and other investigators have shown that A-LAK from peripheral blood of normal donors display substantially higher oncolytic activity than unseparated or nonadherent IL-2-activated lymphocytes (LAK) (9,13). Because

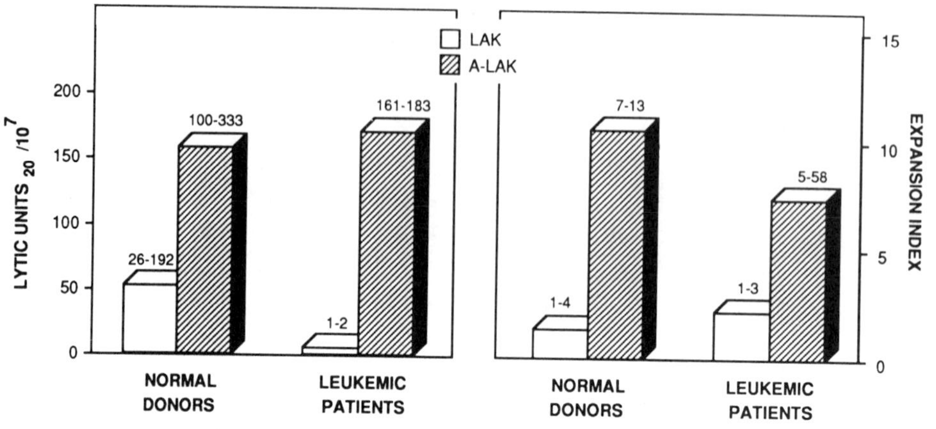

FIGURE 5 Cytolytic and proliferative activity of A-LAK. Peripheral blood was obtained from leukemic patients or from normal donors. A-LAK cultures were prepared as described previously (9,13). LAK cultures consisted of unseparated nylon wool-filtered lymphocytes. Both cultures were tested for cytotoxicity against leukemic blasts in a 3 h ^{51}Cr release assay 7–12 days after culture with 10^3 U/ml of IL-2; the expansion index represents the growth of cells based on the cell counts at culture initiation. Bars represent median of three to five donors; the values above the bars represent the range.

of the high oncolytic activity displayed by A-LAK from normal donors, we examined the possibility of generating this population from AML patients in remission.

Our studies showed that A-LAK with high oncolytic function could be generated from the peripheral blood of AML patients (Fig. 5). Comparative studies of the cytotoxic efficacy of A-LAK and LAK lymphocytes demonstrated that A-LAK was superior in its oncolytic function against AML blasts. As shown in Fig. 5, the unseparated lymphocytes (LAK) mediated lower (normal donors) or no (AML patients) lytic activity against AML targets. Thus, A-LAK represents the lymphocyte population with a high anti-leukemia effect.

Analysis of the growth kinetics of A-LAK versus LAK indicated that A-LAK displayed higher growth patterns in both leukemia patients and normal donors. However, it is important to note that a great degree of variability in the growth kinetics of A-LAK was observed among individual AML patients (Fig. 5).

1. Cell Surface Phenotype Characteristics of A-LAK

In contrast to the cell surface phenotype of A-LAK of normal donors, which has been reported to represent primarily NK cells (13), our studies showed that A-LAK from AML patients represented a heterogeneous lymphocyte population. Although morphologically A-LAK was composed primarily of large granular lymphocytes in 1 day as well as 7–11 day cultures, double-marker analysis of the latter cultures showed variability in the distribution of lymphocyte subsets among individual AML patients. Specifically, the A-LAK of some AML patients were composed of a majority of $CD56^+$, $CD3^-$ NK cells, but in the A-LAK of other patients NK cells were in the minority and $CD3^+$, $CD56^-$ or $CD3^+$, $CD56^+$ T lymphocyte subsets prevailed (Fig. 6). In contrast, LAK cultures were more homogeneous and represented primarily the $CD56^-$, $CD3^+$ subset, although some $CD56^+$, $CD3^+$ and $CD56^+$, $CD3^-$ lymphocytes were also present.

2. *Characterization of Cytotoxic Cells in A-LAK Population*

Because of the heterogeneity of A-LAK cultures, we characterized the oncolytic lymphocyte subset using the complement depletion assay and monoclonal antibodies against NK cells or T cells (Fig. 7). The results of these studies showed that independently of the distribution of lymphocytes in A-LAK cultures (i.e., the prevalence of NK cells or T cells), $CD16^+$ and $CD56^+$ NK cells displayed the highest oncolytic effect. However, the $CD5^+$ T cell subset also participated in cytotoxic function, although to a lesser degree. Thus, NK cells in A-LAK population represent the most oncolytic lymphocyte subset.

3. *Expression of Integrins and Other Surface Molecules on A-LAK: Their Role in Oncolytic Function*

We also analyzed A-LAK for expression of some of the cell surface integrins and other molecules that may be associated with cytotoxic function (Table 1). Moreover, we compared the expression of these molecules on lymphocytes present in A-LAK and LAK cultures. We observed that LAK and A-LAK populations were composed of approximately the same percentage of $CD2^+$ and CD11a $(LFA\text{-}1)^+$ lymphocytes 24 h after activation with IL-2. However, A-LAK contained a higher percentage of the $CD2^+$ and $CD11a^+$ population with bright intensity (i.e., high density of these molecules). The dichotomy between A-LAK and LAK in the expression of the high density of the CD11a molecule remained in 7 day cultures; however, the expression of CD2 bright phenotype-positive cells was high in both LAK and A-LAK cultures at that time. Analysis of the expression of the CD11b molecule showed that A-LAK consistently contained a higher percentage of $CD11b^+$ lymphocytes (Table 1). A-LAK also consisted of a higher percentage of $CD16^+$ and $CD25^+$ (1 day cultures), $CD56^+$, and $HLA\text{-}DR^+$ lymphocytes (in 1 and 7 day cultures).

The importance of the CD11a molecule to A-LAK oncolytic function was demonstrated by significant inhibition of A-LAK cytotoxicity against AML blasts by treatment with anti-CD11a monoclonal antibody (Fig. 8). Blocking the CD2 molecule also partially interfered with A-LAK cytotoxic function, but the anti-CD56 antibody had no effect.

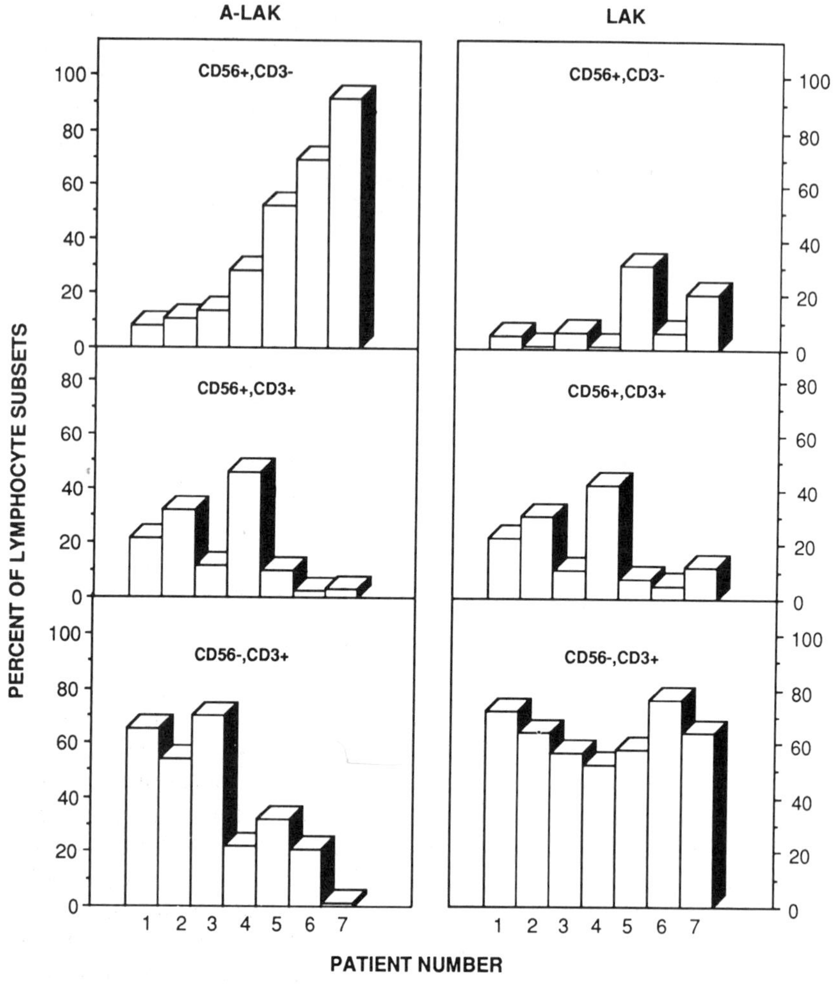

FIGURE 6 Phenotype of A-LAK and LAK cultures of leukemic patients. Nylon wool-filtered lymphocytes (referred to as LAK) and A-LAK populations of seven patients were cultured with IL-2 for 7–11 days; these cultures were then analyzed for the content of $CD56^+$, $CD3^-$; $CD56^+$, $CD3^+$; and $CD56^-$, $CD3^+$ lymphocyte subsets using two-color flow cytometry analysis, as described in Fig. 1.

B. Generation of Highly Oncolytic Lymphocytes Against Leukemia: Stimulation with AML Blasts

Although A-LAK appears to be one of the most oncolytic lymphocyte subsets against AML, we observed that these lymphocytes could not be generated indiscriminately from peripheral blood of all donors. This observation

TABLE 1 Expression of Cell Surface Molecules by A-LAK Cultures

Surface structure[a]	% Positive lymphocytes[b]			
	Day 1		Day 7	
	A-LAK	LAK	A-LAK	LAK
CD2 total	76.0 ± 1.9	78.2 ± 0.1	84.6 ± 1.5	91.8 ± 0.8
CD2 dim[c]	43.4 ± 1.6	68.6 ± 0.5	15.2 ± 2.8	29.4 ± 3.0
CD2 bright	32.5 ± 2.9	9.6 ± 0.5	69.3 ± 4.3	62.4 ± 3.6
CD11a total	96.2 ± 0.1	88.3 ± 0.7	92.1 ± 1.4	89.1 ± 1.1
CD11a dim[c]	17.1 ± 1.5	68.9 ± 2.4	13.3 ± 1.8	34.0 ± 2.2
CD11a bright	79.1 ± 1.5	19.4 ± 2.7	78.8 ± 1.8	55.2 ± 1.7
CD11b	53.9 ± 3.3	10.3 ± 1.2	58.7 ± 3.0	29.7 ± 1.1
CD16	40.2 ± 3.0	5.1 ± 0.2	9.0 ± 0.9	7.9 ± 0.5
CD25	41.1 ± 4.6	11.6 ± 1.4	37.1 ± 6.0	40.9 ± 4.4
CD56	62.9 ± 5.8	11.5 ± 1.4	76.1 ± 5.4	23.5 ± 2.9
HLA-DR	31.4 ± 6.8	7.7 ± 2.4	67.3 ± 6.0	41.1 ± 2.8

[a]Cell surface phenotype of unseparated lymphocytes and A-LAK cultures were analyzed by single- and two-color flow cytometry using phycoerythrin- and fluorescein-conjugated monoclonal antibodies.
[b]Values represent mean ± standard error of the mean (SEM) of three to seven normal donors.
[c]Dim and bright CD2- and CD11a-positive lymphocyte subsets were determined by histogram analysis of fluorescence intensity staining patterns; the populations were defined visually and gated according to natural boundaries between the two populations.

initiated our efforts in developing new ways to generate highly oncolytic lymphocyte subsets.

The first study addressed the question of whether the simultaneous stimulation of lymphocytes with AML blasts and IL-2 would enhance their antileukemia activity. The results of these studies showed that addition of irradiated AML blasts at the initiation of LAK culture resulted in the induction of a highly cytotoxic antileukemia-directed lymphocyte population (Fig. 9). It is of note that both the autologous and allogeneic (in relation to targets) AML blasts were effective in enhancing the antileukemia response. Importantly, these highly oncolytic lymphocytes were induced from the peripheral blood of individuals incapable of generating A-LAK (Fig. 9).

We next examined whether A-LAK activity from the latter group of individuals could be triggered by activation with AML blasts. As shown in Fig. 10, A-LAK activity could be induced by this approach. Similarly to LAK, autologous and allogeneic AML blasts were effective in the induction of A-LAK activity against leukemia. All these data demonstrate that the activation of lymphocytes with IL-2 and AML blasts resulted in the induction of high levels of LAK and A-LAK activity.

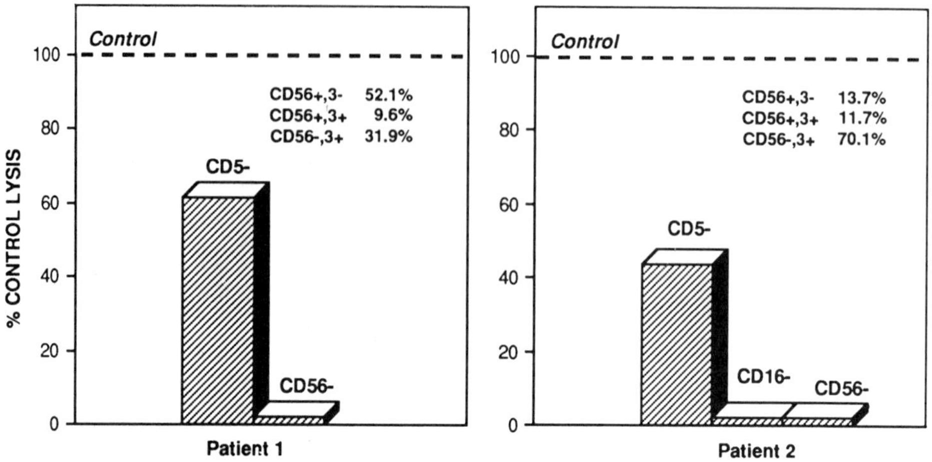

FIGURE 7 Characterization of oncolytic lymphocytes in A-LAK cultures. Peripheral blood A-LAK (7–11 days of culture) of AML patients with a high (patient 1) and low (patient 2) content of $CD56^{+}$, $CD3^{-}$ NK cells were depleted of NK cells and T cells using monoclonal antibodies and a complement-dependent assay, as described in Fig. 4. Depleted lymphocyte populations were then tested for cytotoxicity against Daudi cells in a 3 h ^{51}Cr release assay. Control represents the cell treated with complement only.

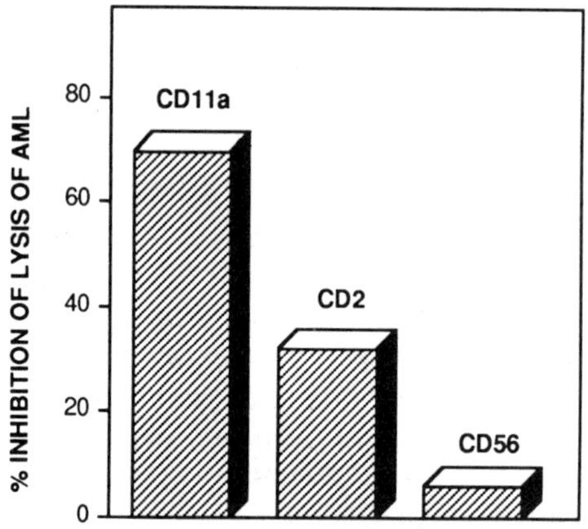

FIGURE 8 Inhibition of A-LAK activity by anti-CD11a (LFA-1) antibody. Peripheral blood A-LAK (8–13 day cultures) of normal donors was incubated with a 1:50 dilution of anti-CD11a, anti-CD2, or anti-CD56 (LFA-1, Leu-5b, and Leu-19, respectively) monoclonal antibodies and tested for cytotoxicity against fresh AML blasts in a 4 h ^{51}Cr release assay. Data are expressed as percentage inhibition of cytotoxicity in comparison to control cells (incubated in medium alone). Bars represent mean of two experiments.

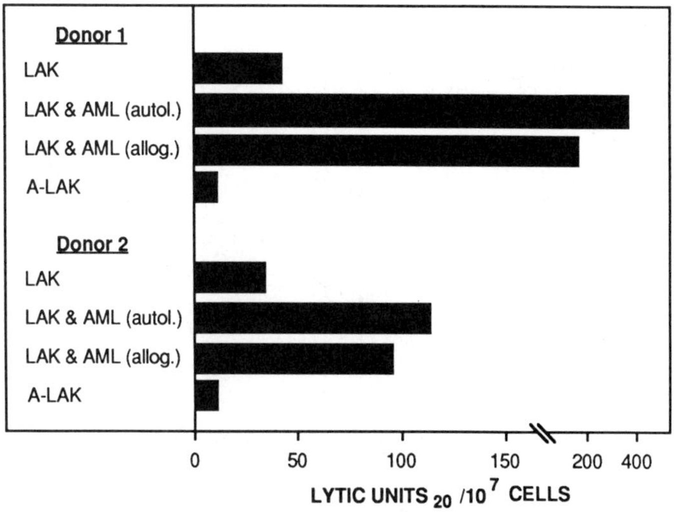

FIGURE 9 Augmentation of lytic activity of peripheral blood LAK cultures by activation with AML. Peripheral blood LAK and A-LAK lymphocytes of two normal donors were cultured for 7–13 days with IL-2 alone. Some LAK cultures were activated simultaneously with IL-2 and 5000 R irradiated (^{137}Cs source) AML blasts (5:1 LAK:AML ratio). All cultures were tested for cytotoxicity against AML target (autologous or allogeneic with the irradiated blasts) in a 4 h ^{51}Cr release assay.

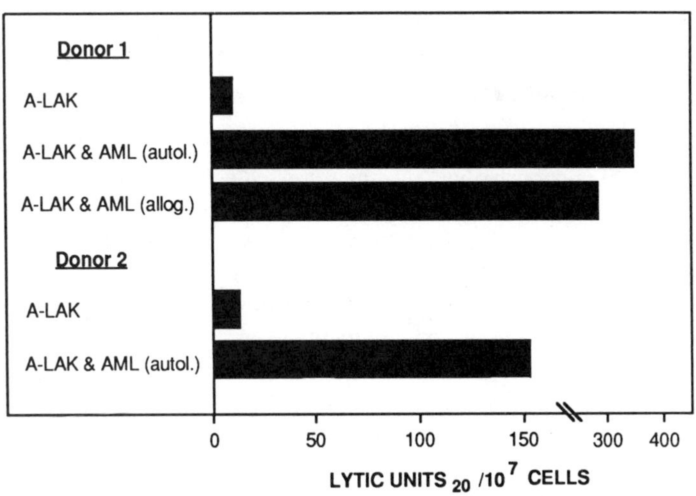

FIGURE 10 Induction of cytotoxic activity of A-LAK by stimulation with AML blasts. Peripheral blood A-LAK of two normal donors were cultured for 8–13 days with IL-2 alone or with IL-2 and irradiated AML blasts (5:1 A-LAK:AML ratio). These cultures were then tested for cytotoxicity to AML targets (autologous or allogeneic to the irradiated blasts) in a 4 h ^{51}Cr release assay.

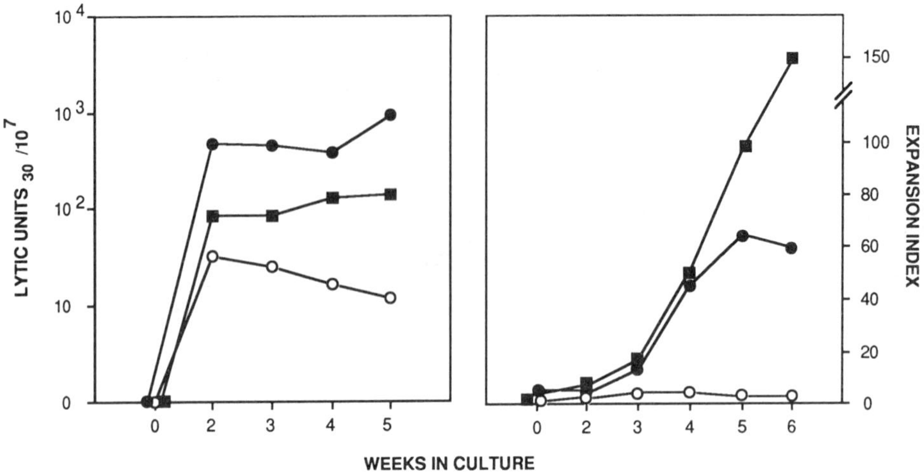

FIGURE 11 Cytolytic and proliferative activity of bone marrow IL-2 cultures stimulated with AML blasts or the Daudi cell line. Bone marrow cells of normal donors were cultured with 10^3 U/ml of IL-2 (o), or with IL-2 and irradiated AML blasts (•) or irradiated Daudi cell line (■) at 5:1 effector-AML (Daudi) ratio. Cytotoxic activity against AML blasts was measured in a 3 h ^{51}Cr release assay. Symbols represent the mean of 4–10 experiments.

C. Bone Marrow: An Alternative Source of Highly Oncolytic Lymphocyte Subsets

1. Oncolytic Activity and Growth Kinetics

We have shown previously that leukemia-directed cytotoxic lymphocytes can be generated from bone marrow tissue (14–16). In the present study, we examined the different pathways of generation of cytotoxic lymphocytes from the bone marrow compartment. Specifically, we compared the cytotoxic efficacy and growth kinetics of lymphocytes generated in conventionally prepared IL-2 cultures (LAK) with those activated by simultaneous exposure to IL-2 and irradiated AML blasts or to IL-2 and the irradiated Daudi cell line (which was shown previously to generate NK cells) (17). The cytotoxicity and growth kinetics of these individual groups of lymphocytes were analyzed at weekly intervals for 5–6 weeks. Figure 11 illustrates that the oncolytic cells against leukemia were induced from all types of cultures within 2 weeks; however, lymphocytes induced by divergent pathways differed in oncolytic efficacy. The highest cytotoxic activity against AML blasts was displayed by lymphocytes from cultures stimulated simultaneously with IL-2 and AML cells. Lymphocytes stimulated with IL-2 and the Daudi cell line also displayed a high lytic activity; however, the cytotoxic levels were 10-fold lower than those displayed by AML-induced

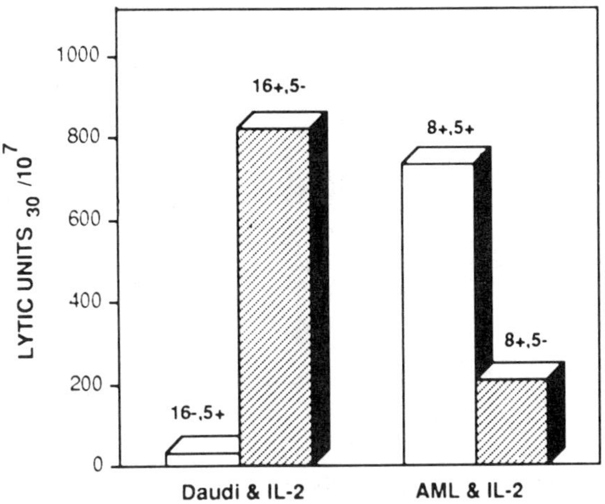

FIGURE 12 Characterization of bone marrow lymphocytes induced by combined activation with IL-2 and AML blasts or the Daudi cell line. Bone marrow cells of normal donors were cultured for 3 weeks with 10^3 U/ml of IL-2 and irradiated Daudi or AML stimulator cells. The individual lymphocyte subsets were then separated by fluorescence-activated cell sorting using a FACStar Plus cell sorter and tested for cytotoxicity against AML blasts in a 3 h ^{51}Cr release assay. Bars represent the mean of two experiments.

lymphocytes. The cytotoxicity of lymphocytes generated from conventional LAK cultures was lowest (Fig. 11). In addition, the lytic activity of these cultures declined after 2 weeks, but the AML- and Daudi-activated lymphocytes retained high and stable levels of lytic activity for at least 5 weeks.

The studies of growth kinetics showed that the Daudi- and AML-activated oncolytic cells displayed superior growth and showed a longer proliferative activity (up to 6 weeks) than the conventional IL-2 cultures.

2. Characterization of Lymphocytes in Bone Marrow Cultures

It has been shown repeatedly that oncolytic cells from peripheral blood, bone marrow, and splenic LAK cultures were NK cells (14–16, 18–21). In the present studies we were interested in identifying the oncolytic lymphocyte subset generated in IL-2 cultures activated with AML blasts or the Daudi cell line. To answer this question, we separated the bone marrow lymphocytes from these cultures by fluorescence-activated cell sorting (FACS) into NK and T cell subsets and tested for cytotoxic activity against AML (Fig. 12). We found that the cytotoxic lymphocytes generated from Daudi-stimulated cultures displayed the $CD16^+$, $CD5^-$ NK cell phenotype. Only very low cytotoxicity was generated from the $CD5^+$, $CD16^-$ T lymphocyte subset. On the contrary, the oncolytic lymphocytes generated from AML-stimulated cultures displayed the $CD5^+$,

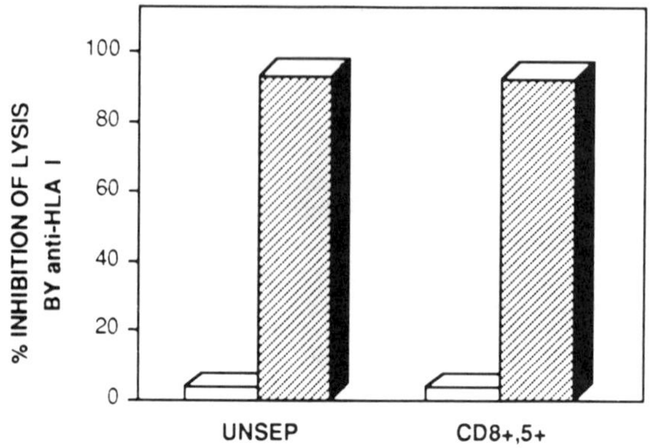

FIGURE 13 Inhibition of lysis of AML blasts by anti-HLA-I antibodies. Bone marrow cells were cultured for 3 weeks with irradiated AML blasts and IL-2 (10^3 U/ml). Unseparated and $CD8^+$, $CD5^+$ lymphocytes (obtained as described in Fig. 12) were then tested for cytotoxicity against AML targets (autologous with irradiated AML blasts) in the presence of 25 μg/ml of anti-HLA-I (▨) or isotype (IgG_{2a}) control (□) antibodies. Bars represent the mean of two experiments.

$CD8^+$ T cell phenotype. Blocking experiments using antibody directed against major histocompatibility complex (MHC) class I antigens indicated that the cytotoxic function of the $CD5^+$, $CD8^+$ T cell subset was restricted by the major histocompatibility complex (Fig. 13). Even though T cells from AML-stimulated bone marrow cultures were the major effector cells in oncolytic activity against leukemia, it is important to note that $CD8^+$, $CD5^-$ NK cells also mediated significant levels of leukemia lysis (Fig. 12).

IV. THERAPEUTIC IMPLICATIONS

We have shown that repeated cycles of continuous infusion of IL-2 in AML patients resulted in the generation of high numbers of NK cells in both peripheral blood and bone marrow. However, this treatment regimen was not effective in inducing NK cell activity against fresh leukemia, despite the generation of high cytotoxic function against the K-562 and Daudi cell lines. The manifestation of cytotoxicity against fresh AML was dependent on additional in vitro stimulation of effector cells with a higher dose of IL-2. Therapeutically, these observations could be interpreted to indicate that continuous infusion of IL-2 is effective in inducing the proliferation and moderate cytotoxicity of effector cells; however, the higher IL-2 serum levels may be necessary for the optimal activation of cytotoxic cells against highly resistant leukemia blasts. Consequently, the combination of continuous IL-2 infusion with occasional bolus injection (generating higher serum levels of IL-2) may represent an approach leading to both the induction of cell growth and high cytotoxic function. Another lesson that could be learned from these studies relates to the in vitro immunologic monitoring of in vivo studies. Our data clearly showed that the Daudi cell line (used routinely as a prototype target reflecting lytic activity against fresh tumors) is not an optimum target for monitoring the lytic response to AML blasts and, most likely, other fresh tumors. In this respect the K-562 cell line, also used for monitoring in vivo cytotoxicity, is even less relevant because of its high sensitivity to lysis. This has been clearly demonstrated by the dichotomy in reactivity of in vivo IL-2-primed lymphocytes against K-562 and Daudi cells (positive response) versus AML blasts (negative response). This discrepancy between lymphocyte reactivity against cultured cell lines as opposed to fresh tumors implies that it is imperative to optimize the in vitro monitoring systems to achieve a true reflection of in vivo antitumor reactivity. One of the steps in this direction is the use of fresh tumor cells as targets in the in vitro cytotoxicity assay. This approach, although more elaborate, may provide more insight into anticancer responses in vivo.

Our studies have also some implications for adoptive therapy with activated lymphocytes. It is clear that adoptive immunotherapy is not optimal in its present form. Very little attention has been given to the sensitivity of individual tumors to a particular lymphocyte subset, although emerging evidence indicates that discriminatory tumor cell susceptibility to lymphocyte subsets may exist (22,23). Thus, it may be beneficial to dissect the most cytotoxic lymphocyte subset reactive against a particular type of cancer, and enrich and propagate these lymphocytes in vitro for use in adoptive therapy. This approach may optimize the anticancer effect. For instance, it would be logical to enrich the NK cell population for the adoptive therapy of NK cell-sensitive tumors and the T cell population in the case of T cell-sensitive tumors. Based on our studies, a high NK cell enrichment (up to 80%) can be accomplished in peripheral blood and bone marrow (up to 60%) after continuous IL-2 infusion. It may thus be possible to collect NK cells after in vivo IL-2 treatment and stimulate these cells additionally with IL-2 in vitro to obtain a highly cytotoxic population for therapeutic use.

Our data showed that highly oncolytic lymphocytes can be obtained not only from peripheral blood but also from bone marrow tissue. It remains to be determined whether bone marrow and peripheral blood compartments are equally effective in mediating antitumor effects. It is plausible that the lymphocyte precursors in bone marrow may after IL-2 activation represent the oncolytic population with a longer life span than the lymphocytes already disseminated into peripheral blood. The use of bone marrow lymphocytes may be beneficial when leukopheresis is not practical or possible.

In our in vitro studies, we have identified various pathways to activation and generation of antileukemia-directed cytotoxic cells. A-LAK is one of the highly oncolytic lymphocyte populations. However, several warnings have to be made concerning A-LAK therapy. First, we and other investigators observed that A-LAK cannot be induced from all patients. Furthermore, the A-LAK from patient population may not contain highly purified NK cells, as has been described in normal donors (13). As we have shown in AML patients, the A-LAK of some patients was composed primarily of NK cells, but in the A-LAK of other patients, T cells represented the major population. If NK cells are shown to be most effective against certain cancers, then the A-LAK would need to be analyzed for the distribution of this population before adoptive therapy. The same argument can be used for T cell-sensitive tumors.

Another way of inducing the highly cytotoxic lymphocytes against leukemia is a combined stimulation with irradiated AML blasts (or the Daudi cell line) and IL-2. As indicated by our studies, both autologous and allogeneic AML stimulators (with regard to the targets) are effective in inducing a high antileukemia effect. This approach, especially that including AML-induced oncolytic lymphocytes, is attractive but needs further experimentation. The analysis of efficacy of these lymphocytes in vivo would be of particular interest.

Despite a number of unresolved questions, it is encouraging to see how much has been learned in the last few years in the immunotherapy arena and how rapidly new information is emerging. It is hoped that this new accumulating knowledge will accelerate and optimize our approaches to cancer immunotherapy.

ACKNOWLEDGMENTS

We thank Drs. P. Fuchshuber and Y. Huh for contribution to some of these studies, Drs. K. McCredie and J. Schachner for providing the samples from leukemia patients, and Pamela Baxter for assistance in the preparation of this manuscript. The IL-2 used in studies in vitro was kindly provided by Cetus Corporation (Emeryville, CA). The experimental part of these studies was supported by Grant CA 39632 from National Cancer Institute and by a generous donation from Olympia & York Development Limited (Toronto, Ontario, Canada). Eva Lotzová is a recipient of the Florence Maude Thomas Cancer Research Professorship.

REFERENCES

1. Kiessling R, Klein E, Wigzell H. Natural killer cells in the mouse. I. Cytotoxic cells with specificity for mouse Moloney leukemia cells. Specificity and distribution according to genotype. Eur J. Immunol 1975; 5:112–7.
2. Kasai M, Yoneda T, Habu S, Maruyama Y, Okumura K, Tokunaga T. In vivo effect of anti-asialo GM-1 antibody on natural killer activity. Nature 1981; 291:334–55.
3. Li LH, Wallace TL, Richard KA, Tracey DE. Mechanism of antitumor action of pyrimidinones in the treatment of B16 melanoma and P388 leukemia. Cancer Res 1985; 45:532–8.

4. Warner J, Dennert F. In vivo function of a cloned cell line with NK activity: effects on bone marrow transplants, tumor development and metastases. Nature 1982; 300:31–4.
5. Lotzová E. Interleukin-2 generated killer cells, their characterization and role in cancer therapy. Cancer Bull 1987; 39:30–8.
6. Lotzová E, McCredie KB, Muesse L, Dicke KA, Freireich EJ. Natural killer cells in man: their possible involvement in leukemia and bone marrow transplantation. In: Baum SJ, Ledney GD, eds. Experimental hematology today, 1979. New York: Springer-Verlag, 1979; 207–13.
7. Lotzová E, Savary CA, Keating MJ. Leukemia diseased patients exhibit multiple defects in natural killer cell lytic machinery. Exp Hematol 1983; 10:83–95.
8. Lotzová E, Savary CA, Herberman RB. Impaired NK cell profile in leukemia-diseased patients. In: Lotzová E, ed. Herberman RB, assoc. ed. Immunobiology of natural killer cells, Vol. II. Boca Raton, FL: CRC Press, 1986; 163–77.
9. Lotzová E, Savary CA. Function of interleukin-2 activated NK cells in leukemia resistance and treatment. In: Lotzová E, ed. Herberman RB, assoc. ed. Interleukin-2 and killer cells in cancer. Boca Raton FL: CRC Press, 1990; 153–61.
10. Hauch M, Gazzola MV, Small T, et al. Anti-leukemia potential of interleukin-2 activated natural killer cells after bone marrow transplantation for chronic myelogenous leukemia. Blood 1990; 75:2250–62.
11. Lotzová E, Savary CA, Herberman RB. Inhibition of clonogenic growth of fresh leukemia cells by unstimulated and IL-2 stimulated NK cells of normal donors. Leuk Res 1987; 11:1059–66.
12. Lotzová E, Savary CA, Herberman RB. Induction of NK cell activity against fresh human leukemia in culture with interleukin-2. J Immunol 1987; 138:2718–27.
13. Melder RJ, Rosenfeld CS, Herberman RB, Whiteside TL. Large-scale preparation of adherent lymphokine-activated killer (A-LAK) cells for adoptive immunotherapy in man. Cancer Immunol Immunother 1989; 29:67–73.
14. Lotzová E, Savary CA. Generation of NK cell activity from human bone marrow. J Immunol 1987; 139:279–94.
15. Lotzová E. Cytotoxicity and clinical application of activated NK cells. Med Oncol Tumor Pharmacother 1989; 6:93–8.
16. Lotzová E, Savary CA, Pollock RE, Fuchshuber P. Immunologic and clinical aspects of natural killer cells in human leukemia. Nat Immun Cell Growth Regul 1990; 9:173–81.
17. Perussia B, Ramoni C, Anegon I, Cuturi MC, Faust J, Trinchieri G. Preferential proliferation of natural killer cells among peripheral blood mononuclear cells cocultured with B lymphoblastoid cell lines. Nat Immun Cell Growth Regul 1987; 6:171–88.
18. Lotzová E, Herberman RB. Reassessment of LAK phenomenology—a review. Nat Immun Cell Growth Regul 1987; 6:109–15.
19. Herberman RB, Balch C, Bolhuis R, et al. Most lymphokine activated killer (LAK) activity mediated by blood and splenic lymphocytes is attributable to stimulation of natural killer (NK) cells by interleukin-2. Immunol Today 1987; 8:178–81.
20. Lotzová E. Analysis of effector mechanisms in cancer. In: Curr Opin Immunol 1989; 5:904–9.

21. Lotzová E. Role of natural killer cells in defense against leukemia: therapeutic considerations. Nat Immun Cell Growth Regul 1988; 7:170–9.
22. Parkinson DR, Lotzová E. Interleukin-2, killer cells and cancer therapy: an overview. Nat Immun Cell Growth Regul 1990; 9:237–41.
23. Lotzová E. Role of human circulating and tumor-infiltrating lymphocytes in cancer defense and treatment. Nat Immun Cell Growth Regul 1990; 9:254–65.
24. Wang A, Lu SD, Mark DF. Site-specific mutagenesis of the human interleukin-2 gene: structure-function analysis of the cysteine residues. Science 1984; 224: 1431–3.
25. Rosenberg SA, Grimm EA, McGrogan M, et al. Biological activity of recombinant human interleukin-2 produced in *Escherichia coli*. Science 1984; 223:1412–5.

9

The Therapeutic Potential of Interleukin-2 in Lymphomas and Leukemias

Carlo Gambacorti-Passerini*, Vera Malkovska, and Paul M. Sondel

University of Wisconsin, Madison, Wisconsin

I. INTRODUCTION

Interleukin 2 (IL-2) is a glycoprotein that regulates a variety of functions of T and B lymphocytes, natural killer (NK) cells, monocytes, and oligodendrocytes (1–3). Recently this molecule has received considerable attention as a potential drug for patients with a variety of tumors, including lymphoma and leukemia (4–8). Although IL-2 is not directly cytotoxic, it plays a crucial role in several cell-mediated antitumor effector systems that can operate both in vitro and in vivo. IL-2 can augment the lytic activity of antigen-specific T lymphocytes, induce major histocompatibility complex (MHC)-unrestricted cytolytic cells known as lymphokine-activated killer (LAK) cells (9), stimulate macrophage cytotoxicity, and induce a variety of cells to produce cytokines with antitumor activity (10). Antigen-specific T lymphocytes recognize peptide antigen in association with MHC determinants and utilize the T cell receptor (TCR) and the CD3 molecules to interact with their targets. Tumor-specific T cells have been detected in many experimental tumors (11,12) and also in some human neoplasias, such as melanomas, sarcomas, and pancreatic carcinomas (13–15). They have been obtained from peripheral blood (13,14) or from tumor-infiltrating

*On leave from the Istituto Nazionale Tumori, Milano, Italy.

TABLE 1 In Vitro Lysis of Leukemia and Lymphoma Cells by Autologous LAK[a]

Type of disease	Lysis	References
Hodgkin's lymphoma	NA	—
Non-Hodgkin's lymphoma	+	4
ANLL	+	4, 5, 20
ALL	+	4, 5, 21
CML	+/−	Foa unpublished,[b] 22
CLL	−	5
HCL	+/−	5, 23

[a](−) Negative data reported in at least one study;
(+/−) negative data and positive data in different reports;
(+) positive data in at least one study.
[b] Allogeneic LAK tested on five different CML cells.

lymphocytes (TIL) (15–17). The biologic significance of tumor-specific lymphocytes in humans remains to be assessed.

Unlike antigen-specific T cell cytotoxicity, LAK cell activity is not restricted by the MHC. Although NK cells are considered major contributors to LAK activity (18), T lymphocytes and other cells can produce a significant amount of IL-2-induced MHC-unrestricted cytotoxicity in vitro (19).

The mechanisms by which activated lymphocytes destroy tumor cells *in vivo* are unknown. In particular, it is not known whether direct lymphocyte-tumor cell contact is necessary or whether the cytotoxic effect is mediated by lymphokines secreted by lymphocytes (10); lymphocyte infiltration is, in fact, not uniformly present in regressing tumor nodules.

The first description of the killing of autologous tumor cells by IL-2-activated human lymphocytes came from acute nonlymphocytic leukemia (ANLL) patients (20).

Table 1 presents the cumulative data from seven studies investigating the in vitro lysis of leukemia and lymphoma cells by autologous LAK cells (4,5,20–23). No data are available, to our knowledge, for Hodgkins's lymphoma because of the difficulty of identifying and isolating the neoplastic cells in this disease. The overall results indicate that leukemia and lymphoma cells are usually lysed by autologous LAK cells and that higher cytotoxicity is usually measured in poorly differentiated types of leukemia. Chronic myelogenous leukemia (CML) and hairy cell leukemia (HCL) seem relatively resistant to both autologous and allogeneic LAK cells in vitro. In each study reported in Table 1, there is considerable variation in the amount of killing between patients. It is not clear whether a higher level of in vitro lysis is related to better therapeutic effects of IL-2; therefore, the clinical relevance of this in vitro information is uncertain.

The commonly used cytotoxic assay employing ^{51}Cr may not be sufficiently sensitive to detect lysis of a minority population of clonogenic neoplastic cells (24,25).

IL-2 can also exert a growth-promoting activity on some differentiated neoplasias, chronic lymphocytic leukemia (CLL) (26,27), in which functional receptors for IL-2 (IL-2R) have been described. If this growth promotion by IL-2 supersedes the antitumor effects of IL-2, this could constitute a potential contraindication to the use of IL-2 in the treatment of these diseases. In contrast, a direct effect of IL-2 on cell growth has not been demonstrated in acute leukemias, with the exception of one study using nonrecombinant IL-2 (28). Moreover, surface high-affinity IL-2R are generally absent from ANLL and acute lymphocytic leukemia (ALL) cells or are nonfunctional (29,30). It therefore seems improbable that IL-2 has a major effect directly on the growth of ALL and ANLL cells.

The drug-resistant phenotype exerted by leukemic cells also constitutes an important variable in relation to the possible therapeutic use of IL-2 in the treatment of leukemias and lymphomas. Adoptive immunotherapy may be most beneficial to patients in the setting of minimal residual disease, that is, after induction and consolidation chemotherapy. It is therefore important to know whether tumor cells surviving intensive chemotherapy that are resistant to cytotoxic drugs also develop resistance to IL-2-activated lymphocytes. Extensive in vitro studies conducted in different laboratories and using both human and murine cell lines or clones have uniformly shown that drug-resistant tumor cells do not develop resistance to activated lymphoctyes (24,31–33). In fact, in many of these experiments drug-resistant tumor cells proved to be even better targets for activated lymphocytes than their drug-sensitive counterparts, thus providing a strong rationale for the use of adoptive immunotherapy in conjunction with or after chemotherapy (34). Similar results have recently been obtained with ANLL cells selected in vivo for drug resistance; ANLL cells obtained from patients in relapse were equally or more sensitive to in vitro lysis by LAK than ANLL cells collected at diagnosis (35).

The mechanisms responsible for augmented susceptibility to the LAK effect are not understood. An increase in sensitivity to cytotoxic molecules released by lymphocytes or an augmented expression of adhesion molecules on drug-resistant tumor cells could be involved (31,36,37). In some systems, the resistance to drugs is explained by the increased expression of p170, the protein responsible for the multidrug-resistant (MDR) phenotype; in other drug-resistant cells, expression of p170 is not increased. It therefore seems unlikely that p170 or the MDR phenomenon plays a significant role in modifying the susceptibility of neoplastic cells to activated lymphocytes. Interestingly, the drug-resistant cells that were easily lysed by LAK cells appeared to have a less differentiated morphology and immune phenotype than drug-sensitive cells. Since this phenomenon was observed in cells derived from different tissues (melanocytes, colon epithelium, and B lymphocytes), it could be hypothesized that the process of differentiation is associated with the reduction in sensitivity to LAK cells, perhaps through the downregulation of adhesion molecule expression. Decreasing the expression of various adhesion molecules described during the differentiation pathway of B lymphocytes may play a role in this phenomenon (38,39). It will be interesting to see if patients with poorly differentiated tumors respond better to therapy with IL-2/LAK cells.

Similar results have been obtained using LAK-resistant tumor cells (37,40) instead of utilizing drug-resistant lines. In these systems, melanoma or lymphoma cells resistant to IL-2-activated lymphocytes were obtained by *in vitro* immunoselection or by simple screening of a large number of tumor clones; therefore, both induced and spontaneous LAK-resistant cells were analyzed (37,40). Also in this reverse situation, LAK-resistant cells proved to be more differentiated and more sensitive to doxorubicin than their LAK-sensitive counterparts (37,40). It is therefore conceivable that there is an inverse relationship between resistance to certain chemotherapeutic drugs and resistance to IL-2-activated cytolytic activity and that the differentiation status of the cells is an important determinant of the sensitivity to activated lymphocytes, perhaps through a differential expression of adhesion molecules.

II. CLINICAL STUDIES OF IL-2 IN LEUKEMIAS AND LYMPHOMAS

The clinical use of IL-2 has thus far been focused on patients with solid tumors, mainly melanoma and renal cancer (6,7,41,42). Some patients affected by Hodgkin's and non-Hodgkin's lymphomas (NHL) were also treated, and occasional responses have been documented (6,7,43). Although it is clear that objective tumor responses can be obtained in advanced NHL patients, they are usually partial and short-lived. It remains uncertain if this treatment will increase the percentage of cure achievable by chemotherapy alone. In leukemic patients, the clinical use of IL-2 has been proposed in three different settings.

A. Patients with Active Disease

In a pilot Italian study, 12 patients affected by relapsing or resistant ANLL (7 patients) or ALL (5 patients) were treated with multiple cycles of IL-2. The results of this study (8,44) can be summarized as follows:

1. The treatment did not enhance the growth of ANLL or ALL cells *in vivo* as judged by clinical observation.
2. The well-described side effects of IL-2 were noted in these patients. In particular, severe thrombocytopenia was frequently recorded.
3. The treatment induced peripheral lymphocytosis with spontaneous LAK activity and the release of tumor necrosis factor α (TNF-α) in the serum.

These phenomena were observed both in the peripheral blood, as previously described (45,46), and in bone marrow (BM) samples obtained during therapy.

4. No antitumor activity was observed in patients with massive (≥30%) leukemic infiltration of the BM.
5. In 3 patients (2 ANLL and 1 ALL) with active but limited disease (≤15% of blasts in the BM) a clinical and histologic complete remission (CR) was obtained. The 2 ANLL patients were still in CR at 6 and 20 months, respectively, while the ALL patient relapsed after 2 months.

Previous in vivo exposure to cytotoxic drugs could enhance the sensitivity of leukemic cells to activated lymphocytes. It is interesting to note that the ANLL patient reported in the study just mentioned to be in CR for ≥20 months after IL-2 treatment was treated with IL-2 after the failure of two autologous bone marrow transplants (ABMT).

Many variables, including disease type, tumor cell load, and in vitro sensitivity of the leukemia to LAK cells, could correlate with the outcome of IL-2 immunotherapy. Although these data demonstrate some clinical activity of IL-2 in advanced leukemia, better therapeutic results might be obtained by combining IL-2 with other therapies.

B. Combination of IL-2 with Conventional Therapy

IL-2 therapy has been tested in the setting of autologous bone marrow transplantation. Brenner and coworkers (47) treated patients with lymphoma or acute leukemia in remission who underwent high-dose chemoradiotherapy and ABMT. Treatment with IL-2 was started when granulocytes exceeded $500/mm^3$ to avoid negative effects on the regenerating BM and possible misinterpretation of fever in these patients. Although no antileukemic effect could be demonstrated in this type of study, the *in vivo* generation of LAK activity and the release of interferon-γ (IFN-γ) and TNF-α in the serum of treated patients were documented.

The timing of chemotherapy and IL-2 therapy may also prove to be important. For example, chemotherapy is immunosuppressive and IL-2 needs to be administered when the cells responsive to IL-2 are present. Current data regarding the recovery of the different antitumor effector mechanisms that could be regulated by IL-2 after ABMT are limited. In one report, IL-2-responsive cells were observed in the peripheral blood of patients as early as 17 days after AMBT (48). This result is in agreement with previous observations indicating that NK cells are the first cells appearing in the circulation after ABMT.

Although data on the combination of ABMT and IL-2 are limited, this therapeutic modality could constitute an ideal setting for maximizing the therapeutic effects of IL-2. The conditioning regimen of ABMT not only diminishes the leukemic cell burden but also places the patient in a particular immunologic situation in which the administration of IL-2 and/or in vitro activated lymphocytes may have greater effects than in a conventional setting. Moreover, IL-2 is administered to the patient *after* ABMT and is therefore potentially active on leukemic cells both surviving chemotherapy and reinfused with the autologous bone marrow.

C. Use of In Vitro IL-2-Activated Lymphocytes for BM Purging

Leukemic relapse in a transplanted patient can originate from cells surviving the conditioning regimen or from cells reinfused with the bone marrow. Although the respective influence of those two sources of leukemic cells on subsequent relapse is difficult to define, it appears that reinfused neoplastic cells could play a significant role in causing clinical relapse (49). A possible approach to BM purging is the in vitro culture of BM with LAK cells before infusion. This would be useful if LAK cells can lyse leukemic cells without seriously affecting the number and function of normal BM stem cells. The potential advantages of in vitro purging by LAK cells are the higher effector-target ratios and better cell-to-cell contact than can be achieved in vivo (50).

Both ANLL and ALL cells contaminating patient BM can be selectively destroyed by LAK-BM coculture (51). In four cases, fresh autologous leukemic cells appeared to be totally eliminated (by Southern blot analysis) from the BM, which contained a low leukemic cell concentration (2%). The use of LAK cells for BM purging, however, needs to be evaluated in the global context of ABMT and IL-2 therapy. In vitro purging would be beneficial only if leukemic cells reinfused with the BM constitute a significant portion of the total neoplastic cells present in the host at the time of immunotherapy and if immunotherapy *in vivo* is not sufficient to eradicate residual leukemic cells.

A final issue for discussion is the involvement of different subpopulations of IL-2-activated lymphocytes that can exert antitumor effects. The most easily detectable antitumor activity elicited by IL-2 is the so-called LAK cell phenomenon, in which MHC-nonrestricted tumor cytotoxicity is generated (9). Aside from these relatively nonspecific killer cells, tumor-specific T cells can be found in animal tumors and in some human neoplasias (13–17). Animal models clearly indicate that LAK cells are much less efficient in eradicating tumor cells in vivo than tumor-specific T lymphocytes (12,52). It is not known whether autologous tumor-specific lymphocytes are present in most patients with acute leukemia (53). However, lymphocytes with an apparently specific recognition of ALL cells have been described in an allogeneic setting (54,55). These have included T cells with α and β T cell receptors and T cells with γ and δ T cell receptors. The isolation of autologous immune effectors from leukemic patients would constitute an important step, not only in understanding the antileukemic immune response but also in the potential clinical use of specific antitumor lymphocytes.

The clear demonstration of an antileukemic "graft-versus-leukemia" (GVL) effect (56,57) associated with clinical allogeneic BMT gives rise to the possibility that the immune components of this GVL effect might be manipulated to allow a more focused immunologic antileukemic approach.

Future research will assess the overall impact of various immunotherapeutic approaches with IL-2 on the treatment of leukemia and lymphoma. Such therapy may involve activation and propagation of antigen-specific and nonspecific lymphoid populations of autologous or even allogeneic origin. We believe that combinations of treatment modalities utilizing other antileukemic agents are most likely to be successful.

ACKNOWLEDGMENTS

The authors thank their colleagues for collaboration and discussion regarding these concepts: Drs. E. C. Borden, P. Fisch, R. Foa, J. Hank, R. Hong, M. Malkovsky, G. Parmiani, J. Sosman, and Kathy Edge for preparing this manuscript. Dr. Gambacorti-Passerini was supported by a fellowship from the European Organization for Research and Treatment of Cancer. Research support was received from the University of Wisconsin Medical and Graduate Schools, American Cancer Society Research Grant CH-237, and NIH Grant CA-32685.

REFERENCES

1. Gillis S. Interleukin biochemistry and biology: summary and introduction. Fed Proc 1983; 42:3635–8.
2. Malkovsky M, Loveland B, North M, et al. Recombinant interleukin 2 directly augments the cytotoxicity of human monocytes. Nature 1987; 325:262–5.
3. Benveniste EN, Merril JE. Stimulation of oligodendroglial proliferation and maturation by interleukin-2. Nature 1986; 321:610–3.
4. Oshimi K, Oshimi Y, Akutsu M, et al. Cytotoxicity of interleukin 2-activated lymphocytes for leukemia and lymphoma cells. Blood 1986; 68:938.
5. Foa R, Fierro MT, Raspadori D, et al. Lymphokine activated killer (LAK) activity in lymphoproliferative disorders. Bone Marrow Transplant 1988; 4:153–5.
6. Rosenberg SA, Lotze MT, Muul LM, et al. A progress report on the treatment of 157 patients with advanced cancer using lymphokine activated killer cells and interleukin-2 or high dose interleukin-2 alone. N Engl J Med 1987; 316:889–97.
7. West WH, Tauer KW, Yannelli JR, et al. Constant-infusion recombinant interleukin-2 in adoptive immunotherapy of advanced cancer. N Engl J Med 1987; 316:898–905.
8. Foa R, Fierro MT, Tosti S, Meloni G, Gavosto F, Mandelli F. Induction and persistence of complete remission in a resistant acute myeloid leukemia patient after treatment with recombinant interleukin-2. Leuk Lymph 1990; 1:113–117.

9. Grimm EA, Mazumder A, Zhang HX, Rosenberg SA. Lymphokine activated killer cell phenomenon. I. Lysis of natural killer-resistant fresh solid tumor cells by interleukin 2-activated autologous human peripheral blood lymphocytes. J Exp Med 1982; 155:1823.
10. Gemlo BT, Palladino MA, Jaffe HS, Espevik TP, Rayner AA. Circulating cytokines in patients with metastatic cancer treated with recombinant interleukin and lymphokine-activated killer cells. Cancer Res 1988; 48:5864–7.
11. Greenberg PD, Cheever MA, Fefer A. Eradication of disseminated murine leukemia by chemoimmunotherapy with cyclophosphamide and adoptively transferred immune syngeneic Lyt-1^+,2^- lymphocytes. J Exp Med 1981; 154:952.
12. Rosenberg SA, Spies P, Lafreniere R. A new approach to the adoptive immunotherapy of cancer with tumor-infiltrating lymphocytes. Science 1986; 233:1318–21.
13. Anichini A, Fossati G, Parmiani G. Heterogeneity of clones from a human metastatic melanoma detected by autologous cytotoxic T lymphocyte clones. J Exp Med 1986; 163:215–20.
14. Slovin SF, Lackman RD, Ferrone S, Kiely PE, Mastrangelo MJ. Cellular immune response to human sarcomas: cytotoxic T cell clones reactive with autologous sarcomas. J Immunol 1986; 137:3042, 3048.
15. Wölfel T, Meyer zum Buschenfelde KH, Knuth A. Cytolytic T lymphocyte (CTL) clones directed against autologous pancreatic carcinoma cells. Effect of gamma-interferon on tumor cell lysis. Eightieth Meeting of the American Association for Cancer Research, San Francisco, May 24–27, 1989, abstract 1360.
16. Muul-Mesler L, Spiess PJ, Director EP, Rosenberg SA. Identification of specific cytolytic immune responses against autologous tumor in humans bearing malignant melanoma. J Immunol 1987; 138:989–95.
17. Itoh K, Platsoucas CD, Balch CM. Autologous tumor-specific cytotoxic T lymphocytes in the infiltrate of human metastatic melanomas. J Exp Med 1988; 168:1419–41.
18. Phillips JH, Lanier LL. Dissection of the lymphokine-activated killer phenomenon. Relative contribution of peripheral blood natural killer cells and T lymphocytes to cytolysis. J Exp Med 1986; 164:814–25.
19. Damle NK, Doyle LV, Bradley EC. Interleukin-2 activated human killer cells are derived from phenotypically heterogeneous precursors. J Immunol 1986; 1337:2814–22.
20. Zarling YM, Bach FH. Continuous culture of T cells cytotoxic for autologous human leukaemia cells. Nature 1979; 280:685.
21. Findley HW, Mageed AA, Nasr SA, Ragab AH. Recombinant interleukin-2 activates peripheral blood lymphocytes from children with acute leukemia to kill autologous leukemic cells. Cancer 1988; 62:1928–31.
22. Verfaillie C, Kay N, Miller W, McGlave P. Diminished NK function accompanies disease progression in CML. Thirty-First Annual Meeting of the American Society of Hematology, Atlanta, Georgia, December 2–5, 1989, abstract 74.
23. Griffiths SD, Cawley JC. α-Interferon and lymphokine activated killer cells in hairy cells in hairy cell leukemia. Leukemia 1988; 2:337–81.
24. Gambacorti-Passerini C, Radrizzani M, Erba E, Fossati G, Parmiani G. Lysis by activated lymphocytes of melanoma and small cell lung cancer cells surviving *in vitro* treatment with Mafosfamide. Cancer Res 1987; 47:2547.

25. Lista P, Fierro MT, Liao SX, *et al.* Lymphokine activated killer (LAK) cells inhibit the clonogenic growth of human leukemic stem cells. Eur J Haematol 1989; 42:425–30.
26. Giovarelli M, Foa R, Benetton G, Lusso P, Fierro MT, Forni G. Release of interleukin 2-like material by B-chronic lymphocytic leukemia cells. An autocrine or paracrine model of production and utilization? Leuk Res 1988; 12:201–9.
27. Malkovska V, Murphy J, Hudson L, Bevan D. Direct effect of interleukin-2 on chronic lymphocytic leukemia B cell function and morphology. Clin Exp Immunol 1987; 68:677–84.
28. Carron JA, Cawley JC. IL-2 and myelopoiesis: IL-2 induces blast cell proliferation in some cases of acute myeloid leukaemia. Br J Hematol 1989; 73:168–72.
29. Yamamoto S, Hattori T, Matsuoka M, et al. Induction of Tac antigen and proliferation of myeloid leukemic cells by ATL-derived factor: comparison with other agents that promote differentiation of human myeloid or monocytic leukemic cells. Blood 1986; 67:1713–20.
30. Estrov Z, Freedman MH. Growth requirements for human acute lymphoblastic leukemia cells: refinement of a clonogenic assay. Cancer Res 1988; 48:5901–7.
31. Gambacorti-Passerini C, Rivoltini L, Supino R, et al. Susceptibility of chemoresistant murine and human tumor cells to lysis by interleukin 2-activated lymphocytes. Cancer Res 1988; 48:2372–6.
32. Gambacorti-Passerini C, Rivoltini L, Supino R, Mariani M, Parmiani G. Differential lysis of melanoma clones by autologous recombinat interleukin-2-activated lymphocytes. Relationship with spontaneous resistance to doxorubicin. Int J Cancer 1988; 42:544–8.
33. Allavena P, Grandi M, D'Incalci M, Geri O, Giuliani FC, Mantovani A. Human tumor cell lines with pleiotropic drug-resistance are efficiently killed by interleukin-2 activated killer cells and by activated monocytes. Int J Cancer 1987; 40:104–7.
34. Gambacorti-Passerini C, Rivoltini L, Radrizzani M, Supino R, Mariani M, Parmiani G. Susceptibility of human and murine drug-resistant tumor cells to the lytic activity of rIL2-activated lymphocytes (LAK). Cancer Metastasis Rev 1988; 7:263–84.
35. Pogliani E, Gambacorti-Passerini C, Supino R, et al. Sensitivity to lymphokine-activated killers (LAK) of relapsing acute nonlymphocytic leukemia (ANLL) cells: comparison with drug sensitivity and P170 expression. Thirty-First Annual Meeting of the American Society of Hematology, Atlanta, Georgia, December 2–5, 1989, abstract 836.
36. Rivoltini L, Gambacorti-Passerini C, Cattoretti G, Parmiani G. Chemoresistant tumor cells are more susceptible to lytic activity of different immunocompetent cells and display a less differentiated phenotype. Biology and Clinical Application of IL2, Sheffield, England October 23–25, 1989, abstract 7.
37. Gambacorti-Passerini C, Cattoretti G, Marinoni A, Parmiani G. Generation of human lymphoma clones with stable resistance to lymphokine activated killer (LAK) cells. Correlation with integrin expression and differentiation status. Thirty-First Annual Meeting of the American Society of Hematology, Atlanta, Georgia, December 2–5, 1989, abstract 837.
38. Boyd AW, Dunn SM, Fecondo JV, et al. Regulation of expression of a human in-

tercellular adhesion molecule (ICAM-1) during lymphohematopoietic differentiation. Blood 1989; 73:1896–03.

39. Ryan DH, Nucci BL, Abboud CL, Liesveld JL. Maturation-dependent adhesion of human B cell precursor to the bone marrow microenvironment. Thirty-First Annual Meeting of the American Society of Hematology, Atlanta, Georgia, December 2–5, 1989, abstract 846.
40. Rivoltini L, Gambacorti-Passerini C, Supino R, Parmiani G. Generation of partial characterization of melanoma sublines resistant to lymphokine activated killer (LAK) cells. Relevance to the drug resistant phenotype. Int J Cancer 1989; 43:880–5.
41. Fisher RI, Coltman CA, Doroshow JD, *et al.* Metastatic renal cancer treated with interleukin 2 and lymphokine activated killer cells. Ann Intern Med 1988; 108:518–23.
42. Sosman JA, Kohler PC, Hank J, et al. Repetitive weekly cycles of recombinant human interleukin 2: responses of renal carcinoma with acceptable toxicity. J Natl Cancer Inst 1988; 80:60–3.
43. Allison MA, Jones SE, McGuffey P. Phase II trial of outpatient interleukin-2 in malignant lymphoma, chronic lymphocytic leukemia, and selected solid tumors. J Clin Oncol 1989; 7:75–80.
44. Foa R, Meloni G, Tosti S, Novarino A, Fenu S, Gavosto F, Mandelli F. Treatment of acute myeloid leukemia patients with recombinant interleukin-2: a pilot study. Brit. J. Haematol. 1991; 77, 491–496.
45. Gambacorti-Passerini C, Radrizzani M, Marolda R, et al. *In vivo* activation of lymphocytes in melanoma patients receiving escalating doses of recolmbinant interleukin 2. Int J Cancer 1988; 41:700–6.
46. Sondel PM, Kohler PC, Hank JA, et al. Clinical and immunological effects of recombinant interleukin-2 given by repetitive weekly cycles in patients with cancer. Cancer Res 1988; 48:2561–7.
47. Gottlieb DJ, Prentice HG, Heslop HE, et al. Effects of recombinant interleukin-2 administration on cytotoxic function following high-dose chemo-radiotherapy for hematological malignancy. Blood 1989; 74:2335–42.
48. Higuchi C, Thompson JA, Cox T, Lindgren CG, Buckner C, Fefer A. Lymphokine-activated killer function following autologous bone marrow transplantation for refractory hematological malignancies. Cancer Res 1989; 49:5509–13.
49. Butturini A, Gale RP. How can we cure leukaemia? Br J Hematol 1989; 72:479–85.
50. Fisher B, Packard BS, Read EJ, et al. Tumor localization of adoptively transferred Indium-111 labeled tumor infiltrating lymphocytes in patients with metastatic melanoma. J Clin Oncol 1989; 7:250–61.
51. Gambacorti-Passerini C, Rivoltini L, Fizzotti M, Rodolfo M, Sensi ML, Castelli C, Orazi A, Polli N, Bregni M, Siena S, Borin L, Pogliani E, Corneo GM, Parmiani G. Selective purging by human interleukin-2 activated lymphocytes of bone marrows contaminated with a lymphoma line or autologous leukemia cells. Brit. J. Haematol. 1991: 78, 197–205.
52. Thompson JA, Peace DJ, Klarnet JP, Kern DE, Greenberg PD, Cheever MA. Eradication of disseminated murine leukemia by treatment with high-dose interleukin 2. J Immunol 1986; 137:3675–80.

53. Fisch P, Weil-Hillman GW, Uppenkamp M, et al. Antigen specific recognition of autologous leukemia cells and allogeneic class I MHC antigens by IL-2 activated cytotoxic T cells from a patient with acute T-cell leukemia. Blood 1989; 74:343–53.
54. Sosman JA, Oettel KR, Hank JA, Fisch P, Sondel P. Specific recognition of human leukemic cells by allogeneic T cell lines. Transplantation 1989; 48:486–95.
55. Fisch P, Malkovsky M, Braakman E, et al. Gamma/delta T cell clones and natural killer cell clones mediate distinct patterns of non-MHC restricted cytolysis. J Exp Med 1990; 171:1567–1569.
56. Sosman JA, Sondel PM. The graft versus leukemia effect following bone marrow transplantation (BMT): a review of laboratory and clinical data. Hematol Rev 1987; 2:77–91.
57. Horowitz MM, Gale RP, Sondel PM, et al. Graft versus leukemia reactions following bone marrow transplantation in humans. Blood 1990; 75:555–62.

III

HEMATOPOIETIC GROWTH FACTORS

10

Molecular Control of Normal and Abnormal Hematopoiesis

Leo Sachs

Weizmann Institute of Science, Rehovot, Israel

> The described cultures thus seem to offer a useful system for a quantitative kinetic approach to hematopoietic cell formation and for experimental studies on the mechanism and regulation of hematopoietic cell differentiation. (1)

I. INTRODUCTION

The formation of different types of blood cells is essential for the development of a normal individual. New blood cells belonging to different cell lineages are formed from stem cells during embryogenesis and during the lifetime of the adult. Abnormalities in the normal developmental program for the formation of blood cells result in various types of hematologic diseases. Understanding the molecular control of normal development makes it possible to answer questions about the origin and possible treatment of these diseases. What are the molecular regulators that control the normal developmental program of cell multiplication and differentiation to different blood cell lineages? How do these regulators interact to give the correct balance between the number of immature and mature cells? What changes cause hematologic diseases, including leukemia, and can normal blood cell development be restored in hematologically abnormal individuals by treatment with normal regulators of development? I mainly describe results obtained with cells of the myeloid

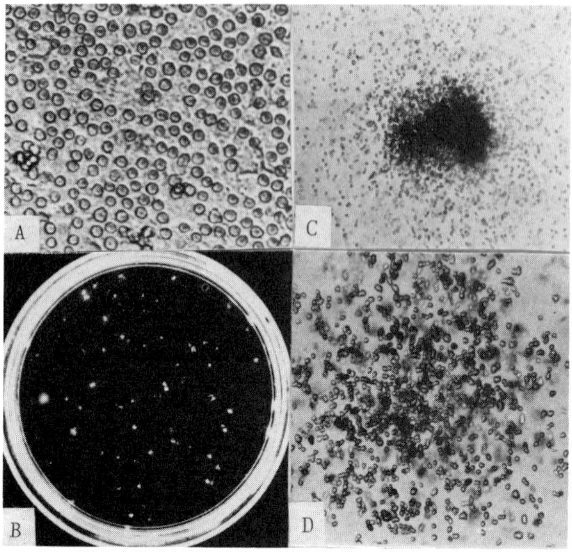

FIGURE 1 (A). Culture of mouse mast cells that have multiplied and differentiated on a feeder layer of mouse embryo cells (1). (B–D) Clones of macrophages and granulocytes in cultures of normal blood cell precursors incubated with the appropriate myeloid cell regulatory protein. (B) Petri dish with clones (3). (C) Granulocyte clone and (D) macrophage clone (5).

blood cell lineages, which have been used as a model system to answer these questions.

To analyze the controls that regulate the multiplication and differentiation of normal blood cells to different cell lineages and the changes in these controls in disease, it is desirable and convenient to study the entire process in cell culture starting from single cells. The analysis therefore began with the development of a cell culture system for the cloning and clonal differentiation of different types of normal blood cells. This cell culture system was then used to discover a family of protein hormones that regulates cell multiplication and differentiation of specific blood cell lineages, to analyze the origin of some hematologic diseases, including leukemia, and to identify ways of treating these diseases with normal regulatory molecules.

II. CLONING AND CLONAL DEVELOPMENT OF NORMAL HEMATOPOIETIC CELLS IN CULTURE

In the cell culture system that was developed, normal cells from blood-forming tissues from mice were first cultured with feeder layers of other cell types, such as normal embryo fibroblasts. These other cell types were chosen as possible candidates for cells that produce the inducers required for the cloning and clonal differentiation of different blood cell lineages. The first such system (1,2), using cells cultured in liquid medium (Fig. 1A), showed that it was possible to obtain by this procedure clones containing mast cells or granulocytes in various stages of differentiation. To make it simpler to distinguish and isolate separate clones, this system was then applied to the cloning of different blood cell lineages in semisolid medium containing agar (3,4). An analysis of the first types of clones obtained in agar with these feeder layers showed (Fig. 1B–D) clones containing macrophages, granulocytes, or both macrophages and granulocytes, in various stages of differentiation. The macrophage clones in agar contained many metachromatic granules, giving them an apparent morphologic resemblance to mast cells (3,4). These granules were not present when the cells were cloned in methylcellulose (5), however, and electron microscopy also clarified that these cells in agar were really macrophages that had phagocytosed agar (6). The experiments also showed that these clones could originate from single cells (3,4,7). This assay in agar (3,4) or methylcellulose (Table 1) (5) was then applied to the cloning and clonal differentiation of normal human macrophages and granulocytes (8,9) and to the cloning of all the other blood cell lineages, including erythrocytes (10), B lymphocytes (11), and T lymphocytes (12).

III. PROTEINS THAT CONTROL THE DEVELOPMENT OF DIFFERENT CELL LINEAGES

When cells were cloned in a semisolid substrate, such as agar, there was a more solid agar layer between the feeder layer cells and the cells seeded for cloning. This showed that the inducers required for the formation of macrophage and granulocyte clones were secreted by the feeder layer cells and could diffuse through agar (3). It was discovered that the inducers required for the formation of macrophage and granulocyte clones are present in conditioned medium produced by the feeder cells (5,7). These inducers were found in the conditioned medium from different types of normal and malignant cells (see Refs. 13 and 14). These media were then used to purify the inducers, which were shown to be glycoproteins or proteins without detectable sugars (15–19). Sugars do not seem

TABLE 1 Establishment of the Cell Culture System for Cloning and Clonal Differentiation of Normal Hematopoietic Cells and Discovery of the Molecular Regulators of This Clonal Development in Cell Culture Supernatants

Cloning and differentiation in liquid medium (mast cells and granulocytes) (1)
Cloning and differentiation in agar (macrophages and granulocytes) (3,4)
Inducer(s) for cloning and differentiation secreted by cells (3)
Inducer(s) in cell culture supernatants (macrophages and granulocytes) (5,7)
Cloning and differentiation in methylcellulose (macrophages and granulocytes) (5)

to be necessary for biologic activity (18). A similar approach was later used to identify the protein inducers for cloning of T lymphocytes (20) and B lymphocytes (see Ref. 21). When cells were washed at various times after initiating the induction of clones, there was no further development of either macrophage or granulocyte clones unless the inducer was added again (22). The development of clones with differentiated cells thus requires both an initial and continued supply of inducer.

In cells belonging to the myeloid cell lineages, four different proteins that induce cell multiplication and can thus induce the formation of clones (growth-inducing proteins) have been identified (reviewed in Refs. 23–25). The same proteins have been given different names. After they were first discovered in cell culture supernatant fluids (5,7), the first inducer identified was called mashran gm from the Hebrew word meaning "to send forth" with the initials for granulocytes and macrophages (26). This and other growth-inducing proteins were then renamed and are now called colony-stimulating factors (CSF) (27) or macrophage and granulocyte inducers (MGI) (15), type 1 (MGI-1), and one protein is called interleukin-3 (IL-3) (Table 2) (19). Of these four growth inducers, one protein (M) induces the development of clones with macrophages, another (G) clones with granulocytes, and third (GM) clones with granulocytes, macrophages, or both macrophages and granulocytes; the fourth (IL-3) clones with macrophages, granulocytes, eosinophils, mast cells, erythroid cells, or mega-

TABLE 2 Induction of Growth and Differentiation of Normal Myeloid Precursor Cells by Different Hematopoietic Regulatory Proteins

Nomenclature	Location on chromosome: Mouse	Location on chromosome: Human	Induction of colonies[a]	Induction of differentiation: Direct	Induction of differentiation: Indirect[b]
MGI-1M = CSF-1 = M-CSF	3	5	+ (M)	–	+
MGI-1G = G-CSF	11	17	+ (G)	–	+
MGI-1GM = GM-CSF	11	5	+ (G, M)	–	+
IL-3	11	5	+ (G, M, others)	–	+
MGI-2 = IL-6	5	7	–	+ (G, M)	–
IL-1	2	2	–	–	+ (G, M)
D-factor = LIF = HILDA	?	22	–	CD	CD
DIF = TNF	17	6	–	CD	CD

[a]Colonies with macrophages (M), granulocytes (G), granulocytes and macrophages (G, M), and granulocytes, macrophages, eosinophils, mast cells, megakaryocytes, and erythroid cells (G, M, others).

[b]The four growth-inducing proteins and IL-1 activate production of MGI-2/IL-6. References in text. CD = cell death.

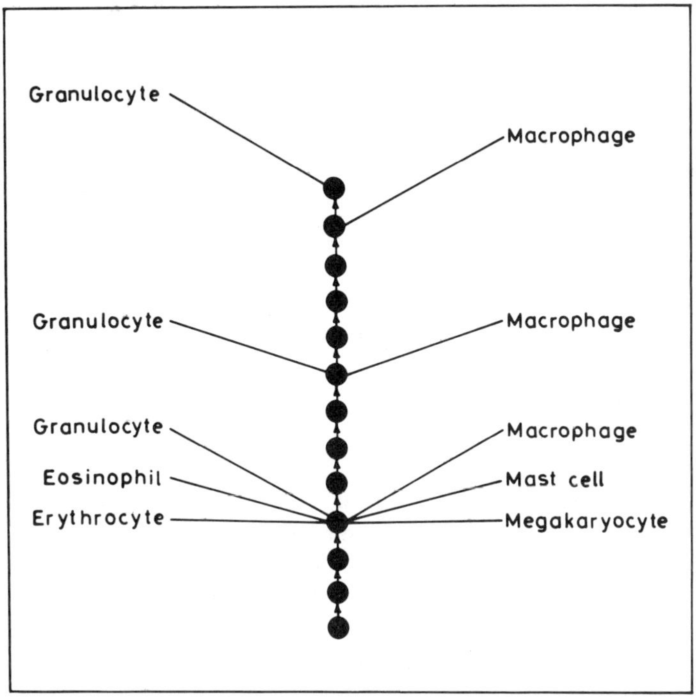

FIGURE 2 Myeloid precursor cells can be induced to multiply by four different growth-inducing proteins. One (IL-3) induces growth in precursors that have the potential to develop into six cell types, the second (GM) induces growth in precursors that develop into two cell types, and the third (G) and fourth (M) in precursors that develop into one cell type.

karyocytes (Table 2 and Fig. 2). These proteins induce cell viability and cell multiplication (28–30) and enhance the functional activity of mature cells (reviewed in Ref. 27). Cloning of genes from mice and humans for the IL-3, GM, M, and G growth inducers has shown that these genes are unrelated in their nucleotide sequence (reviewed in Ref. 31). The production of mRNA and protein for these four growth inducers has been analyzed at various stages of fetal development. The results show that the M growth inducer was the only gene for which mRNA and protein were detected in fetal development (32).

How do normal myeloid precursor cells induced to multiply by these growth inducers develop into clones containing mature cells that stop multiplying when they terminally differentiate? It appears unlikely that a growth inducer that induces cell multiplication is also a differentiation inducer whose action stops cell multiplication in mature cells. Indeed, proteins that act as myeloid cell

```
m-MGI-2A          . . . . . . M N N D D A L A E N N L K L P E I Q R N D G . . . . . .
                              | | | | | | | | | | | | | | | | | | | | | |
m-IL-6        67  N G N S D C M N N D D A L A E N N L K L P E I Q R N D G C Y Q T G Y   100
                  |         |           | | | | | | |   | |           | | |   |   |
h-IL-6        73  N K S N M C E S S K E A L A E N N L N L P K M A E K D G C F Q S G F   106
```

FIGURE 3 Amino acid sequence of CNBr-cleaved peptide from purified MGI-2A. The 22 amino acid sequence of the CNBr-cleaved mouse MGI-2A peptide (top line) is shown to be matched with the amino acids sequence of mouse IL-6 (middle line) and human IL-6 (bottom line). Matching amino acids are indicated by vertical bars (40).

differentiation inducers and do not have growth-inducing activity have been identified (18,33–38), and these have been called macrophage and granulocyte inducers type 2 (MGI-2) (34,35), D factor (37), and differentiation-inducing factor (DIF) (38). The myeloid growth and differentiation-inducing proteins are produced by various cell types and induce growth and differentiation when supplied externally to target cells (see Refs. 24 and 25). Studies on amino acid sequence, neutralization by monoclonal antibody (39), and myeloid cell differentiation-inducing activity of recombinant protein have shown that MGI-2 is interleukin 6 (IL-6) (Fig. 3) (40,41). D factor was identified (42) as a protein that has also been called LIF (43) and HILDA (44), and DIF was found to be a form of tumor necrosis factor (TNF) (45). IL-1 can also induce the differentiation of myeloid cells without inducing growth (see Ref. 46). MGI-2/IL-6, IL-1, D factor/LIF, and TNF are coded for by different genes. MGI-2/IL-6 (47,48) and IL-1 (46) can induce the differentiation of normal myeloid precursors, but D factor/LIF and TNF, which induce differentiation in certain clones of myeloid leukemic cells (see later), do not induce the differentiation of normal myeloid cells (Table 2).

IV. CASCADE OF INTERACTIONS BETWEEN PROTEINS IN DEVELOPMENT

Experiments with normal myeloid precursor cells, which can be separated from other cell types in the bone marrow (49), have shown that in these cells any one of the four growth-inducing proteins induces cell viability, cell multiplication, and also production of differentiation-inducing protein MGI-2/IL-6 (28,29,35,36,50). This myeloid differentiation inducer activates differentiation directly, whereas the myeloid growth inducers activate differentiation indirectly by inducing the production of differentiation inducer (Table 2 and Figs. 4 and 5). This induction of differentiation inducer by growth inducer serves as an effective mechanism to couple growth and differentiation, a mechanism that may also apply to other cell types. Differences in the time of switch-on of the differentiation inducer would produce differences in the amount of cell multiplication before differentiation. IL-1 also induces myeloid cell differentiation indirectly

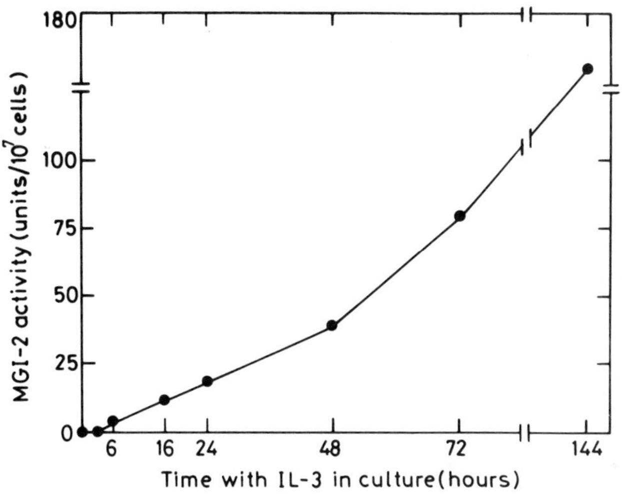

FIGURE 4 Induction of differentiation-inducing protein MGI-2/IL-6 by growth-inducing protein IL-3 in normal myeloid precursors (29).

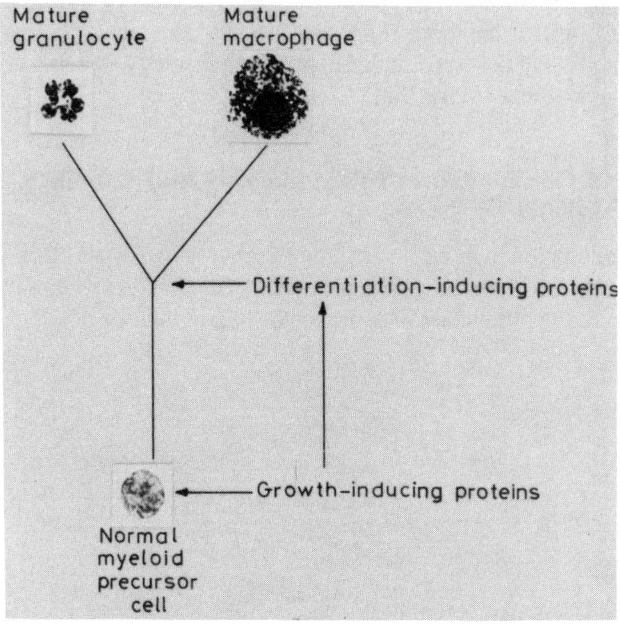

FIGURE 5 Growth of normal myeloid precursor cells and their differentiation to macrophages or granulocytes are induced by different proteins, growth-inducing proteins and differentiation-inducing proteins. The growth-inducing proteins induce cell viability and multiplication of normal precursors and production in these cells of differentiation-inducing protein. The induction of differentiation inducer by growth inducer provides a mechanism to couple the multiplication of normal precursor cells and their differentiation.

by activating the production of MGI-2/IL-6 (Table 2) (46), and the same applies to the induction of megakaryocyte development by IL-3 (51). The differentiation inducer MGI-2/IL-6 can also switch on production of the growth inducer GM-CSF in myeloid cells (46,52), and this may then enhance the function of mature cells.

Studies of myeloid regulatory proteins have shown that different growth and differentiation inducers participate in development and there is a network of interactions between these proteins (Fig. 6) (reviewed in Refs. 41 and 53). Interpretation of experimental data on the effects of each of these regulators or their combination must take into account this network of interactions to avoid an incorrect assignment of a specific effect to the direct action of a particular protein. The genes for the myeloid regulatory proteins are located on various chromosomes (Table 2) (54–60), and the cascade of interactions between different regulatory proteins include interactions between proteins whose genes are located on different chromosomes. This shows that there is trans-regulation between different proteins. In addition to this trans-regulation between different proteins (28,29,46,52,53,61,62), MGI-2/IL-6 and GM-CSF can positively autoregulate their own gene expression (63), and this has also been reported for IL-1 (64) and TNF (Fig. 6) (65). It has been suggested that this autoregulation may serve to enhance and prolong the signal induced in cells transiently exposed to these proteins from an external source (63).

V. CONTROL OF LEUKEMIA BY THE PROTEINS THAT CONTROL NORMAL HEMATOPOIESIS

Normal myeloid growth inducers are produced by various types of cells (see Ref. 25), but not by the normal myeloid precursor cells (28,29), so that normal precursors require the production of growth-inducing protein by other cell types for

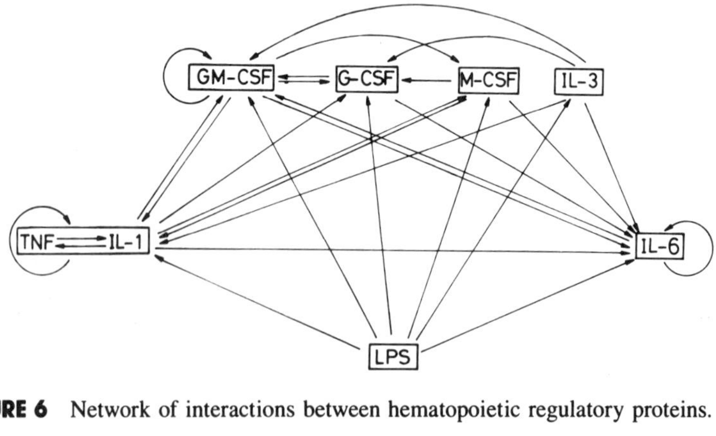

FIGURE 6 Network of interactions between hematopoietic regulatory proteins.

cell viability and growth. There are myeloid leukemic cells from patients with myeloid leukemia that still require an external source of myeloid growth-inducing protein for cell viability and growth (8,66), but other leukemic cells have become independent of a growth inducer for cell viability and multiplication (see Refs. 24 and 25) because of changes from an induced to a constitutive expression of certain genes (see Refs. 24, 35, 36, and 67). This gives the leukemic cells a growth advantage over the normal cells when there is a limiting amount of growth inducer in the body. There are also leukemic clones in which growth inducer no longer switches on the production of differentiation inducer (28,29, 35). Can myeloid leukemic cells still be induced to differentiate to mature nondividing cells by the normal protein regulators of differentiation? This question has been answered by showing that there are clones of myeloid leukemic cells that can be induced to differentiate normally to mature macrophages or granulocytes through the normal sequence of gene expression by incubation with the normal myeloid differentiation-inducing protein MGI-2/IL-6 (Fig. 7) (see Refs. 14, 24, 25, 36, 67, and 68). These are called D^+ clones (D for differentiation) (69). The mature cells, which can be formed from all the cells of a leukemic clone, then stop multiplying like normal mature cells and are no longer malignant in vivo (70–72).

In addition to the D^+ clones from the M1 myeloid leukemia that can be induced to differentiate by MGI-2/IL-6, other D^+ clones from other myeloid leukemias, like normal myeloid cells, can be induced to differentiate by incubating the leukemic cells with a normal myeloid growth-inducing protein (Table 3). Different clones can be induced to differentiate by incubation with GM-CSF (73,74), IL-3 (74), or G-CSF (see Refs. 25 and 27). In these clones, the growth inducers presumably induce the production of an appropriate differentiation inducer and thus induce differentiation indirectly. This was confirmed in WEHI-3B cells in which G-CSF was shown to induce differentiation indirectly mediated by factor(s), thus far unidentified, induced by G-CSF at high cell densities (75). D^+ leukemic cells that respond to MGI-2/IL-6 can also be induced to differentiate by IL-1α and IL-1β, and this is mediated by the endogenous production of MGI-2/IL-6 (Table 3) (46). Various clones derived from the M1 leukemia, such as clone 11, that are induced to differentiate by MGI-2/IL-6 are not induced to differentiate with D factor/LIF (76). M1 clone T22, which is also derived from the M1 leukemia (42), is a special clone that is induced to differentiate by D factor/LIF and by MGI-2/IL-6 (Table 3) (76). Induction of differentiation by D factor/LIF may also be indirect.

Studies in animals and humans have shown that normal differentiation of D^+ myeloid leukemic cells to mature nondividing cells can be induced not only in culture but also in vivo (62,73,74,77–81). These leukemias therefore grow progressively when there are too many leukemic cells for the normal amount of differentiation inducer in the body. The development of leukemia can be

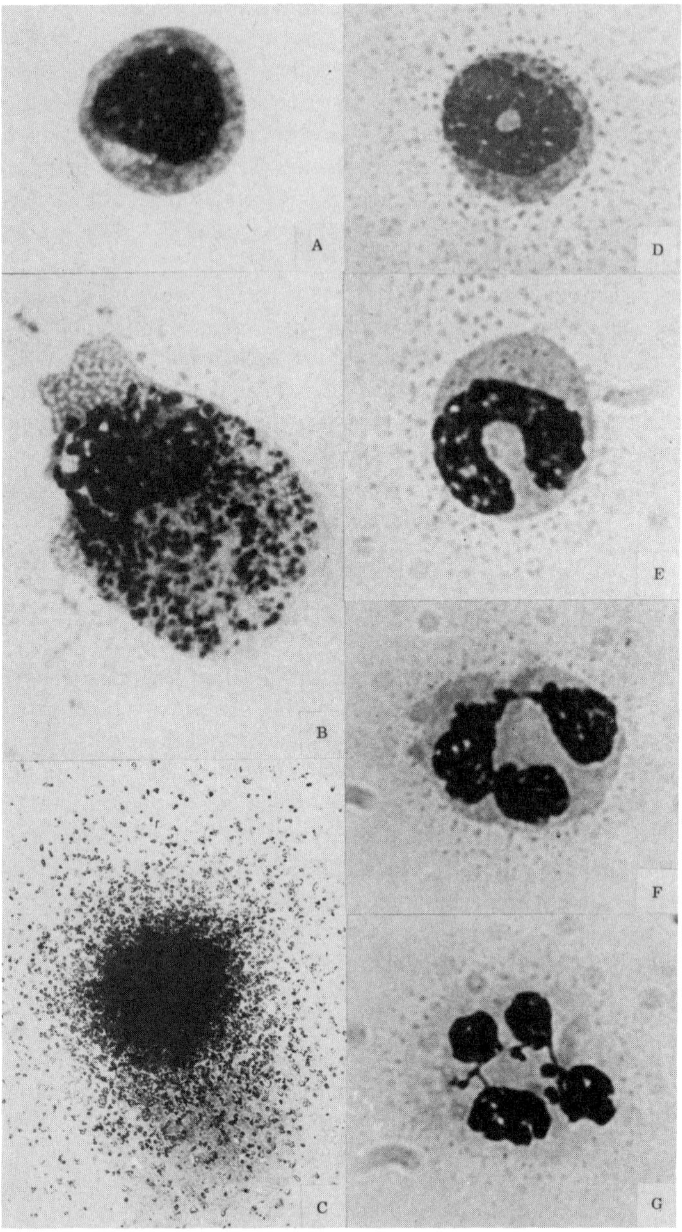

FIGURE 7 Differentiation of myeloid leukemic cells to nonmalignant mature macrophages or granulocytes by the normal myeloid differentiation-inducing protein MGI-2/IL-6: (A) leukemic cell; (B) macrophage; (C) colony of cells with macrophages; (D–G) stages in differentiation to granulocytes (68).

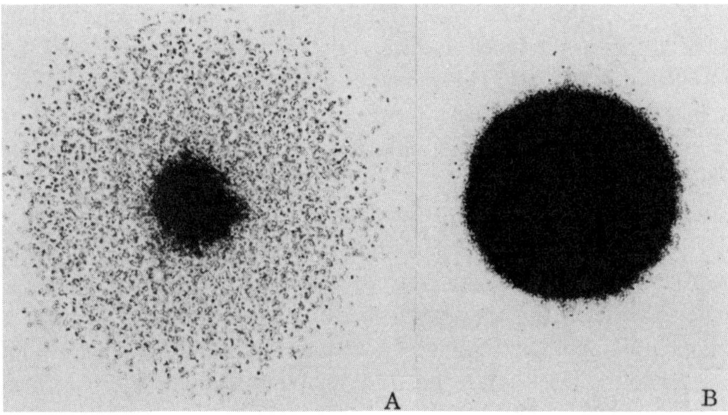

FIGURE 8 Colony of cells from (A) D^+ clone and (B) D^- clone of myeloid leukemic cells cultured with MGI-2/IL-6 (94). The differentiated cells in the D^+ clone migrate from the colony when the cells are induced to respond to chemotactic stimuli (88).

inhibited in mice with these D^+ leukemic cells by increasing the amount of differentiation-inducing protein, either by injecting it or by injecting a compound that induces its production by cells in the body (71,72). This in vivo differentiation is controlled by the host's helper T lymphocytes (77,81), which can produce MGI-2/IL-6 (81) as well as GM-CSF and IL-3. Injection of MGI-2/IL-6, GM-CSF, IL-3, or IL-1 induced the in vivo differentiation of D^+ myeloid leukemic cells that are also induced to differentiate with these proteins in vitro

TABLE 3 Differentiation of Myeloid Leukemic Cells by Different Hematopoietic Regulatory Proteins

Myeloid leukemic clone	Differentiation after culture with							
	MGI-2/ IL-6	IL-1	D factor/ LIF	TNF	IL-3	GM-CSF	G-CSF	M-CSF
M1-clone 11	+	+[a]	−	−	−	−	±[a]	−
M1-clone T22	+	+[a]	+[a]	−	−	−	±[a]	−
7-M12	−	−	−	−	+[a]	+[a]	−	−
WEHI-3B	−	−	−	−	−	−	+[a]	−
HL-60	−	−	−	+[a]	−	−	±[a]	−

[a]IL-1 and G-CSF induce differentiation indirectly in clones 11 and WEHI-3B, respectively (46,75). It is suggested that the induction of differentiation in clone 7-M12 by GM-CSF or IL-3, in clone T22 by D factor/LIF, in HL-60 by TNF and partial differentiation by G-CSF in some clones may also be indirect.

(62,74). However, GM-CSF and IL-3 also induce in vivo differentiation of D^+ leukemic cells that are induced to differentiate in vitro with MGI-2/IL-6 but not with GM-CSF or IL-3 (74). This shows that induction of differentiation in vivo like that in vitro can occur directly or by an indirect mechanism that involves induction of the appropriate differentiation-inducing protein either by the same cells or by other cells in the body. The results indicate (Table 3) that there is a clonal distribution of response of myeloid leukemic cells to different myeloid regulatory proteins (24,25,50,53), and there is presumably also a clonal distribution in the response of normal myeloid precursor cells to these regulators. Most and possibly all the physiologic regulatory proteins of normal myeloid blood cell development can regulate the differentiation of D^+ myeloid leukemic cells (50) (Table 3). Injection of myeloid leukemic cells into fetuses has shown that after such injection the leukemic cells can participate in blood cell development in apparently healthy adult animals (79,80). In one of these clones (Table 23, WEHI-3B) the genetic abnormalities include a rearrangement of the Hox 2.4 homeobox gene (82,83), and in other clones with a deletion in one chromosome 2 (84) there is a deletion of one copy of Hox 4.1 (85).

The study of different clones of myeloid leukemic cells has also shown that in addition to D^+ clones there are differentiation-defective clones (8,14,24, 25,69,86), D^- clones (Fig. 8) (69). Some D^- clones are induced by MGI-2/IL-6 to an intermediate stage of differentiation that then slows the growth of the cells,

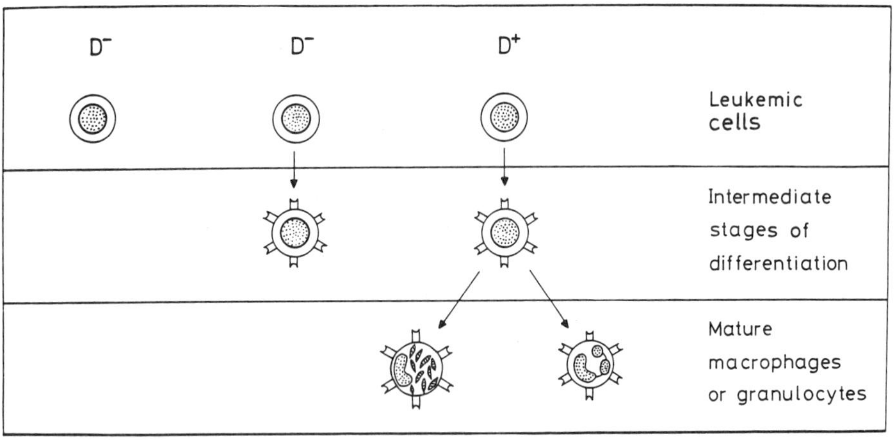

FIGURE 9 Classification of different types of myeloid leukemic cell clones according to their ability to be induced to differentiate by normal differentiation-inducing protein MGI-2/IL-6. Some differentiation-defective (D^-) clones can be induced by this protein to intermediate stages by differentiation, whereas other D^- clones are not induced to differentiate by this protein even to an intermediate stage (24,36).

and others cannot be induced to differentiate even to this intermediate stage by the normal myeloid regulatory proteins (Fig. 9) (see Refs. 24, 25, and 86–88). Since normal regulatory proteins induce differentiation to mature nondividing cells in the D^+ clones, it has been suggested that D^+ clones are the early stages of leukemia and that the formation of different types of D^- clones may be later stages in the progression of malignancy (87). There are D^- clones of myeloid leukemic cells that can no longer be induced to differentiate by proteins that regulate normal blood cell development but that can be induced to differentiate by other compounds (36,86,87), including such hormones as certain steroids (86,89) and insulin (90,91), which induce differentiation by alternative pathways (see Refs. 24, 25, 92, and 93). Although the cell response to induction of differentiation by normal myeloid regulatory proteins has been altered, these D^- clones have not lost all the genes for differentiation.

VI. CHROMOSOME CHANGES AND BYPASS OF GENETIC DEFECTS IN THE SUPPRESSION OF LEUKEMIA

Myeloid leukemic cells in mice (84,94) and humans (95) have chromosomal abnormalities, and the most common chromosomal change in mouse myeloid leukemias is a deletion in one chromosome 2 (84,85). The D^+ myeloid leukemic cells also have an abnormal chromosomal composition (84,94), and suppression of malignancy in these cells was not associated with chromosomal changes: it was obtained by induction of the normal sequence of cell differentiation by a normal myeloid regulatory protein. In this suppression, the stopping of cell multiplication by inducing differentiation to mature cells bypasses genetic changes such as changes in the requirement for the normal growth inducer and a block in the ability of growth inducer to induce differentiation inducer, that produced the malignant phenotype. Genetic changes that make cells defective in their ability to be induced to differentiate by the normal differentiation inducer occur in the evolution of myeloid leukemia. Even these D^- cells can be induced to differentiate by other compounds, however, either singly or in combination, that can induce the differentiation program by alternative pathways. Also in these cases, the stopping of cell multiplication by inducing differentiation by these alternative pathways bypasses the genetic changes that inhibit the response to the normal differentiation inducer.

Studies of the chromosomes of myeloid leukemic cells have shown that the change from D^- to D^+ and vice versa, that is, the ability to be induced to differentiate to mature nondividing cells by a normal myeloid regulatory protein, is controlled by the balance between genes that allow induction of differentiation and genes that suppress differentiation (84). Chromosomal changes can thus change leukemic cells from D^- to D^+, so that the cells can then be induced to differentiate when exposed to normal differentiation inducer. It can therefore be

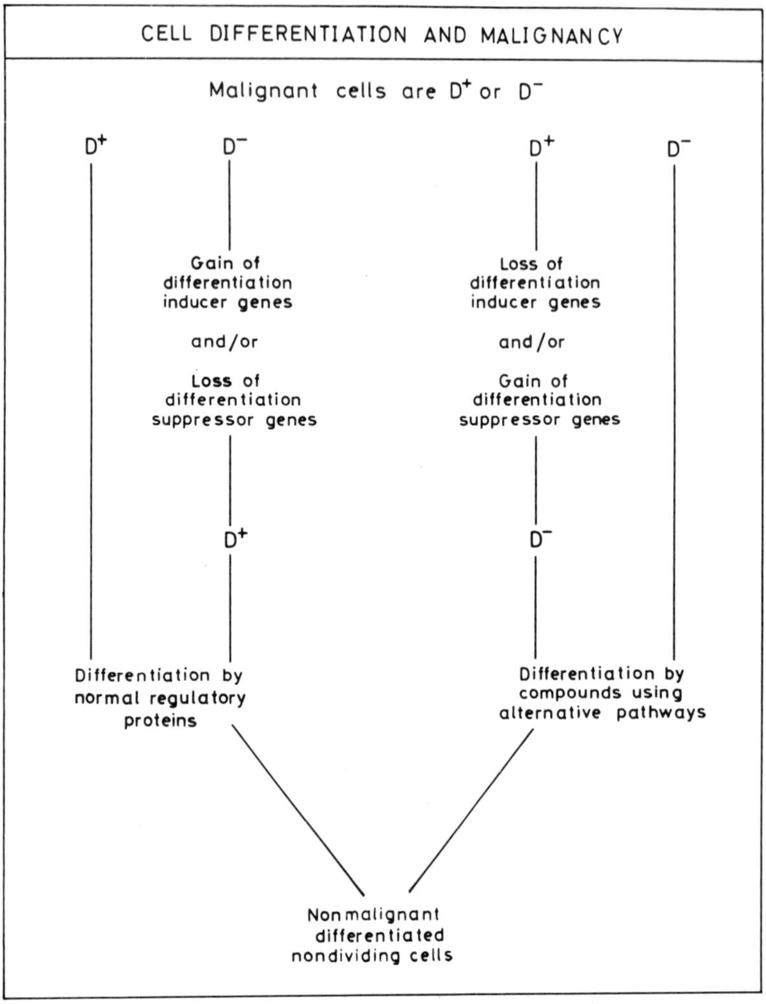

FIGURE 10 Suppression of malignancy by inducing differentiation can be achieved in different ways. Leukemic cells can (D^+) or cannot (D^-) be induced to differentiate to mature nondividing cells by normal regulatory proteins. The D^- cells can, however, be induced to differentiate by compounds that induce differentiation by alternative pathways. Chromosomal changes that change the balance between genes for induction and genes for suppression of differentiation can change cells from D^- to D^+ and vice versa (96).

concluded from studies of the molecular regulators of growth and differentiation in normal development, changes in the normal development program in leukemic cells, and suppression of leukemia that (A) malignancy can be suppressed by inducing differentiation either with or without genetic changes in the malignant cells (Fig. 10), (B) this suppression does not have to restore all the normal controls, and (C) genetic defects that give rise to malignancy can be bypassed and their effects nullified by inducing differentiation, which stops cells from multiplying (23–25,53,92,96).

VII. CLINICAL APPLICATIONS

Identification of the myeloid cell regulatory proteins has suggested novel possibilities for the therapy of nonmalignant and malignant hematologic disease (24,25,87). The concentration of these proteins can be increased in vivo either by injecting the protein (71–73,97) or by injecting one of the compounds that induces their production (98–101), reviewed in Ref. 41. Injection of protein stimulated myelopoiesis (71,72,97), reviewed in Ref. 41, under normal circumstances and after suppression of myelopoiesis induced by such compounds as cyclophosphamide, with minimal side effects. In nonmalignant hematologic abnormalities, myeloid regulatory proteins were shown to be clinically useful in more quickly restoring the normal number and function of the myeloid blood cell population in patients with suppressed myelopoiesis, such as that after treatment for transplantation and after cytotoxic cancer therapy (102,103). These treatments not only suppress myelopoiesis but also destroy cells that produce the regulatory proteins. Addition of these proteins in vitro to bone marrow cells before grafting and/or their injection in vivo (24,25,87,104,105), reviewed in Ref. 41, can also increase the success of bone marrow transplant grafts and increase survival in patients deficient in these proteins and the cells that produce them in the bone marrow. Because of the many functions of mature cells, such as granulocytes and other myeloid cells, the increased function of mature cells induced by these regulatory proteins can also be clinically helpful to patients with deficiencies in myeloid cell functions, such as acquired immunodeficiency syndrome (AIDS) patients (106). The finding that granulocyte development can be induced in culture in cells from patients with congenital agranulocytosis (8,107) has led to promising clinical results in children with this genetic disease (108). It has also been shown that injection of the protein erythropoietin, which stimulates the production of erythrocytes, can correct the anemia in patients with end-stage renal disease or progressive renal failure (109).

In the therapy of malignant disease, suppression of malignancy by inducing differentiation (87) is an alternative approach to the use of cytotoxic doses of compounds that, with the compounds used thus far, kill many normal cells as well as tumor cells. Results showing that the development of myeloid leukemia can be inhibited in mice with D^+ leukemic cells by injecting MGI-2/IL-6 or GM-CSF or injecting a compound that induces the production of these proteins in vivo (71,72) indicate a therapeutic potential for normal hematopoietic regulatory proteins in myeloid leukemia. There are leukemic cells from patients with myeloid leukemia that still require a myeloid growth-inducing protein for cell viability and multiplication, so that injection of one of these proteins may possibly stimulate the growth of these leukemic cells. However, the D^+ myeloid leukemic cells that no longer require normal growth inducer again require it for cell viability and growth after induction of differentiation (28,29,110,111). Despite the requirement of a myeloid growth inducer for growth, the further induction of differentiation can change the balance between multiplying cells and nonmultiplying differentiated cells sufficiently to inhibit the development of leukemia (71,72). Restoration of the requirement for a myeloid growth inducer for viability and growth in these D^+ myeloid leukemic cells also suggests that induction of differentiation to this stage may result in the loss of viability of the induced leukemic cells in vivo if there is not enough growth inducer present.

It can be concluded that with the availability of human recombinant myeloid regulatory proteins (31) the study of myeloid blood cell regulatory proteins has now progressed from the original cell culture assays (1–4) and discovery of these regulators in cell culture supernatants (5,7) to their application in the clinic.

VIII. SUMMARY

The establishment of a cell culture system for the clonal development of hematopoietic cells has made it possible to discover the proteins that control the growth and differentiation of different hematopoietic cell lineages and the molecular basis of normal and abnormal cell development in blood-forming tissues. A model system with myeloid cells has shown that normal hematopoietic cells require different proteins to induce cell multiplication and cell differentiation and that a cascade of interactions between proteins determines the correct balance between immature and mature cells in normal development. Gene cloning has shown that there is a family of different genes for these proteins. Normal protein regulators of hematopoiesis can control the abnormal growth of certain types of leukemic cells and suppress malignancy by inducing differentiation to mature nondividing cells. Genetic abnormalities that give rise to malignancy in these leukemic cells can be bypassed and their effects nullified by inducing differentiation, which stops cells from multiplying. These hematopoietic regulatory proteins are active in culture and in vivo and have been used clinically to correct defects in blood cell development. The results provide new approaches to therapy.

ACKNOWLEDGMENTS

This work was supported by the National Foundation for Cancer Research, Bethesda, the Ebner Foundation for Leukemia Research, and the Jerome A. and Estelle R. Newman Assistance Fund.

REFERENCES

1. Ginsburg H, Sachs L. Formation of pure suspension of mast cells in tissue culture by differentiation of lymphoid cells from the mouse thymus. *J Natl Cancer Inst* 1963; **31:**1–40.
2. Sachs L. The analysis of regulatory mechanisms in cell differentiation. In: Sela M, ed. New perspectives in biology. Amsterdam: Elsevier, 1964; 246–60.
3. Pluznik DH, and Sachs L. The cloning of normal "mast" cells in tissue culture. *J Cell Comp Physiol* 1965; **66:**319–24.
4. Bradley TR, Metcalf D. The growth of mouse bone marrow cells in vitro. *Aust J Exp Biol Med Sci* 1966; **44:**287–300.
5. Ichikawa Y, Pluznik DH, Sachs L. In vitro control of the development of macrophage and granulocyte colonies. *Proc Natl Acad Sci U S A* 1966; **56:**488–95.
6. Lagunoff D, Pluznik DH, Sachs L. The cloning of macrophages in agar: identification of the cells by electron microscopy. *J Cell Physiol* 1966; **68:**385–8.
7. Pluznik DH, Sachs L. The induction of clones of normal "mast" cells by a substance from conditioned medium. *Exp Cell Res* 1966; **43:**553–63.
8. Paran M, Sachs L, Barak Y, Resnitzky P. *In vitro* induction of granulocyte differentiation in hematopoietic cells from leukemic and non-leukemic patients. *Proc Natl Acad Sci U S A* 1970; **67:**1542–9.
9. Pike B, Robinson WA. Human bone marrow growth in agar gel. *J Cell Physiol* 1970; **76:**77–84.
10. Stephenson JR, Axelrad AA, McLeod DL, Shreeve MM. Induction of colonies of hemoglobin-synthesizing cells by erythropoietin *in vitro*. *Proc Natl Acad Sci U S A* 1971; **68:**1542–6.
11. Metcalf D, Nossal GJV, Warner NL, et al. Growth of B lymphocyte colonies *in vitro*. *J Exp Med* 1975; **142:**1534–49.
12. Gerassi E, Sachs L. Regulation of the induction of colonies in vitro by normal human lymphocytes. *Proc Natl Acad Sci U S A* 1976; **73:**4546–50.
13. Sachs L. In vitro control of growth and development of hematopoietic cell clones. In: Gordon AS, ed. Regulation of hematopoiesis, Vol. 1. New York: Appleton-Century-Crofts, 1970; 217–33.
14. Sachs L. Regulation of membrane changes, differentiation and malignancy in carcinogenesis. Harvey Lec New York: Academic Press, 1974; **68:**1–35.
15. Landau T, Sachs L. Characterization of the inducer required for the development of macrophage and granulocyte colonies. *Proc Natl Acad Sci U S A* 1971; **68:**2540–4.

16. Burgess AW, Camakaris J, Metcalf D. Purification and properties of colony-stimulating factor from mouse lung conditioned medium. *J Biol Chem* 1977; **252:**1998–2003.
17. Stanley ER, Heard PM. Factors regulating macrophage production and growth. Purification and some properties of the colony stimulating factor from medium conditioned by mouse cells. *J Biol Chem* 1977; **252:**4305–12.
18. Lipton J, Sachs L. Characterization of macrophage and granulocyte inducing proteins for normal and leukemic myeloid cells produced by the Krebs ascites tumor. *Biochim Biophys Acta* 1981; **673:**552–69.
19. Ihle JN, Keller J, Henderson L, Klein F, Palaszinski E. Procedures for the purification of interleukin-3 to homogeneity. *J Immunol* 1982; **129:**2431–6.
20. Mier JW, Gallo RC. Purification and some characteristics of human T-cell growth factor from phytohemagglutinin-stimulated lymphocyte-conditioned media. *Proc Natl Acad Sci U S A* 1980; **77:**6134–8.
21. Kishimoto T, Hirano T. Molecular regulation of B lymphocyte response. *Ann Rev Immunol* 1988; **6:**485–512.
22. Paran M, Sachs L. The continued requirement for inducer for development of macrophage and granulocyte colonies. *J Cell Physiol* 1968; **72:**247–50.
23. Sachs L. Growth, differentiation and the reversal of malignancy. *Sci Am* 1986; **254**(1): 40–7.
24. Sachs L. The molecular regulators of normal and leukaemic blood cells. The Wellcome Foundation Lecture 1986. *Proc R Soc Lond [Biol]* 1987; **231:**289–312.
25. Sachs L. The molecular control of blood cell development. *Science* 1987; **238:**1374–9.
26. Ichikawa Y, Pluznik DH, Sachs L. Feedback inhibition of the development of macrophage and granulocyte colonies. I Inhibition by macrophages. *Proc Natl Acad Sci U S A* 1967; **58:**1480–6.
27. Metcalf D. The granulocyte-macrophage colony-stimulating factors. *Science* 1985; **199:**16–22.
28. Lotem J, Sachs L. Mechanisms that uncouple growth and differentiation on myeloid leukemia cells. Restoration of requirement for normal growth-inducing protein without restoring induction of differentiation-inducing protein. *Proc Natl Acad Sci U S A* 1982; **79:**4347–51.
29. Lotem J, Sachs L. Coupling of growth and differentiation in normal myeloid precursors and the breakdown of this coupling in leukemia. *Int J Cancer* 1983; **32:**127–34.
30. Tushinski RJ, Oliver IT, Guilbert LJ, Tynan PW, Warner JR, Stanley ER. Survival of mononuclear phagocytes depends on a lineage-specific growth factor that the differentiated cells selectively destroy. *Cell* 1982; **208:**71–81.
31. Clark SC, Kamen R. The human hematopoietic colony-stimulating factors. *Science* 1987; **236:**1129–37.
32. Azoulay M, Webb CG, Sachs L. Control of hematopoietic cell growth regulators in mouse fetal development. *Mol Cell Biol* 1987; **7:**3361–4.
33. Fibach E, Sachs L. Control of normal differentiation of myeloid leukemic cells. XI. Induction of a specific requirement for cell viability and growth during the differentiation of myeloid leukemic cells. *J Cell Physiol* 1976; **89:**259–66.

34. Lotem J, Lipton JH, Sachs L. Separation of different molecular forms of macrophage and granulocyte inducing proteins for normal and leukemic myeloid cells. *Int J Cancer* 1980; **25:**763–71.
35. Sachs L. Constitutive uncoupling of pathways of gene expression that control growth and differentiation in myeloid leukemia: a model for the origin and progression of malignancy. *Proc Natl Acad Sci U S A* 1980; **77:**6153–6.
36. Sachs L. Normal development programmes in myeloid leukaemia: regulatory proteins in the control of growth and differentiation. *Cancer Surv* 1982; **1:**321–42.
37. Tomida M, Yamamoto-Kamaguchi Y, Hozumi M. Purification of a factor inducing differentiation of mouse myeloid leukemic M1 cells from conditioned medium from mouse fibroblast L929 cells. *J Biol Chem* 1984; **259:**10978–82.
38. Olsson I, Sarngadharan MG, Breitman TR, Gallo RC. Isolation and characterization of a T lymphocyte-derived differentiation inducing factor for the myeloid leukemic cell line HL-60. *Blood* 1984; **63:**510–7.
39. Shabo Y, Sachs L. Inhibition of differentiation and affinity purification with a monoclonal antibody to a myeloid cell differentiation-inducing protein. *Blood* 1988; **72:**1543–9.
40. Shabo Y, Lotem J, Rubinstein M, et al. The myeloid blood cell differentiation-inducing protein MGI-2A is interleukin 6. *Blood* 1988; **72:**2070–3.
41. Sachs L, Lotem J, Shabo Y. The molecular regulators of macrophage and granulocyte development: role of MGI-2/IL-6ln. Regulation of the acute phase and immune responses: interleukin 6. *Ann N Y Acad Sci* 1989; **557:**417–37.
42. Lowe DG, Nunes W, Bombara M, et al. Genomic cloning and heterologous expression of human differentiation-stimulating factor. *DNA* 1989; **8:**351–9.
43. Gearing DP, Gough NM, King JA, et al. Molecular cloning and expression of cDNA encoding a murine myeloid leukaemia inhibitory factor. *EMBO J* 1987; **6:**3995–4002.
44. Moreau JF, Donaldson DD, Bennett F, Witek-Giannoti J, Clark SC, Wong GG. Leukaemia inhibitory factor is identical to the myeloid growth factor human interleukin for DA cells. *Nature* 1988; **336:**690–2.
45. Gullberg, V, Lantz M, Nilsson E, Peetre C, Adolf G, Olsson I. Characterization of a relationship between the T-lymphocyte derived differentiation inducing factor (DIF) and lymphotoxin: a common receptor system for DIF, lymphotoxin and tumor necrosis factor downregulated by phorbol diesters. *Eur J Haematol* 1987; **39:**241–51.
46. Lotem J, Sachs L. Indirect induction of differentiation in normal and leukemic myeloid cells by recombinant interleukin 1. *Leuk Res* 1989; **13:**13–21.
47. Liebermann D, Hoffman-Liebermann B, Sachs L. Regulation and role of different macrophage and granulocyte inducing proteins in normal and leukemic myeloid cells. *Int J Cancer* 1982; **29:**159–61.
48. Shabo Y, Lotem J, Sachs L. Target cell specificity of hematopoietic regulatory proteins for different clones of myeloid leukemic cells: two regulators secreted by Krebs cells. *Int J Cancer* 1988; **41:**622–8.
49. Lotem J, Sachs L. Control of normal differentiation of myeloid leukemic cells. XII. Isolation of normal myeloid colony-forming cells from bone marrow and the

sequence of differentiation to mature granulocytes in normal and D^+ myeloid leukemic cells. *J Cell Physiol* 1977; **92:**97–108.

50. Lotem J, Shabo Y, Sachs L. Role of different normal hematopoietic regulatory proteins in the differentiation of myeloid leukemic cells. *Int J Cancer* 1988; **41:**101–7.
51. Lotem J, Shabo Y, Sachs L. Regulation of megakaryocite development by interleukin 6. *Blood* 1989; **74:**1545–51.
52. Lotem J, Sachs L. Regulation of cell surface receptors for different hematopoietic growth factors on myeloid leukemic cells. *EMBO J* 1986; **5:**2163–70.
53. Sachs L. The proteins that control haemopoiesis and leukaemia. In. Molecular control of haemopoiesis. *Ciba Found Symp,* 1990; **148:**5–19.
54. Pettenati MJ, Le Beau MM, Lemons RS, et al. Assignment of CSF-1 to 5q33.1: evidence for clustering of genes regulating hematopoiesis and for their involvement in the deletion of the long arm of chromosome 5 in myeloid disorders. *Proc Natl Acad Sci U S A* 1987; **84:**2970–4.
55. Yang Y-C, Kovacic S, Kriz R, et al. The human genes for GM-CSF and IL 3 are closely linked in tandem on chromosome 5. *Blood* 1988; **71:**958–61.
56. Ferguson-Smith AC, Chen Y-F, Newman MS, May LT, Sehgal PB, Ruddle FH. Regional localization of the interferon-β_2/B-cell stimulatory factor 2/hepatocyte stimulating factor gene to human chromosome 7p15-p21. *Genomics* 1988; **2:**203–8.
57. Peters J. Mouse gene list. *Mouse News Lett* 1989; **83:**19–64.
58. Mock BA, Nordan RP, Justice MJ. et al. The murine IL-6 gene maps to the proximal region of chromosome 5. *J Immunol* 1989; **142:**1372–6.
59. Sutherland GR, Baker E, Hyland VJ, Callen DF, Stahl J, Gough, NM. The gene for human leukemia inhibitory factor (LIF) maps to 22q12. *Leukemia* 1989; **3:**9–13.
60. Gisselbrecht S, Sola B, Fichelson S, et al. The murine M-CSF gene is localized on chromosome 3. *Blood* 1989; **73:**1742–6.
61. Shabo Y, Lotem J, Sachs L. Regulation of the genes for interleukin 6 and granulocyte-macrophage colony stimulating factor by different inducers of differentiation in myeloid leukemic cells. *Leukemia* 1989; **3:**859–65.
62. Lotem J, Sachs L. In vivo control of differentiation of myeloid leukemic cells by cyclosporin A and recombinant interleukin 1α. *Blood* 1988; **72:**1595–1601.
63. Shabo Y, Lotem J, Sachs L. Autoregulation of interleukin 6 and granulocyte-macrophage colony stimulating factor in the differentiation of myeloid leukemic cells. *Mol Cell Biol,* 1989; **9:**4109–4112.
64. Warner SJC, Auger KR, Libby P. Human interleukin 1 induces interleukin 1 gene expression in human vascular smooth muscle cells. *J Exp Med* 1987; **165:**1316–1331.
65. Niitsu Y, Watanabe N, Neda H, Yamauchi N, Maeda M, Sone H, Kuriyama H. Induction of synthesis of tumor necrosis factor in human and murine cell lines by exogenous recombinant human tumor necrosis factor. *Cancer Res.* 1988; **48:**5407–5410.
66. Griffin JD, Lowenberg B. Clonogenic cells in acute myeloblastic leukemia. *Blood* 1986; **68:**1185–119.
67. Liebermann JD, Hoffman-Liebermann B, Sachs L. Molecular dissection of differentiation in normal and leukemic myeloblasts. Separately programmed pathways of gene expression. *Dev Biol* 1980; **79:**46–63.

68. Fibach E, Landau T, Sachs L. Normal differentiation of myeloid leukemic cells induced by a differentiation-inducing protein. *Nature* 1972; **237:**276–278.
69. Fibach E, Hayashi M, Sachs L. Control of normal differentiation of myeloid leukemic cells to macrophages and granulocytes. *Proc Natl Acad Sci USA* 1973; **70:**343–346.
70. Fibach E, Sachs L. Control of normal differentiation of myeloid leukemic cells. VIII. Induction of differentiation to mature granulocytes in mass culture. *J Cell Physiol* 1975; **86:**221–30.
71. Lotem J, Sachs L. In vivo inhibition of the development of myeloid leukemia by injection of macrophage and granulocyte inducing protein. *Int J Cancer* 1981; **28:**375–86.
72. Lotem J, Sachs L. Control of in vivo differentiation of myeloid leukemic cells. IV. Inhibition of leukemia development by myeloid differentiation-inducing protein. *Int J Cancer* 1984; **33:**147–54.
73. Lotem J, Sachs L. In vivo induction of normal differentiation in myeloid leukemic cells. *Proc Natl Acad Sci U S A* 1978; **75:**3781–5.
74. Lotem J, Sachs L. In vivo control of differentiation of myeloid leukemic cells by recombinant granulocyte-macrophage colony stimulating factor and interleukin 3. *Blood,* 1988; **71:**375–82.
75. Bohmer RM, Burgess AW. Granulocytic colony stimulating factor (G-CSF) does not induce differentiation of WEHI 3B (D^+) cells but is required for the survival of the mature progeny. *Int J Cancer* 1988; **42:**53–8.
76. Lotem J, Shabo Y, Sachs L. Clonal variation in susceptibility to differentiation by different protein inducers in the myeloid leukemia cell line M1. *Leukemia* 1989; **3:**804–7.
77. Lotem J, Sachs L. Control of in vivo differentiation of myeloid leukemic cells. III. Regulation by T lymphocytes and inflammation. *Int J Cancer* 1983; **32:**781–91.
78. Fearon ER, Burke PJ, Schiffer CA, Zehnbauer BA, Vogelstein B. Differentiation of leukemia cells to polymorphonuclear leukocytes in patients with acute nonlymphocytic leukemia. *N Engl J Med* 1986; **315:**15–24.
79. Gootwine E, Webb CG, Sachs L. Participation of myeloid leukaemic cells injected into embryos in haematopoetic differentiation in adult mice. *Nature* 1982; **299:**63–5.
80. Webb CG, Gootwine E, Sachs L. Developmental potential of myeloid leukaemic cells injected into mid-gestation embryos. *Dev Biol* 1984; **101:**221–4.
81. Lotem J, Ben-Nun A, Sachs L. Regulation of in vivo differentiation of myeloid leukemic cells by antigen-specific helper T lymphocytes. *Leuk Res* 1986; **10:**1165–8.
82. Blatt C, Goldberg R, Aberdam D, Sachs L. Homeobox gene rearrangement in myeloid leukemic cells. *Third Annual Meeting on Oncogenes,* Fredrick, MD 1987; 364.
83. Blatt C, Aberdam D, Schwartz R, Sachs L. DNA rearrangement of a homeobox gene in myeloid leukemic cells. *EMBO J* 1988; **7:**4283–90.
84. Azumi J, Sachs L. Chromosome mapping of the genes that control differentiation and malignancy in myeloid leukemic cells. *Proc Natl Acad Sci U S A* 1977; **74:**253–7.

85. Blatt C, Sachs L. Deletion of a homeobox gene in myeloid leukemias with a deletion in chromosome 2. *Biochem Biophys Res Commun* 1988; **156:** 1265–70.
86. Lotem J, Sachs L. Different blocks in the differentiation of myeloid leukemic cells. *Proc Natl Acad Sci U S A* 1974; **71:**3507–11.
87. Sachs L. Control of normal cell differentiation and the phenotypic reversion of malignancy in myeloid leukaemia. *Nature* 1978; **274:**535–9.
88. Symonds G, Sachs L. Activation of normal genes in malignant cells: activation of chemotaxis in relation to other stages of normal differentiation in myeloid leukemia. *Somat Cell Genet* 1979; **5:**931–44.
89. Lotem J, Sachs L. Induction of specific changes in the surface membrane of myeloid leukemic cells by steroid hormones. *Int J Cancer* 1975; **15:**731–40.
90. Symonds G, Sachs L. Modulation of cell competence for induction of differentiation in leukemic cells. *J Cell Physiol* 1982; **111:**9–14.
91. Symonds G, Sachs L. Cell competence for induction of differentiation by insulin and other compounds in myeloid leukemic clones continuously cultured in serum-free medium. *Blood* 1982; **60:**208–12.
92. Sachs L. Cell differentiation and tumour suppression. In. Genetic analysis of tumour suppression. *Ciba Found Symp* 1989; **142:**217–31.
93. Cohen L, Sachs L. Constitutive gene expression in myeloid leukemia and cell competence for induction of differentiation by dexamethasone. *Proc Natl Acad Sci U S A* 1985; **78:**353–7.
94. Hayashi M, Fibach E, Sachs L. Control of normal differentiation of myeloid leukemic cells V. Normal differentiation in aneuploid leukemic cells and the chromosome banding pattern of D^+ and D^- clones. *Int J Cancer* 1974; **14:**40–8.
95. Rowley JD. Chromosome abnormalities in leukemia. Karnofsky Memorial Lecture. *J Clin Oncol* 1988; **6:**194–202.
96. Sachs L. Cell differentiation and by-passing of genetic defects in the suppression of malignancy. *Cancer Res* 1987; **47:**1981–6.
97. Kindler V, Thorens B, De Kossodo S, et al. Stimulation of hematopoieis *in vivo* by recombinant bacterial murine interleukin 3. *Proc Natl Acad Sci U S A* 1986; **83:**1001–5.
98. Fibach E, Sachs L. Control of normal differentiation of myeloid leukemic cells. IV. Induction of differentiation by serum from endotoxin treated mice. *J Cell Physiol* 1974; **83:**177–85.
99. Weiss B, Sachs L. Indirect induction of differentiation in myeloid leukemic cells by lipid A. *Proc Natl Acad Sci U S A* 1978; **75:**1374–8.
100. Falk A, Sachs L. Clonal regulation of the induction of macrophage and granulocyte inducing proteins for normal and leukemic myeloid cells. *Int J Cancer* 1980; **26:**595–601.
101. Lotem J, Sachs L. Independent regulation of myeloid cell growth and differentiation-inducing proteins. *In vivo* regulation by compounds that induce inflammation. *Int J Cancer* 1985; **35:**93–100.
102. Antman KS, Griffin JD, Elias A, et al. Effect of recombinant human granulocyte-macrophage colony-stimulating factor on chemotherapy-induced myelosuppression. *N Engl J Med* 1988; **319:**593–8.

103. Brandt SJ, Peters WP, Atwater SK, et al. Effect of recombinant human granulocyte-macrophage colony-stimulating factor on hematopoietic reconstitution after high-dose chemotherapy and autologous bone marrow transplantation. *N Engl J Med* 1988; **318:**869–76.
104. Monroy RL, Skelly RR, MacVittie TJ, et al. The effect of recombinant GM-CSF on the recovery of monkeys transplanted with autologous bone marrow. *Blood* 1987; **70:**1696–9.
105. Blazar BR, Widmer MB, Soderling CCB, et al. Augmentation of donor bone marrow engraftment in histoincompatible murine recipients by granulocyte/macrophage colony-stimulating factor. *Blood* 1988; **71:**320–8.
106. Groopman JE, Mitsuyasu RT, DeLeo MJ, Oette DH, Golde DW. Effect of recombinant human granulocyte-macrophage colony-stimulating factor on myelopoiesis in the acquired immunodeficiency syndrome. *N Engl J Med* 1987; **317:**593–8.
107. Barak Y, Paran M, Levin S, Sachs L. *In vitro* induction of myeloid proliferation and maturation in infantile genetic agranulocytosis. *Blood* 1971; **38:**74–80.
108. Bonilla MA, Gillio AP, Ruggeiro M, et al. Effects of recombinant human granulocyte colony-stimulating factor on neutropenia in patients with congenital agranulocytosis. *N Engl J Med* 1989; **320:**1574–80.
109. Eschbach JW, Egrie JC, Downing MR, Browne JK, Adamson JW. Correction of the anemia of end-stage renal disease with recombinant human erythropoietin. *N Engl J Med* 1987; **316:**73–8.
110. Lotem J, Sachs L. Induction of dependence on hematopoietic proteins for viability and receptor upregulation in differentiating myeloid leukemic cells. *Blood* 1989; **74:**579–85.
111. Lotem J, Cragoe EJ, Sachs L. Rescue from programmed cell death in leukemic and normal myeloid cells. *Blood* 1991; **78:**953–60.

11

Granulocyte-Macrophage Colony-Stimulating Factor in Myelodysplastic Syndromes and Aplastic Anemia

Razelle Kurzrock, Elihu H. Estey, Moshe Talpaz, and Jordan U. Gutterman

University of Texas, M. D. Anderson Cancer Center, Houston, Texas

I. INTRODUCTION

Hematopoietic growth factors are generally produced at multiple sites in the body by a few different cell types. They interact in protean ways with specific blood target cells at various levels in the cascade of cell differentiation. First, colony-stimulating factors (CSFs) are necessary to enhance cell survival; the in vitro life span of blood neutrophils, eosinophils, and monocytes is extended by the appropriate growth factor, such as granulocyte-macrophage CSF (GM-CSF). Second, the continuous presence of CSF is required for the proliferation of hematopoietic precursor cells and their progeny. Finally, CSFs can induce differentiation and functional activation of mature hematopoietic cells. GM-CSF, for instance, increases the capacity of neutrophils to phagocytose and kill organisms and to participate in antibody-dependent cell killing (reviewed in Ref. 1).

The biologic effects of the CSFs, as measured by the stimulation of cell growth in vitro, have been the basis for isolation of the genes that encode them. GM-CSF is located on the long arm of chromosome 5 (Table 1). It is produced predominantly by T lymphocytes but also by monocytes, fibroblasts, and endothelial cells (1–3). Its progenitor cell targets include CFU-blasts, CFU-GEMM, CFU-GM, CFU-G, CFU-M, CFU-EO, CFU-MEG, and BFU-E (3).

Different target cells may be stimulated at varying concentrations of CSF (1,2). GM-CSF stimulates macrophages and granulocytes at very low concentrations

TABLE 1 Characteristics of GM-CSF

Molecular mass	Chromosomal location of gene[a]	Cellular source	Progenitor cell target[b]	Mature cell target
14–35	5q23–31	T lymphocytes, monocytes, fibroblasts, endothelial cells	CFU blast, CFU-GEMM, CFU-GM, CFU-G, CFU-M, CFU-Eo, CFU-MEG, BFU-E	Granulocytes, eosinophils, monocytes

[a]The chromosomal localization is designated by arm (q denotes long arm) and band number.
[b]CFU-blast, colony-forming unit blast; CFU-GEMM, colony-forming unit granulocyte, erythrocyte, monocyte, megakaryocyte; CFU-GM, colony-forming unit granulocyte and macrophage; CFU-Eo, colony-forming unit eosinophil; CFU-MEG, colony-forming unit megakaryocyte; BFU-E, burst-forming unit erythroid, CFU-G, colony-forming unit granulocyte; CFU-M, colony-forming unit macrophage.

of 5–20 pg/ml; at higher concentrations of 20–2000 pg/ml, eosinophils, megakaryocytes, and multipotential cells are stimulated in vitro (2). The effects of GM-CSF are mediated through specific binding to high-affinity receptors on the surface of the target cells.

The availability of recombinant hematopoietic growth factors for clinical studies has stimulated enthusiasm for trials of these physiologic regulators of blood cell production in bone marrow failure states. Recombinant hematopoietins are generally derived from one of several sources, that is, yeast, bacteria, or mammalian cells. Yeast-derived GM-CSF is glycosolated, whereas *Escherichia coli*-derived GM-CSF is not. Preliminary studies suggest that the glycosolated and nonglycosolated materials have comparable activity and toxicity profiles. In general, trials of GM-CSF have several potential objectives: a decrease in the morbidity and mortality associated with prolonged neutropenia and, perhaps, in vivo induction of cellular differentiation. To date, GM-CSF therapy has been applied to several clinical conditions, including neutropenia complicating the acquired immunodeficiency syndrome, cancer chemotherapy, bone marrow transplantation, and primary bone marrow failure states. We review the current status of GM-CSF treatment in myelodysplastic syndromes and aplastic anemia.

II. MYELODYSPLASTIC SYNDROMES

A. Background

Myelodysplastic syndromes are a heterogeneous group of hematopoietic stem cell disorders characterized by ineffective and dysplastic hematopoiesis (4–6). Most patients are over the age of 60 years and characteristically have moderate to severe pancytopenia with a normocellular or hypercellular bone marrow. Although the natural history of these syndromes is variable, several factors appear to be of prognostic importance, including the French-American-British (FAB) classification and karyotype.

Numerous terms have been applied to the myelodysplastic syndromes and include pre-leukemia, oligoblastic leukemia, dysmyelopoietic syndromes, smoldering leukemia, primary acquired panmyelopathy with myeloblastosis, subacute myeloid leukemia, and hematopoietic dysplasia. In 1982, the FAB cooperative group addressed the problem of the diverse terminology and proposed a morphologic classification system encompassing this spectrum of diseases (Table 2). The myelodysplastic syndromes now include five well-defined pathologic entities: refractory anemia (RA), refractory anemia with ringed sideroblasts (RARS), refractory anemia with excess blasts (RAEB), refractory anemia with excess blasts and transformation (RAEBT), and chronic myelomonocytic leukemia (CMML). This classification scheme has become widely accepted because of its reproducibility and clinical relevance.

Leukemic transformation in patients with myelodysplastic syndromes is not uncommon and varies from 10–20% for RA to 60–75% for RAEBT. The distinction between myelodysplastic syndrome and acute myelogenous leukemia is not always clear. Even without leukemic transformation, myelodysplastic syndromes are generally fatal disorders because of progressive pancytopenia leading to death from infection or hemorrhage.

Chromosomal aberrations have been detected in up to 50% of patients with de novo myelodysplasia. Some of the more common chromosomal abnormalities include monosomy of chromosome 5 or loss of the long (q) arm of

TABLE 2 Characteristics of the Myelodysplastic Syndromes[a]

Myelodysplastic syndromes	Blast cells (%)		Progression to leukemia (% of patients)	Median survival (months)
	Peripheral blood	Bone marrow		
RA	<1	<5	15	65
RARS	<1	<5	10	70
RAEB	<5	5–20	40	10
RAEBT	≥5	20–30	60	5
CMML	<5	<20	30	10
	>1.0 × 10^9 monocytes/L in peripheral blood			

[a]CMML = chronic myelomonocytic leukemia; RA = refractory anemia; RAEB = refractory anemia with excess blasts; RAEBT = refractory anemia with excess blasts in transformation; RARS = refractory anemia with ringed sideroblasts.

chromosome 5 ($5q^-$; 10–20% of patients), monosomy of chromosome 7, or $7q^-$ (15–20% of patients), trisomy 8 (15–20% of patients), and $20q^-$ (7–10% of patients). Those patients who developed myelodysplastic syndromes because of previous exposure to radiation, chemotherapy, or some other mutagen have a higher incidence of cytogenetic abnormalities. Chromosomal abnormalities in patients with myelodysplasias are associated with an increased risk of hematologic progression to leukemia and a short survival independent of FAB type (7). Abnormalities of the long arm of chromosome 5 are of special interest because a cluster of hematopoietic growth factor-related genes reside in this area of the genome and include GM-CSF, interleukin-3, (IL-3), IL-4, IL-5, platelet-derived growth factor (PDGF) receptor, M-CSF, and the M-CSF receptor (c-*fms* oncogene).

Therapeutic agents that have been used in the myelodysplastic syndromes include cytotoxic therapy, bone marrow transplantation, differentiation agents, and, most recently, the growth factors. Treatment with conventional cytarabine and anthracycline combinations have yielded remission rates of about 25%. There is generally a high morbidity and mortality, however, perhaps because of the advanced age of many of the patients. Among younger patients with a compatible marrow donor, bone marrow transplantation is a potentially curative mode of therapy in about 40–60% of cases. Unfortunately, myelodysplastic syndromes predominantly affect patients over the age of 60, and allogeneic bone marrow transplantation is therefore not usually applicable. Low doses of cytarabine have also been used and yield an overall remission rate of about 20%, with a median duration of approximately 8 months. An increase in survival has not been demonstrated, however. A variety of other agents, including thioguanine, interferons, and retinoids, have activity in vitro as inducers of leukemic cell differentiation but have demonstrated limited success in uncontrolled trials in myelodysplasia (reviewed in Ref. 7). In regard to retinoic acid analogs, some trials have demonstrated significant hematologic responses and an improvement in survival, whereas others have not been able to confirm these results (8–15). Overall, the results of conventional therapies are poor and leave much room for improvement.

B. GM-CSF Therapy of Myelodysplastic Syndromes

The first study of GM-CSF demonstrated that doses between 30 and 500 $\mu g/m^2$ by continuous infusion were able to raise the neutrophil count in all of eight patients with myelodysplastic syndrome (16). Improvement in neutrophil counts were often noted within 24–48 h after starting GM-CSF; changes in blood counts were dependent on continued GM-CSF therapy, and counts returned to baseline within 48–72 h after discontinuing therapy. Follow-up studies (Table 3) have shown that both subcutaneous injection of GM-CSF and shorter IV

TABLE 3 GM-CSF Therapy in Myelodysplastic Syndromes[a]

No. of patients	Dose and schedule[b]	Response (% of patients)			Increased bone marrow blasts (% of patients)	Reference
		Neutrophil	Hb	Plt		
8	30–500 μg/m²/day (CI) × 14 days, then 14 days rest	100	38	38	0	Vadhan-Raj et al. (16)
7	15–480 μg/m²/day (IV 1–12 h) × 7–14 days, every 4 weeks	85	0	0	0	Antin et al. (17)
11	15–150 μg/m²/day (IV, 8 h) × 7–14 days, every 4 weeks	90	0	0	36	Ganser et al. (18)
16	0.3–10 μg/kg/day SC (equivalent to about 10–350 μg/m²/day)	75	0	19	6	Thompson et al. (19)
11	30–480 μg/m²/day SC	90	0	9	18	Rifkin et al. (20)
4	5–750 μg/m²/day (IV 30 minutes) × 5 days, then 5 days rest	100	0	0	100	Herrmann et al. (21)
22	120 μg/m²/day (CI)	100	0	9	18	Estey et al. (22)
29	5–10 μg/m²/day SC	48	0	4	17	Estey et al. (23)

[a]CI = continuous infusion; Hb = hemoglobin; IV = intravenous; plt = platelets; SC = subcutaneous
[b]The 2.5 μg/kg is approximately equivalent to 100 μg/m².

infusions (2–4 h) can also raise neutrophil counts. The doses used most commonly are 100–200 μg/m^2 day (2.5–5.0 μg/kg/day). Overall, about 80–90% of patients show an increase in neutrophil counts. Interestingly, about 10% of cases show an increase in other lineages. Therefore, some patients achieve platelet recovery or an increase in reticulocytes and hemoglobin. Unfortunately, a decrease in platelet counts has also been noted and probably occurs in about 20% of patients. This can at times be associated with clinical bleeding. As with the increase in neutrophil counts, GM-CSF-induced platelet rises or thrombocytopenia are reversible within several days after stopping treatment.

Because published studies of GM-CSF have not been randomized, it is unclear whether the increase in neutrophil counts translates to a decrease in rates of infection. Further, neutrophils from many patients with myelodysplastic syndromes function abnormally (24,25) and the functional capacity of neutrophils induced by growth factors in patients with myelodysplastic syndromes is not yet well defined. Peters and coworkers (26) studied neutrophil function in patients with breast cancer or melanoma who received high-dose chemotherapy and autologous bone marrow transplantation followed by GM-CSF injections. Phagocytosis, neutrophil oxidative metabolism, and margination were unaffected by the growth factor, but the ability of neutrophils to migrate to inflammatory skin windows was significantly impaired. Our clinical impression is that the incidence of infection in GM-CSF-treated patients is decreased below that expected in neutropenic patients but not to the level that would be seen in normal individuals. Therefore, sepsis can still occasionally occur in patients who have physiologic levels of neutrophils on GM-CSF therapy. The incidence of infection may be higher in patients on continuous IV infusion because of the presence of a catheter with an attendant risk of bacterial entry into the bloodstream. We therefore treat febrile (temperature ≥ 101°F or 38.3°C) myelodysplastic syndrome patients with intravenous antibiotics if their neutrophils are GM-CSF supported.

Because hematopoietic growth factors can stimulate the proliferation of leukemic blasts in vitro, the question of stimulation of leukemic growth in patients has arisen. Overall, at least 10–20% of patients treated with GM-CSF show an increase in blasts after treatment (reviewed in Ref. 24). Whether these blasts are leukemic or normal is not known at present. However, about half the patients with an increase in bone marrow blasts show a return to baseline levels within 1–2 weeks after GM-CSF is discontinued (Kurzrock, unpublished data). In the other patients, the elevation of blasts is not reversible. It appears that progression to acute leukemia is more frequent in patients who start therapy with ≥15% bone marrow blasts. An increment in peripheral blood blasts is not always accompanied by an increase in bone marrow blasts, and therefore patients should have a bone marrow biopsy performed on a regular basis when on GM-CSF therapy. Whether the rate of leukemic evolution is greater than that expected considering the natural history of the disease can only be addressed by a randomized trial. Preliminary observations of such a multicenter trial in which patients were randomly assigned to observation or GM-CSF therapy for 3 months (after which a crossover was permitted) suggests that GM-CSF does not increase the rate of development of acute leukemia in patients with myelodysplastic syndromes (Bonnem, personal communication). Even so, our experience suggests that patients with chronic myelomonocytic leukemia can progress on GM-CSF therapy, and we therefore avoid treatment of patients suffering from this disorder with GM-CSF.

Investigations at our institute also indicate that maturation of both the leukemic and normal blasts can occur during GM-CSF therapy. Indeed, when patients with mixed diploid and abnormal bone marrow metaphases were studied before and after therapy using peripheral chromosomal condensation analysis of neutrophil chromosomes, it was evident that the ratio of normal to abnormal karyotypes in the mature neutrophils after GM-CSF therapy was similar to that in the bone marrow before GM-CSF therapy (27).

Finally, we recently investigated the therapeutic potential of very low doses of GM-CSF. We treated 29 patients with myelodysplastic syndromes with 5–10 $\mu g/m^2/day$ (0.125–0.25 $\mu g/kg/day$) of subcutaneous GM-CSF (23). Increases in neutrophil counts to levels of over $1.0 \times 10^9 L^{-1}$ were observed in about half of these severely neutropenic patients. Furthermore, although other patients required higher doses of GM-CSF, most were able to achieve physiologic neutrophil counts with doses still well below the conventional 120 $\mu g/m^2/day$. Very low doses of GM-CSF were virtually devoid of constitutional side effects. Therefore, our current approach to the management of these neutropenic patients consists of initiating therapy with very low doses of GM-CSF (10 $\mu g/m^2/day$) and then titrating the dose upward every 5–7 days until neutrophil counts $\geq 1.0 \times 10^9 L^{-1}$ are reached. In patients with persistent thrombocytopenia or excess blasts, low doses of cytarabine are added, because there are data suggesting that the hematopoietins may sensitize malignant cells to the cytotoxic effects of this drug (28–31).

III. APLASTIC ANEMIA

A. Background

Aplastic anemia was first described in 1888 by Ehrlich, who reported a postmortem study of a young, pregnant woman who died of pronounced anemia and neutropenia (32). In 1904, Chauffard coined the term "aplastic anemia" for this condition (33). Aplastic anemia is now considered a group of disorders characterized by peripheral blood pancytopenia, variable bone marrow hypocellularity, and the absence of an underlying malignant or myeloproliferative disease (34).

Underpopulation of the marrow cavity with progeny of all hematopoietic cell lines—granulocytes, erythroblasts, monocytes, and megakaryocytes—is the cardinal feature. The reduced total volume of hematopoietic cells leads to pancytopenia, but the reduction in numbers of various blood cell types may be quite uneven. The disease is likely to be fatal as a result of infection or bleeding. Some patients recover spontaneously, however (35). The annual new case incidence of aplastic anemia ranges from 5 to 10 per million in populations in the Western nations. In the United States, there is an annual incidence of approximately 1200–2400 cases. In Korea and Japan, aplastic anemia is four to five times more frequent than in the West.

The vast majority of aplastic anemias are acquired, and from 40 to 70% of these are idiopathic. Secondary aplastic anemia can be associated with exposure to certain chemicals, radiation, and viruses. In general, a causative agent is often found in patients under the age of 30 but not in older individuals. The best documented chemical cause of marrow suppression in benzene. It is a commercial reagent employed in the manufacture of drugs, dyes, rubber goods, linoleum, waterproof fabrics, enamels, lacquers, and varnishes and is a solvent for degreasing waxes, resins, and tars. Idiopathic aplastic anemia is unrelenting and progressive in 80–90% of cases; in patients with aplastic anemia due to benzene exposure, however, up to 85% of patients have a partial or complete recovery within 2–10 years. Arsenic exposure can also lead to chronic hematologic poisoning with pancytopenia and fatal aplasia. In addition, 400 chemicals and drugs have been suspected of causing aplastic anemia unpredictably or occasionally. About 90% of these secondary aplastic anemias are in the idiosyncratic category. Only several drugs or drug families cause aplastic anemia sufficiently often to want routine consideration. These drugs include chloramphenicol, quinacrine, hydrochloride, phenylbutazone, anticonvulsants, and carbonic anhydrase inhibitors. Radiation is another important source of aplasia, and there is a 50% mortality after exposure to 500 rem. Finally, certain types of infection may trigger aplasia. For instance, the viruses incriminated include human parvovirus and hepatitis B virus. Posthepatitis aplastic anemia may also follow non-A, non-B hepatitis. Finally, aplastic anemia may be a sporadic but rare complication of pregnancy. There is also a group of hereditary aplastic anemias, which includes Fanconi's anemia, dyskeratosis congenita, and Bloom's syndrome (36).

Multiple pathogeneses for aplastic anemia have been postulated. Early reports of hematopoietic recovery after infusion of bone marrow from a normal identical twin without a preparative regimen suggested that aplastic anemia may be due to an agent that damages or destroys hematopoietic stem cells, rather than a disorder of the microenvironment or the immune system (37). It soon became apparent, however, that many patients with aplastic anemia do not recover following simple infusion of syngeneic bone marrow (38). When these patients were conditioned with an immunosuppressive regimen, implantation of a second infusion of syngeneic marrow was successful. This observation suggested that aplastic anemia may be an autoimmune disorder. Further, demonstrations that marrow engraftment may include the grafting of macrophages, fibroblasts, and other cells that constitute the stromal marrow culture in vitro opened up the possibility that marrow transplantation may actually restore a damaged microenvironment in vivo (35). To further confuse the issue, it is known that antilymphocyte globulin can result in the recovery of approximately 50% of patients with severe aplastic anemia (reviewed in Ref. 35) (39). The apparent response of some patients treated with antilymphocyte globulin or antithymocyte globulin lent credence to the theory of an autoimmune etiology for aplastic anemia. In addition, several in vitro studies of aplastic anemia indicate that T lymphocytes suppress hematopoietic stem cell colony formation and that this suppression may be mediated by a cytokine and can be reversed by removal of the inhibitory T cells. Moreover, treatment with a T cell-selective immunosuppressive agent (cyclosporine) may be beneficial in some patients with aplastic anemia (40). Synthesis of the known data leads one to suspect that aplastic anemia is heterogeneous in etiology, with possible defects including loss of pluripotent stem cells, dysfunction of progenitor cells, a perturbed marrow microenvironment, abnormalities in humoral regulators of hematopoiesis, and autoimmune-mediated inhibition of hematopoiesis.

The diagnosis of aplastic anemia should be reserved for patients having pancytopenia and reduced marrow cellularity unassociated with marrow infiltration by non-hematopoietic or neoplastic cells. Even so, 1–5% of patients presenting with aplastic anemia eventually develop acute myelogenous leukemia. This range of leukemic incidence is seen in both idiopathic aplasia and in aplastic anemia secondary to benzene or choramphenicol. In some series in which aplastic anemia patients survived and were followed for 2 years or longer, the incidence of acute anemia is from 5 to 10%. This suggests that kinetically frustrated stem cells may, if they survive long enough, engender a clonal population that is not susceptible to the underlying hematosuppressive process. The association of aplasia with a clonal disorder of pluripotent stem cells (paroxysmal nocturnal hemoglobulinuria) has also encouraged the view that some forms of aplastic anemia are either clonal or preleukemic disorders. Finally, some patients with myelodysplastic syndrome eventually develop a severe peripheral pancytopenia accompanied by a profound decrease in marrow cellularity mimicking aplastic anemia.

B. GM-CSF Therapy of Aplastic Anemia

Several studies of GM-CSF have been conducted in patients with aplastic anemia (Table 4). Vadhan-Raj and colleagues (42) treated patients with continuous infusions of GM-CSF (60–500 $\mu g/m^2/day$) for 2 weeks with a 2 week rest

TABLE 4 GM-CSF Therapy of Aplastic Anemia[a]

No. of evaluable patients	Dose and schedule[b]	Neutrophil response (% of patients)	Comment	Reference
7	15–480 μg/m^2/day × 7–14 days, every 4 weeks (IV 1–12 h)	86		Antin et al. (17)
4	4–32 μg/kg/day × 14 days sc or CI	25	Patients had severe disease	Nissen et al. (41)
10	60–500 μg/m^2/day × 14 days every 4 weeks (CI)	100	Bone marrow cellularity increased in 7 of 10 patients	Vadhan-Raj et al. (42)
11	4–64 μg/kg/day CI	90	One patient had increase in hemoglobin from 7 to 11 g/dl and an increase in platelets from 25 to 45 × 10^9 L^{-1}	Champlin et al. (43)
8	10–20 μg/m^2/day SC	75	One patient showed an increase in platelets from 10 to 169 × 10^9 L^{-1} and a decrease in RBC transfusion requirements	Kurzrock et al. (manuscript submitted and unpublished data)

[a]CI = continuous infusion; IV = intravenous; SC = subcutaneous.
[b]The 2.5 μg/kg approximately equivalent to 100 μg/m^2.

period. The majority of these individuals had disease of moderate severity. All patients showed a rise in white counts that was mainly due to increases in neutrophils, eosinophils, and, to a lesser extent, monocytes. Rates of hydrogen peroxide production in purified granulocyte fractions were also enhanced during GM-CSF therapy, indicating functional activation. Increases in bone marrow cellularity, myeloid precursor cells, and myeloid-erythroid cell ratios accompanied the white cell response. Despite the in vivo response of the white cells, the concentration of colony-forming cells remained the same. There were no significant changes in the erythroid or megakaryocytic lineage. Similar results were obtained in other trials. Antin and coworkers (17) treated seven patients with aplastic anemia with GM-CSF. Doses ranged from 15 to 240 $\mu g/m^2$/day with IV infusions lasting between 1 and 12 h. Increases in neutrophils were seen in all patients, although the count reached $>1.0 \times 10^9$ cells L^{-1} in only two individuals. The majority of subjects also showed an increase in reticulocytes; however, hemoglobin responses were not generally seen. There were no changes in platelet counts. The study was designed so that patients received infusions for 7–14 days every 4 weeks and then a repeat infusion at a higher dose level. Interestingly, the peak responses were often observed during the first or second infusion. It is unclear if the decrease in responsiveness with successive courses indicated some type of marrow "burnout" or, possibly, if lower doses of GM-CSF resulted in better responses than the higher doses given later. In this regard, we treated eight aplastic anemia patients (moderate severity) with 10–20 $\mu g/m^2$/day (SC) of GM-CSF. Of eight patients six have shown a rise in neutrophils to physiologic levels. Interestingly, one patient also demonstrated a dramatic platelet recovery (from 10 to 169×10^9 L^{-1}) accompanied by a bone marrow monocytosis. This last observation suggests that the increase in platelets may have been caused by induction of monocyte proliferation and subsequent activation of these cells to release thrombopoietic factors.

In severe aplastic anemia, GM-CSF may not be as effective, perhaps because of a lack of stem cells. In this regard, Nissen and coworkers (41) gave GM-CSF to 4 patients with severe aplastic anemia. One patient with residual hematopoiesis responded with an increase in neutrophil count, as well as with resolution of septicemia and bilateral pneumonia. Three patients with no evidence of myelopoiesis did not respond. These investigators concluded that GM-CSF does not induce hematopoiesis in long-standing, severe, treatment-resistant aplastic anemia with complete myelopoietic failure. Champlin and colleagues (43) treated 11 patients with refractory aplastic anemia with GM-CSF by continuous intravenous infusion; 10 patients had substantial increments of granulocytes, monocytes, and eosinophils associated with myeloid and eosinophilic hyperplasia in the bone marrow. Patients with pretreatment granulocytes $\geq 0.3 \times 10^9$ L^{-1} had greater increments in circulating myeloid cells than patients with more severe granulocytopenia. Only 1 patient had improvement in erythrocytes and platelets. This patient showed an increase in hemoglobin from 7 to 11 g/dl and an increase in platelets from 25 to 45 × $10^9/L^{-1}$.

Only one group investigated the effects of GM-CSF on lymphoid cells in detail. Apparently, an increase in B cell numbers, together with an increase in natural killer cytotoxicity, was seen in a group of 14 aplastic anemia patients (44).

Based on the studies performed, it appears that GM-CSF can be used successfully to increase granulocyte counts in aplastic anemia patients with moderate to severe disease (reviewed in Ref. 45). Future trials of GM-CSF in combination with other growth factors and as an adjuct to antithymocyte globulin therapy or bone marrow transplantation are warranted.

IV. TOXICITY OF GM-CSF IN PATIENTS WITH MYELODYSPLASTIC SYNDROME AND APLASTIC ANEMIA

The constitutional side effects of GM-CSF are generally mild (Table 5). At standard doses of 100–200 μg/m²/day (2.5–5.0 μg/kg/day), low-grade fever is common. Patients also occasionally experience myalgia, headaches, and flulike symptoms. In neutropenic patients, fever can be confusing to the clinician, as infection is a constant risk. However, most GM-CSF-induced temperatures are <101°F (38.3°C). In patients with temperatures above these levels, we generally initiate intravenous antibiotic therapy and, if necessary, reduce the GM-CSF dose. Bone pain is also seen occasionally. Because this discomfort can localize in the sternum, it may be difficult to differentiate this symptom from cardiac pain. Local erythema at the injection site has been observed in about 20–30% of our patients. This side effect often improves with time. It is our clinical impression that it occurs more often in patients who develop an increase in eosinophils rather than in neutrophils after GM-CSF therapy. Thrombocytopenia has occurred in about 20% of our patients treated with GM-CSF. This side effect is

TABLE 5 Side Effects of GM-CSF

Side effect[a]	% of patients
Low-grade fever	60–80
Bone pain	30
Local erythema at injection site	20–30
Fluid retention	20
Thrombocytopenia	20
Eosinophilia	20
Dyspnea	10–20
Pleuritis, pericarditis	10

[a]Most side effects are mild and reversible when GM-CSF is discontinued. Toxicity appears to be more common and more severe in patients over the age of 70 years.

almost always reversible once GM-CSF is discontinued. Furthermore, in many patients the degree of thrombocytopenia seems to be inversely related to the increase in neutrophil count. Therefore, in some individuals, decreasing the GM-CSF dose can lead to a balance between the positive effect of GM-CSF on neutrophils and the negative effect on platelets. The mechanism by which thrombocytopenia occurs is not clear, but the inverse relationship with myeloid responses suggests the possibility of a "steal" phenomenon. We have also noted that about 15–20% of patients have an increase in eosinophils rather than in neutrophil counts. The reason for this heterogeneity in response is also unclear, but we are currently analyzing patient characteristics to determine if the response to GM-CSF reflects an underlying biologic heterogeneity in myelodysplastic syndromes that is not clarified by FAB type. If so, it is conceivable that the response to GM-CSF may be a prognostic factor. Fluid retention, pleuritis, and pericarditis are occasionally seen. All these side effects appear to be more common and more severe in patients over the age of 70 years. Younger individuals tolerate GM-CSF with few adverse effects. As mentioned earlier, we have noted that many patients respond to very low doses of GM-CSF (5–10 $\mu g/m^2$/day). These doses are virtually free of side effects. Finally, the toxicities seen in transgeneic mice expressing the GM-CSF genes—accumulation of macrophages, blindness, and a fatal tissue damage syndrome (46)—have not been observed in any patients on either conventional or low-dose GM-CSF, even after 1–2 years of therapy.

V. PHARMACOKINETICS OF GM-CSF

After subcutaneous administration of 3–10 μg/kg (120–400 $\mu g/m^2$) of GM-CSF in patients with myelodysplastic syndrome, GM-CSF levels are measurable for 14–24 h. Peak serum levels achieved are between 4 and 16 ng/ml (19). In contrast, the half-life of GM-CSF after intravenous (IV) bolus administration is measured in minutes. These data suggest that GM-CSF should be administered by the subcutaneous route or by prolonged (>2 h) infusions for adequate exposure times to be achieved. Clinically, subcutaneous GM-CSF appears to be as potent as IV infusions. Furthermore, the subcutaneous route is more convenient for patients and is not complicated by catheter-induced sepsis.

VI. FUTURE DIRECTIONS

A. Myelodysplastic Syndromes

Combination growth factor therapy, titrated to individual patient needs, is an appealing approach to the future management of myelodysplastic syndromes. In these disorders, however, the potential for eventual leukemic transformation needs to be dealt with appropriately. A possible strategy involves synchronization of malignant cells with a growth factor followed by treatment with an S phase-specific agent, such as cytarabine. This approach leads to increased cell killing in vitro with a differential effect on neoplastic versus normal cells (28–31). In light of these observations, we are currently carrying out a study in which patients are begun on low doses of GM-CSF. The doses are titrated to achieve a neutrophil count in the physiologic range. After 1 month of treatment, if the patient remains anemic, erythropoietin is added. If, however, the patient is thrombocytopenic or if an increase in blasts has been observed, then low-dose cytarbine therapy is initiated (15 $\mu g/m^2$/day subcutaneously in three divided doses for 14 days every 5 weeks). Preliminary data suggest that about 40% of patients benefit from this therapy, with about 15% maintained for prolonged periods on GM-CSF alone and about 25% achieving a complete remission on the GM-CSF–cytarabine combination. Toxicity is mild.

Comparative trials of G-CSF and GM-CSF should also be performed because some data indicate that G-CSF enhances neutrophil function in myelodysplasia. Further, its preferential specificity for late myeloid progenitors suggests comparatively less stimulatory effect on existing leukemic clones. However, current clinical studies with this molecule do not permit an assessment of its relative advantages and disadvantages compared to GM-CSF therapy.

Finally, combination growth factor therapy is an appealing option for the future. We recently studied the effects of GM-CSF, IL-3, and combinations of these two molecules in the colony/culture assay (Estrov et al., manuscript submitted). When used singly, each growth factor stimulated myelodysplastic syndrome-derived CFU-GM and BFU-E in a dose-dependent fashion in vitro. IL-3 was a more potent stimulus in some individuals, GM-CSF in others. When used in combination, IL-3 plus GM-CSF was more effective than each growth factor by itself in five of six patients. These data indicate heterogeneity in response between patients; combining IL-3 and GM-CSF appears to enhance activity, however, and such an approach may be exploitable in the clinic.

B. Aplastic Anemia

GM-CSF may be a useful management strategy in several settings. Antithymocyte globulin is an effective treatment for about half of newly diagnosed patients with this disease. However, there is a 1–3 month period before peripheral blood counts rise. A course of GM-CSF treatment following antithymocyte globulin could conceivably induce a more prompt granulocytosis or enhance recovery. Bone marrow transplantation is considered the preferred treatment for young patients with aplastic anemia. Even so, only one-third of patients have a HLA-identical sibling donor. Registries for HLA-matched unrelated donors are available, but several months are generally required to identify a histocompatible individual and to procure bone marrow for transplantation. GM-CSF therapy may be useful to support myelopoiesis during this period. Further, GM-CSF may be exploited to accelerate hematopoietic recovery after allogeneic bone marrow transplant. It will be necessary, however, to determine if this type of therapy can adversely affect graft rejection, graft-versus-host disease, or other complications. Finally, hematopoietic growth factor therapy alone may ultimately be an effective treatment for patients with aplastic anemia. It is obvious that, in many cases, myeloprogenitors are present and are capable of proliferating in response to stimulatory agents. Since GM-CSF often does not affect erythroid and megakaryocyte lineages, future trials should include concomitant administration of other hematopoietic growth factors. In vitro data suggest that many growth factors have additive or synergistic activity. Indeed, in vitro and monkey modeling studies indicate that the use of interleukin-1 or interleukin-3 (which affects more primitive hematopoietic progenitors), followed sequentially by the use of GM-CSF, may result in synergistic hematopoietic responses. GM-CSF administered together with erythropoietic or thrombopoietic growth factors may aid in alleviating both neutropenia and anemia. Eventually, combination therapy tailored to individual needs should be the most effective approach to the management of aplastic anemia.

ACKNOWLEDGMENTS

Research supported in part by the Schering-Plough Corporation and the Occidental Petroleum Corporation for Cancer Research. Research conducted in part by the Clayton Foundation for Research. Dr. Gutterman is a Senior Clayton Foundation Investigator.

REFERENCES

1. Nicola NA. Hematopoietic cell growth factors and their receptors. Annu Rev Biochem 1989; 58:45–77.
2. Metcalf D. The colony stimulating factors. Discovery, development, and clinical applications. Cancer 1990; 65:2185–95.
3. Groopman JE, Molina J-M, Scadden DT. Hematopoietic growth factors. Biology and clinical applications. N Engl J Med 1989; 321:1449–59.
4. Doll DC. Myelodysplastic syndromes. West J Med 1989; 151:161–7.
5. Koeffler HP. Myelodysplastic syndromes (preleukemia). Semin Hematol 1986; 23:284–99.
6. Bennett JM, Catovsky D, Daniel MT, et al. Proposals for the classification of the myelodysplastic syndromes. Br J Haematol 1982; 51:189–99.
7. List AF, Garewal HS, Sandberg AA. The myelodysplastic syndromes: biology and implications for management. J Clin Oncol 1990; 8:1424–41.

8. Besa EC, Hyzinski M, Nowell PC, Itri LM, Abrahm J. Clinical trials and in vitro evaluation of 13-cis retinoic acid in myelodysplastic syndrome (abstract). Proc Am Soc Clin Oncol 1985; 4:216.
9. Greenberg BR, Durie BGM, Barnett TC, Meyskens FL Jr. Phase I–II study of 13-cis-retinoic acid in myelodysplastic syndrome. Cancer Treat Rep 1985; 69:1369–74.
10. Picozzi VJ Jr, Swanson GF, Morgan R, Hecht F, Greenberg PL. 13-Cis retinoic acid treatment for myelodysplastic syndromes. J Clin Oncol 1986; 4:589–95.
11. Gold EJ, Mertelsmann RH, Itri LM, et al. Phase I clinical trial of 13-cis-retinoic acid in myelodysplastic syndromes. Cancer Treat Rep 1983; 67:981–6.
12. Kerndrup G, Bendix-Hansen K, Pedersen B, Ellegaard J, Hokland P. 13-Cis retinoic acid treatment of myelodysplastic syndromes. Leuk Res 1987; 11:7–16.
13. Leoni F, Ciolli S, Longo G, Messori A, Ferrini PR. 13-Cis retinoic acid treatment in patients with myelodysplastic syndrome. Acta Haematol (Basel) 1988; 80:8–12.
14. Clark RE, Jacobs A, Lush CJ, Smith SA. Effect of 13-cis retinoic acid on survival of patients with myelodysplastic syndrome. Lancet 1987; 1:763–5.
15. Koeffler HP, Heitjan D, Mertelsmann R, et al. Randomized study of 13-cis retinoic acid v placebo in the myelodysplastic disorders. Blood 1988; 71:703–8.
16. Vadhan-Raj S, Keating M, LeMaistre A, et al. Effects of recombinant human granulocyte-macrophage colony-stimulating factor in patients with myelodysplastic syndromes. N Engl J Med 1987; 317:1545–52.
17. Antin JH, Smith BR, Holmes W, Rosenthal DS. Phase I/II study of recombinant human granulocyte-macrophage colony-stimulating factor in aplastic anemia and myelodysplastic syndrome. Blood 1988; 72:705–13.
18. Ganser A, Volkers B, Greher J, et al. Recombinant human granulocyte-macrophage colony-stimulating factor in patients with myelodysplastic syndromes—a phase I/II trial. Blood 1988; 73:31–7.
19. Thompson JA, Lee DJ, Kidd P, et al. Subcutaneous granulocyte-macrophage colony-stimulating factor in patients with myelodysplastic syndrome: toxicity, pharmacokinetics, and hematological effects. J Clin Oncol 1989; 7:629–37.
20. Rifkin RM, Hersh EM, Hultquist KN, Salmon SE. Therapy of the myelodysplastic syndrome (MDS) with subcutaneously (sc) administered recombinant human granulocyte-macrophage colony-stimulating factor (GM-CSF) (abstract). Proc Am Soc Clin Oncol 1989; 8:178.
21. Herrmann F, Lindemann A, Klein H, Lubbert M, Schultz G, Mertelsmann R. Effect of recombinant human granulocyte-macrophage colony-stimulating factor in patients with myelodysplastic syndrome with excess of blasts. Leukemia 1989; 3:335–8.
22. Estey E, Kurzrock R, Talpaz M, et al. Therapy of myelodysplastic syndromes (MDS) with GM-CSF. Proc Am Soc Clin Oncol 1989; 8:200.
23. Estey EH, Kurzrock R, Talpaz M, et al. Effects of low-doses of recombinant human granulocyte-macrophage colony-stimulating factor (GM-CSF) in patients with myelodysplastic syndromes. Br J Haematol 1991; 77:291–295.
24. Cheson BD. The myelodysplastic syndromes: current approaches to therapy. Ann Intern Med 1990; 112:932–41.
25. Boogaerts MA, Nelissen V, Roelant C, Goossens W. Blood neutrophil function in primary myelodysplastic syndromes. Br J Haematol 1983; 55:217–27.

26. Peters WP, Stuart A, Affronti ML, Kim CS, Coleman RE. Neutrophil migration is defective during recombinant human granulocyte-macrophage colony-stimulating factor infusion after autologous bone marrow transplantation in humans. Blood 1988; 72:1310–5.
27. Hittelman WN, Tigaud J-D, Estey E, Gutterman JU, Vadhan-Raj S. Relative maturation of aneuploid and diploid elements in patients with myelodysplasia treated with granulocyte-macrophage colony-stimulating factor. Blood 1988; 72:121a.
28. Lista P, Porcu P, Avanzi GC, Pegoraro L. Interleukin 3 enhances the cytotoxic activity of 1-beta-D-arabinofuranosylcytosine (ara-C) on acute myeloblastic leukaemia (AML) cells. Br J Haematol 1988; 70:121–3.
29. Miyauchi J, Kelleher CA, Wang C, Minkin S, McCulloch EA. Growth factors influence the sensitivity of leukemic stem cells to cytosine arabinoside in culture. Blood 1989; 73:1272–8.
30. Bhalla K, Birkhofer M, Arlin Z, Grant S, Lutzky J, Graham G. Effect of recombinant GM-CSF on the metabolism of cytosine arabinoside in normal and leukemic human bone marrow cells. Leukemia 1988; 2:810–3.
31. Cannistra SA, Groshek P, Griffin JD. Granulocyte-macrophage colony-stimulating factor enhances the cytotoxic effects of cytosine arabinoside in acute myeloblastic leukemia and in the myeloid blast crisis phase of chronic myeloid leukemia. Leukemia 1989; 3:328–34.
32. Ehrlich P. Uber einen Fall von Anamie mit Bemerkungen uber regenerative Veranderugen des Knochenmarks. Charite-Annalen 1888; 13:300.
33. Chauffard M. Un cas d'anemie pernicieuse aplastique. Bull Soc Med Hop Paris 1904; 21:313.
34. Camitta BM, Storb R, Thomas ED. Aplastic anemia. Pathogenesis, diagnosis, treatment, and prognosis. N Engl J Med 1982; 306:645–52.
35. Thomas ED, Storb R. Acquired severe aplastic anemia: progress and perplexity. Blood 1984; 64:325–8.
36. James H, Jandl MD, eds. Blood. Boston: Little, Brown, 1987.
37. Robins MM, Noyes WD. Aplastic anemia treated with bone-marrow transplantation from an identical twin. N Engl J Med 1961; 265:974.
38. Appelbaum FR, Fefer A, Cheever MA, et al. Treatment of aplastic anemia by bone marrow transplantation in identical twins. Blood 1980; 55:1033.
39. Speck B, Gluckman E, Haak HL, van Rood JJ. Treatment of aplastic anaemia by antilymphocyte globulin with and without allogeneic bone-marrow infusions. Lancet 1977; 2:1145.
40. Totterman TH, Hoglund M, Bengtsson M, Simonsson B, Almqvist D, Killander A. Treatment of pure red-cell aplasia and aplastic anemia with ciclosporin: long-term clinical effects. Eur J Haematol 1989; 42:126–33.
41. Nissen C, Tichelli A, Gratwohl A, et al. Failure of recombinant human granulocyte-macrophage colony-stimulating factor therapy in aplastic anemia patients with very severe neutropenia. Blood 1988; 72:2045–7.
42. Vadhan-Raj S, Buescher S, Broxmeyer HE, et al. Stimulation of myelopoiesis in patients with aplastic anemia by recombinant human granulocyte-macrophage colony-stimulating factor. N Engl J Med 1988; 319:1628–34.

43. Champlin RE, Nimer SD, Ireland P, Oette DH, Golde DW. Treatment of refractory aplastic anemia with recombinant human granulocyte-macrophage colony-stimulating factor. Blood 1989; 73:694–9.
44. Faisal M, Cumberland W, Champlin R, Fahey JL. Effect of recombinant human granulocyte-macrophage colony-stimulating factor administration on the lymphocyte subsets of patients with refractory aplastic anemia. Blood 1990; 76:1580–5.
45. Gutterman J, Vadhan-Raj S, Logothetis C, et al. Effects of granulocyte-macrophage colony-stimulating factor in iatrogenic myelosuppression, bone marrow failure, and regulation of host disease. Semin Hematol 1990; 27:15–24.
46. Lang RA, Metcalf D, Cuthbertson RA, et al. Transgenic mice expressing a hemopoietic growth factor gene (GM-CSF) develop accumulations of macrophages, blindness, and a fatal syndrome of tissue damage. Cell 1987; 51:675–86.

12

Use of Colony-Stimulating Factors in the Treatment of AML

Elihu H. Estey

University of Texas, M. D. Anderson Cancer Center, Houston, Texas

I. INTRODUCTION

The availability of hematopoietic growth factors (CSFs) has two broad ramifications for patients with acute myelogenous leukemia (AML). First, the molecules might have therapeutic potential. Second, they might serve as tools to permit the elucidation of the underlying cellular changes that characterize AML.

Appreciation of the potential role of CSFs is abetted by some understanding of normal hematopoiesis. All circulating hematopoietic cells are derived from pluripotent ''stem cells,'' also known as CFU-S, and defined by their ability to form colonies containing representatives of all hematopoietic lineages (granulocytic, megakaryocytic, erythroid, and others) in cultures in vitro (1). Stem cells, a tiny minority of nucleated hematopoietic cells, are typically resting (G_0) cells. Evidence exists suggesting that stem cell behavior is in part random or ''stochastic.'' For example, which of a number of stem cells leaves the stem cell compartment, thereby becoming committed to a pathway of differentiation that will result in the production and release of mature cells, may be randomly determined under basal conditions. However two pieces of evidence suggest that stem cell behavior is also determined by external events, a situation that might be predicted from the variations in the need for blood cell production that arise physiologically. First, the surface of stem cells has growth factor receptors (2).

Second, although stem cells die if placed in culture without growth factors, they can survive and proliferate for long periods of time (long-term cultures) in intimate contact with stromal cells, which form a so-called adherent layer (3). Under basal conditions the stromal cell is believed to send an anti-proliferative message to the stem cell and thus to "protect" the stem cell from differentiation. Addition of certain molecules, such as the pleiotrophic growth regulator interleukin-1 (IL-1), to the culture alters the message sent by the stromal cell from negative to positive, resulting in stem cell proliferation. IL-1 may act by causing production of other molecules from stromal cells, for example IL-6 and IL-3, which act synergistically in shortening the time stem cells spend in G_0 (4). In fact, molecules with CSF activity (see later) can be detected in long-term cultures after addition of IL-1. The need for intimate contact between stromal cell and stem cell suggests that growth factors are not released by stromal cells but rather are "presented" by the stromal cell to the stem cell. Membrane-bound extracellular matrix molecules, in particular heparin sulfate (found in stromal but not stem cells), which can bind such molecules as IL-3, may play a role in this presentations (2). As there are molecules like IL-1 that alter the proliferative signal sent by stromal to stem cell from negative to positive, there are also molecules that reinforce the negative message and thus "deepen" quiescence. Transforming growth factor β (TGF-β) and a macrophage inflammatory protein (5) are examples of such inhibitors of stem cell proliferation.

Either randomly or more rapidly after a positive proliferative signal from the coupled stromal cell, stem cells become more restricted in the types of colonies they can give rise to in culture in vitro; that is, they become committed to become a particular type of cell. By virtue of this commitment they cease being a stem cell but remain defined by the types of colonies to which they can give rise. For example, CFU-GEMM can give rise to granulocytes, erythrocytes, monocytes, and megakaryocytes but not lymphocytes. Another defining characteristic of the committed cell (e.g., CFU-GEMM) is that it has less self-renewal capacity than the stem cell. For example, when cells are removed from one agar culture system and replated in another the cells that give rise to a full range of colonies in the first system do so in the second system while the cells that only gave rise to certain types of colonies in the first system die in the second.

As more primitive, more totipotent, cells give rise to CFU-GEMM, CFU-GEMM gives rise to cells that are more lineage restricted than themselves, that is, CFU-GM, which can only form colonies of granulocytes and monocytes; CFU-MEG, which can only form megakaryocyte colonies; and BFU-E, which can only form erythroid colonies. CFU-GM in turn give rise to CFU-G and CFU-M. The former are the immediate source of myeloblasts, promyelocytes, myelocytes, metamyelocytes, bands, and neutrophils and the latter the immediate source of monocytes. In the sense that at successive steps in hemopoiesis cells are more lineage restricted with less self-renewal capacity, hematopoiesis is said to be hierarchic.

Like stem cells, CFU-GEMM, CFU-GM, CFU-G, CFU-M, CFU-MEG, BFU-E, and CFU-E have extensive proliferative capacity. As described for stem cells, there appear to be negative and positive regulators of this capacity. Relatively little is known about negative regulators, but products of myelogenous leukemia cells may be able to mimic the actions of some of these. Positive regulators include the CSFs IL-3, GM-CSF, G-CSF, and M-CSF (6–8). Each is a glycoprotein with similar polypeptide chain size although the constituent amino acids differ considerably. The genes for GM-CSF and IL-3 are adjacent on chromosome 5 and are similarly organized. The gene for M-CSF and its receptors are also on chromosome 5; that for G-CSF is on chromosome 17. Different CSFs appear to target different hematopoietic cells as judged by the presence of different CSF receptors on the different cells. Although IL-3 and GM-CSF receptors appear to be present on a wide range of cells from the more primitive through neutrophils, eosinophils, and monocytes, G-CSF receptors appear limited to CFU-G and morphologically recognizable myeloid cells, and M-CSF receptors seem limited to CFU-M and to mature monocytes and macrophages. The affinity of a receptor for its CSF may differ depending on cell type, perhaps explaining the concentration-dependent effects of growth factors. For example, as its concentration is raised, GM-CSF stimulates the proliferation of a wider variety of cells. The affinity and/or number of receptors for a CSF may also differ if other CSFs are present. For example, such upregulation of G-CSF receptors by GM-CSF may account for synergism between GM-CSF and G-CSF in increasing the number, size, and survivability of CFU-G (9).

In addition to their roles as proliferative stimuli, CSFs also stimulate differentiation and functional activation. The precise action of the CSF appears to depend on the maturational status of the target: for example, GM-CSF stimulates proliferation in CFU-GM and functional activation in neutrophils. This may imply that the GM-CSF receptor is linked to different signaling sequences in the two cells.

The principal sources of CSFs are monocytes, T cells, endothelial cells, and mesenchymal cells, such as fibroblasts, the last, as noted, located in juxtaposition to stem cells. The stimuli for CSF release suggest that CSFs are important in the physiologic response to stress. For example, endotoxin exposure causes monocytes to release G-CSF and exposure to antigens induces T cells to produce GM-CSF and IL-3. IL-1, itself released by monocytes, may play a central role in affecting CSF release. Under basal conditions CSF concentrations are undetectable, and thus it has been difficult to establish a role for CSFs in basal hematopoiesis. However, the striking increases in neutrophil, monocyte, or eosinophil count observed following administration of CSFs to patients leaves little doubt about the ability of these molecules to affect hematopoiesis in vivo (10–12).

II. ROLE OF CSFs IN AML

Only a small minority of the myeloblasts in bone marrow from patients with AML appear capable of self-renewal upon replating in agar culture (13). In analogy to normal bone marrow, this suggests that these myeloblasts serve as leukemia stem cells ("clonogenic cells" or "AML-CFU"). Comparison of the surface antigen phenotype of AML-CFU with phenotypes of normal progenitors, analysis of glucose-6-phosphate dehydrogenase (G-6-PD) isoenzymes in (female) G-6-PD heterozygotes (14), and simultaneous determination of karyotype and lineage (erythroid, megakaryocytic, or granulocytic) in single cells (15) suggest that AML-CFU originate from malignant transformation of CFU-GM in some patients, CFU-GEMM in others, and CFU-S in yet others.

Despite their malignant character, the majority of AML-CFU remain responsive to CSFs. Early studies revealed that in most patients GM-CSF, G-CSF, or IL-3 enhanced colony formation by AML-CFU (16–21). M-CSF was generally a less effective proliferative stimulus for these cells (21). More recent studies have focused on IL-1, IL-6, and TNF. IL-1 stimulates the proliferation of AML-CFU, an effect that can be blocked by anti-GM-CSF antibody (22–24). Furthermore, blast cell-conditioned medium prepared in the presence of IL-1 contains GM-CSF. These observations suggest that the effect of IL-1 is mediated by GM-CSF produced by the AML-CFU in response to IL-1. Others have found that IL-1 by itself has no effect on AML-CFU but acts synergistically with GM-CSF or G-CSF in promoting the proliferation of these cells, possibly either through inducing expression of receptors for these CSFs or through shortening of the G_0 period (25). These findings have also been reported with IL-6 (26). TNF serves as a stimulator of AML-CFU colony formation if GM-CSF is also added to the culture but serves as an inhibitor if G-CSF is added (27,28). These findings have been interpreted in terms of TNF effects on GM-CSF (upregulation) or G-CSF (downregulation) receptors.

The most striking finding that has emerged from all the work just described is the great variability observed when blasts from different patients are explanted in the presence of CSFs. At one extreme, enhancement of AML-CFU colony formation may not occur even after exposure to a combination of CSFs at high concentration; at the other extreme, the number of colonies formed after exposure to a low concentration of a single CSF approaches that formed after exposure to fully conditioned media. Colony formation is most enhanced by one CSF in some patients and by another CSF in others. Combinations of, for example, G-CSF and GM-CSF are synergistic in some patients but less than additive in others.

One possible explanation for this heterogeneity is interpatient variability in the number of receptors for a given CSF and in affinity of the receptors for the ligand; accordingly, characterization of CSF receptors on explanted AML cells has received considerable attention. Certain themes have emerged. Thus it appears that AML blasts contain these receptors for GM-CSF and IL-3: (1) high-affinity IL-3 receptors that do not bind GM-CSF, (2) dual high-affinity IL-3/GM-CSF receptors, and (3) low-affinity GM-CSF receptors that do not bind IL-3 (29). The GM-CSF concentrations needed to trigger AML-CFU proliferation appear to be in the affinity range of a high-affinity GM-CSF receptor (30), and thus the role of the low-affinity GM-CSF receptor is unclear. The G-CSF receptor appears to be of a single-affinity type (31) and is thus perhaps a simpler structure than the GM-CSF or IL-3 receptors.

Despite these generalizations about CSF receptors on explanted AML cells, there appears to be a marked patient-to-patient heterogeneity in these receptor numbers and affinities (32,33). For example, the number of high-affinity GM-CSF sites per cell has varied from not detectable to above 1000, and their K_d has varied from about 60 to about 400 pmol/L. Analyses of binding curves before and after acid-wash techniques that remove bound GM-CSF without altering the GM-CSF receptors indicate that variations in the binding of GM-CSF to its receptor are not due to occupancy of the receptor by an endogenous source of GM-CSF (30). There is similar variability in numbers and affinities of IL-3 and G-CSF receptors. There has been no obvious pattern in numbers of GM-CSF, IL-3, and G-CSF receptors relative to each other.

Does the (variable) number of CSF receptors parallel the (variable) in vitro proliferative response of AML-CFU to the CSFs? There appears to be no necessary correlation between receptor number and the ability of blasts to respond to a growth factor. For example, in only one of five patients whose explanted blasts failed to show an increase in DNA synthesis following exposure to IL-3 receptors was there an absence of IL-3 receptors and receptor numbers were normal in the other 4 (32) tritiated thymidine ([^{3}H]-TdR) uptake may provide a more sensitive assay for mitogenic potential of AML cells than a clonogenic assay (31). Similarly, four of six patients whose blasts failed to proliferate after exposure to GM-CSF had detectable GM-CSF receptors (32). A similar phenomenon has been reported with G-CSF (31). It appears that relatively few CSF receptors are required to permit a brisk proliferative response (31–33). The reason(s) for the failure of blast populations containing significant numbers of CSF receptors to proliferate following CSF exposure are unclear. Receptor numbers are measured using whole leukemia cell populations, and these may not reflect the number on rarer clonogenic cells. Some clonogenic cells may require a combination of CSFs. Perhaps most likely are alterations in postreceptor (signal transduction) pathways. Such pathways are beginning to be investigated. After binding to their receptors, GM-SCF, G-CSF, and TNF all appear to rapidly trigger phosphorylation of tyrosine and serine residues on a 75 kD protein (34). Thus receptors for these CSFs may at least in part be tyrosine-specific phosphokinases (TPK) (34). The target of the receptor TPK may be the *raf* oncogence, a cytoplasmic serine/threonine protein kinase (J. Griffin, personal communication). Activation of *raf* presumably ultimately leads to activation of specific genes. Phosphatases may provide a "negative check" on this system. Indeed, blocking phosphatase function with orthovanadate leads to an increased GM-CSF-induced proliferative response (Griffin, personal communication).

Do CSFs play a role in the proliferative advantage that AML cells enjoy over normal myeloid progenitors? Such a role might be envisioned if CSF receptors were overexpressed on AML cells or the affinity of a receptor for its ligand were greater in AML cells. Alternatively, CSFs may play a role in the pathogenesis of AML if AML cells produced CSFs, thus setting up an autocrine loop that does not exist in similar normal myeloid progenitors or if paracrine loops existed between AML cells and accessory cells for which there is no normal counterpart. The great variability in receptor numbers and affinities in AML blasts alluded to previously would seem to make differences in receptors between these blasts and comparable normal cells an unlikely cause of the proliferative advantage enjoyed by the AML population. This question is very difficult to address directly because it is difficult to obtain the large number of normal myeloblasts (at a similar stage of differentiation as the relevant AML myeloblasts) needed to perform receptor studies. The question has been approached indirectly by using autoradiography to compare [^{125}I] G-CSF grain counts over blast cells in patients with leukemia and normal volunteers (35). The range of grain counts was similar in the "leukemia" and "normal" blasts, as was the range in counts over normal myelocytes, metamyelocytes, and neutrophils compared to the range over comparable cells in patients with AML, which may or may not have been derived from the leukemic clone. Further evidence that receptor properties are similar in AML myeloblasts and comparable normal populations are results indicating that the modulation of response to GM-CSF or G-CSF induced by TNF (upregulation and downregulation, respectively) occurs in highly purified CD34$^+$ normal populations as well as AML clonogenic blast populations (presumably also CD34$^+$) (27). Neutrophils from normal volunteers have been directly demonstrated to have a greater number of GM-CSF and G-CSF receptors than myeloblasts from patients with AML (32). Furthermore, although GM-CSF downregulates GM-CSF receptor number in normal neutrophils, it does not do so in AML blasts (Cannistra, personal communication). Such differences in receptor properties may explain how GM-CSF affects proliferation in blasts but functional activation in neutrophils. It would be of obvious interest to compare receptor number and properties in normal neutrophils with those in neutrophils containing a residual cytogenetic abnormality (demonstrated by, for example, premature chromosome condensation or restriction fragment length polymorphism techniques) obtained from patients with AML in remission.

Although most AML-CFU require CSFs to proliferate in vitro, some do not suggest that these may produce CSFs autonomously (36). Supporting this suggestion, messenger (m) RNA for GM-CSF, G-CSF, and M-CSF but not IL-3 has been detected in explanted blasts from some patients with AML (37–39). Sorting experiments using antibodies to CD33, CD13, and CD14 suggest that blasts of both early and late stages of differentiation can secrete GM-CSF (37). Transcripts do not appear to be derived from accessory cells (e.g., "normal" T cells and monocytes, which are removed before testing for message) as evidenced by failure to identify messages specific for these accessory cells, for example the α chain of the T cell receptor in the case of T cells. However, some evidence suggests that the frequent (>50%) detection of transcripts in blasts results from the processing of samples to remove accessory cells, processing that may result in the release of paracrine factors by the accessory cells (40). The genetic mechanism(s) responsible for the expression of the transcripts is unclear. Although explanted blasts have been found to contain rearrangements of the GM-CSF or G-CSF genes (38), this finding appears to be the exception rather than the rule (39–41).

There is some but by no means a perfect correlation between detection of message for GM-CSF or G-CSF in blasts and their ability to proliferate autonomously (37–39). In some cases it has been demonstrated that, despite the presence of message, CSF is not secreted, although it might still theoretically be produced and used inside the cell to drive proliferation. In other cases autonomous proliferation occurs despite the absence of message for GM-CSF or G-CSF, suggesting that AML cells secrete other factors that could induce cells of the marrow microenvironment to release CSFs that would then drive blast proliferation in a paracrine fashion. This possibility seems likely given the demonstration in blasts of message (without evidence of gene arrangements or amplification) for IL-1, IL-6, and TNF (41,42). These factors are present in medium conditioned by the blasts and have been demonstrated to induce the expression of message for GM- and G-CSF by endothelial cells with subsequent release of these CSFs by these accessory cells. The IL-6 secreted by the blasts appears to synergize with GM-CSF and G-CSF in stimulating proliferation. There is also evidence to suggest that there may be at least two blast subpopulations in AML: an adherent, phagocytic, nonclonogenic population that produces CSFs and a nonadherent, nonphagocytic clonogenic population that proliferates in response to the CSFs (43). Evidence also suggests that the adherent cells are generated in parallel with the clonogenic cells in the presence of CSFs (17).

There is considerable interpatient variability in the expression of transcripts for the different CSFs. The basis for this heterogeneity, at least for GM-CSF, G-CSF, and M-CSF, appears to be variability in the posttranscriptional stability of the message rather than variability in gene transcription itself (44). The heterogeneity itself appears to be difficult to account for if some of the autocrine and paracrine pathways just described play a major role in pathogenesis. However, it is quite possible that more sensitive techniques, such as S_1 protection, would permit more frequent detection of transcripts.

Message for M-, G-, or GM-CSF has not been detected in normal marrow cells despite (presumed) processing of these cells in an identical fashion as leukemia blasts (37–39). Normal blasts do not appear to proliferate in the absence of CSFs as leukemia blasts do on occasion (37–39). Although there is thus evidence that expression of CSFs, IL-1, TNF, and IL-6 is a distinctive property of leukemia cells and hence may be relevant to AML, unequivocal proof of this awaits demonstration that genes for those factors are not expressed in the normal *counterparts* of the leukemia cells. Because it is difficult to obtain the large number of these normal cells for northern analysis, in situ hybridization techniques may be helpful in resolving this issue. The hypothesis that aberrant growth factor gene activation is an important factor in the pathogenesis of AML is strengthened by results following retroviral insertional mutagenesis in a myeloid precursor cell line (45). This technique increases the frequency of mutation to growth factor autonomy by about 20-fold compared to the spontaneous frequency. Of 11 factor-independent mutants recovered, 10 secreted either IL-3 or GM-CSF, or a perhaps novel hematopoietic factor. All factor-independent mutants were tumorigenic in nude mice. Nonetheless, although growth factor autonomy may be crucial to the excessive cellular proliferation characteristic of AML, it seems a block in differentiation would also have to be imposed to account completely for the pathogenesis of AML.

As previously noted, growth factors probably provide stimuli for differentiation in normal hematopoiesis. Some leukemia cell lines differentiate in the presence of G-CSF, losing self-renewal capacity in the process (46,47). However, only limited differentiation occurs after exposure of myeloblasts from most patients to CSFs (21). M-CSF may be most effective in this regard, but induction of differentiation was observed in samples from only 6 of 25 patients after exposure to this CSF (21).

III. CSFs IN THE THERAPY OF AML

CSFs could be used in three different ways in the therapy of AML. These correspond to the roles of CSFs as (1) proliferative stimuli for *normal* progenitors, such as stem cells, CFU-GEMM, CFU-GM, and CFU-G, and functional activators of the mature progeny of these cells; (2) proliferative stimuli for AML-CFU; and (3) stimuli of differentiation for AML-CFU. As proliferative stimuli for normal myeloid progenitors, CSFs would be given after chemotherapy in the expectation that chemotherapy had altered the balance between AML-CFU and normal progenitors such that use of CSFs would result in the more rapid appearance of normal neutrophils. Accelerated recovery of neutrophils, particularly those with CSF-enchanced capabilities of chemotaxis, phagocytosis, superoxide production, and antibody-dependent cellular cytotoxicity (ADCC), might be useful in reducing the frequency of major or fatal infections that are prone to occur in settings of profound neutropenia. This approach has been thought to potentially be particularly useful in elderly or bed-ridden patients. The results of two studies in which GM-CSF was given to elderly patients after induction chemotherapy have been reported. Estey et al. treated 12 consecutive patients with newly diagnosed AML at a high risk of death during induction as judged by a statistical model in which performance status, bilirubin, and age were the dominant variables (48). Chemotherapy consisted of Ara-C (cytarabine, 6.0 g/m^2) given over 96 h by continuous intravenous (IV) infusion. Recombinant GM-CSF, expressed in *E. Cóli* and supplied by Schering-Plough/Sandoz, 120 μg/m^2 daily by continuous IV infusion, began 2 days after completion of chemotherapy and continued until the neutrophil count was ≥1000 μl-^{1}. This dose was chosen because it consistently produced a rise in neutrophil count in patients with myelodysplastic syndromes. The rates of fatal infection (42%), pneumonia and/or sepis (83%), and remission (50%) were similar to those seen in patients at similar risk of death during induction treated in the past with the same dose and schedule of Ara-C without GM-CSF. Given the possibility of a false negative result in light of the small number of patients treated, there was no evidence that GM-CSF accelerated neutrophil recovery in comparison to the historical group. Four patients died of infection before the earliest rise in neutrophil count as judged in patients who entered CR. In some contrast to these results are those of Buechner et al., who treated 16 patients over age 65 (15 previously untreated) and 7 patients irrespective of age (all in relapse) (49). Chemotherapy consisted of "TAD 9" (9 days of "conventional-dose" Ara-C with thioguanine and 3 days of daunorubicin) in the first group and S-HAM ("high-dose" Ara-C + mitoxantrone) in the second. GM-CSF (250 μg/m^2 daily by continuous IV infusion) began 4 days after chemotherapy was completed provided the marrow was hypoplastic and continued until neutrophil recovery when the dose was reduced and later discontinued. A statistically significant increase in neutrophil recovery rate occurred in the TAD 9 group compared to TAD 9 historical controls (median 23 days from onset of TAD-9 in the GM-CSF group versus 28 days in the controls) and in the S-HAM group also compared to historical controls (median 25 days in the GM-CSF group versus 34 days in the controls). Patients who died during induction were "censored" for purposes of analysis, and comparisons of infection, death, or complete remission (CR) rates between GM-CSF and historical patients have not been formally provided. In both the Estey et al. and Buechner et al. studies regrowth of leukemia following administration of GM-CSF was uncommon, occurring in only 1 of the 8 patients who survived long enough for response to induction therapy to be fully evaluated in the former study and in 3 of 23 patients in the latter; these rates of regrowth are not different from those expected without GM-CSF. Similarly, the duration of remission at least in the Buechner et al. study seemed comparable to that expected without GM-CSF (59% probability of CR at $1\frac{1}{2}$ years). The failure to observe an obvious acceleration of leukemia in either study suggests that it might be reasonable to undertake larger studies to definitively determine whether GM-CSF given after chemotherapy accelerates neutrophil recovery and, more importantly, decreases the rates of major and/or fatal infection. However, the Estey et al. observation that 33% of their patients died of infection before the earliest neutrophil recovery observed in patients who entered CR suggests that earlier administration of GM-CSF might be advisable. Even if this is done, it is possible that an elderly AML population is so prone to die of infection so early during induction therapy that improvements in outcome might not be forthcoming even if statistically significant, several-day decreases in neutropenia occur following GM-CSF. Under these circumstances it might be reasonable to emphasize the use of GM-CSF as a supportive care measure in patients in remission undergoing high-dose postremission therapy. The data of Wolff et al. suggest that such therapy produces cure rates of 50%, comparable to those seen after allogeneic marrow transplantation (50). However, the therapy is often associated with prolonged myelosuppression and infections. Although infections are much less frequently fatal than observed in elderly patients during induction (probably because patients who would die during high-dose postremission therapy have already died during induction), they frequently cause sufficient morbidity to prevent the administration of more than one or two courses of such therapy and probably to prevent many physicians from referring patients for the therapy at all. Nonetheless, administration of high-dose postremission therapy, particularly more than one or two courses, might improve the long-term remission rate (particularly in patients with drug-sensitive disease, e.g. those with cytogenetic abnormality with inversion of the long arm of chromosome 16, INV 16). The use of GM-CSF might permit this to be done. Certainly a beneficial effect of GM-CSF on morbidity might be easier to detect in the healthier remission population than the elderly induction population.

The therapeutic use of CSFs before chemotherapy rests on the hypothesis that such manipulations increase the chemosensitivity of AML-CFU, the fate of which may dictate the curability of AML. Most simply this increase could occur because of an increase in the fraction of cells in S phase or a decrease in the fraction in G_0. That such changes in cell cycle parameters can be accompanied by increases in clonogenic cell kill by Ara-C has been demonstrated by work of Cannistra et al. (51) and Tafuri et al. (52). Nonetheless, there is by no means a perfect correlation between "recruitment" and "cell kill." Explanation for this phenomenon may come from data of Miyauchi et al. demonstrating that sensitivity of AML-CFU to Ara-C is dictated by the balance between self-renewal and differentiation in culture independent of cell cycle parameters (53). Alterations that shift the balance in favor of differentiation decrease Ara-C sensitivity; alterations that shift the balance toward self-renewal increase sensitivity. This suggests that it may be necessary to measure the effect of CSFs on both cell cycle parameters and the self-renewal–differentiation balance to predict effect in Ara-C sensitivity.

Another consideration in the use of CSFs to "prime" the AML-CFU to Ara-C is that this might also prime the normal counterparts of the leukemia stem cells to the drug, resulting in prolonged myelosuppression. Comparison of dose-response curves of AML-CFU and normal myeloid progenitors to CSFs indicate that similar concentrations of GM-CSF or G-CSF promote the proliferation of both the leukemia and normal progenitors (35). In the clinical setting, however, leukemia cell inhibitory activities might "protect" normal cells from the CSF effects. Relevant to the possibility of increased cytotoxicity toward normal progenitors are the Bhalla et al. observations that following exposure of normal marrow mononuclear cells on the one hand and myeloblasts from patients with AML on the other to Ara-C, the ara-CTP to dCTP ratio increased more in the malignant than the normal cells (54). The expected result would be that the increase in Ara-C-induced cell kill after GM-CSF exposure (mediated by an increased incorporation of Ara-C into DNA) would occur disproportionally in the malignant rather than the normal population.

These in vitro observations have sparked interest in the clinical use of CSFs to sensitize leukemia cells to chemotherapy. The first such clinical trial was conducted in Austria (Ref. 55 and Andreef, personal communication) in patients with newly diagnosed AML. Six patients received GM-CSF, 250 $\mu g/m^2$ daily by continuous infusion for 2 days, before standard daunorubicin + "conventional"-dose Ara-C chemotherapy with GM-CSF continuing until neutrophil recovery. Three patients received the same dose and schedule of GM-CSF for 1 day before chemotherapy with GM-CSF, discontinued after completion of chemotherapy and resumed 1 week later. Three patients presenting with white cell counts above 30,000 did not receive a GM-CSF "prephase" but received GM-CSF only simultaneously with, and after, chemotherapy. Changes in blast count during the prephase were variable, ranging from no change after 2 days of GM-CSF to a quadrupling. Increases in the percentage of cells in S phase (measured by bromodeoxy-uridine [BUDR] incorporation) occurred in all patients in whom this was measured. This was marked (1.9–10.2%) in 1 patient, whose blasts rise from 8400 to 16,200 during the GM-CSF, but less marked in the other patients (1.4–3.3% after 2 days of GM-CSF; 1.1–1.7% and 1.5–3.9% after 1 day of GM-CSF) whose blasts went from 13,000 to 176,000, 100 to 100, and 1700 to 2600, respectively. A decrease in the fraction of cells in G_0 from 71 to 56% occurred in the only patient studied, the first patient just described. Once chemotherapy began, the circulating blast count fell as rapidly as it had in historical controls, with similar blast counts in patients who had not received GM-CSF before chemotherapy. Of the 12 patients 10 entered CR. Neutrophil recovery occurred on average about 4 days earlier than in historical controls and was not demonstrably quicker in the patients who received continuous GM-CSF than in those in whom GM-CSF was discontinued for a week after completion of chemotherapy. Five patients developed manifestations of the capillary leak syndrome, but this produce no fatalities.

M. D. Anderson Hospital investigators have also administered GM-CSF before and during chemotherapy in newly diagnosed patients (Estey et al., unpublished data). Patients under age 60 received GM-CSF, 125 $\mu g/m^2$ once daily SC, until the circulating blast cell count rose to 50,000 or above or for 8 days, whichever came first. Older patients received 10 $\mu g/m^2$ once daily SC with escalation of the dose to 20, then 40, and then 80 $\mu g/m^2$ if the blast count had not risen within 4 days at the previous dose. Although significant rises in blast count occurred in some patients at <20 $\mu g/m^2$, they did not occur in others at 125 $\mu g/m^2$. Despite occasional rapid rises during the prephase, blast counts fell rapidly once chemotherapy began and the CR rate appears comparable to that expected if the patients had received chemotherapy without GM-CSF (or course, since the CR rate is already reasonably high, a detection of clinical benefit from administration of GM-CSF before chemotherapy will depend on lengthening of the duration of the remission). Increases in the percentage of cells in S phase (measured by flow cytometry on biopsies) only rarely occurred, and although increases in marrow thymidine incorporation did occur on occasion, these were only rarely more than fivefold. Both the Austrian and M. D. Anderson studies have established that the use of GM-CSF before chemotherapy can be safe. Both studies have demonstrated considerable patient-to-patient variability in hematologic response during the GM-CSF prephase reminiscent of the variability demonstrated in the in vitro studies just discussed. Future attention should probably focus on the following. First, it should actually be demonstrated that administration of CSFs to patients increases clonogenic cell kill by Ara-C ex vivo, as has been demonstrated in vitro. Second, a readily measurable biologic parameter that correlates with an increase in clonogenic cell kill should be identified, such as an ex vivo increase in thymidine incorporation after CSF administration that may parallel an increase in colony formation by AML-CFU. Third, it would be helpful if a clinical parameter that correlates with the biologic parameter could be identified to provide a readily measurable end point for CSF therapy. The data of Estey et al. suggest that an increase in circulating blast cell count, which could reflect accelerated release from the marrow rather than an increase in proliferation, may be an inappropriate end point; changes in the marrow blast count can be difficult to detect in patients with AML, whose marrow initially contains a high percentage of blasts. Finally, the ex vivo response to the CSF should be correlated with the in vitro response. The variability in response to CSFs noted in both in vitro and clinical studies suggests that the approach to CSF therapy may need to differ in different patients. For example, in some patients the appropriate CSF would be GM-CSF and in others a combination of IL-3, GM-CSF, and G-CSF. If the in vitro response can be correlated with the ex vivo response, it might be possible in the future to test patient responses to a panel of growth factors in vitro and to use the results to select the appropriate factor to administer to the patient.

The variability in response to CSFs, which has been stressed throughout, may provide a tool to increase our understanding of AML. First, the variability could be used to further characterize the different known variants of AML that are currently best defined, certainly prognostically, by karyotype. For example, it has been suggested that karyotype is a reflection of the stage of differentiation of the cell that has undergone malignant transformation; for example, when a multipotent stem cell is the target of the malignant process, monosomy 7 may result. If this were true one might expect AML-CFU from patients with monosomy 7 to be poorly responsive to a factor like G-CSF, which targets relatively late progenitors. Should this be the case, it might be possible to use the response to G-CSF as a tool to recognize patients who, although a cytogenetic abnormality cannot be detected, have the same prognosis as patients with monosomy 7 based on their response to G-CSF. That is, the response to CSFs may provide a basis for a new classification system that perhaps would reflect "biology" better than the current systems. Based on what we know to date, such a system would likely be quite complex; for example, the no response category would include patients who do not respond on the basis of receptor number and/or affinity as well on the basis of alterations in one of several possible points in the signal transduction pathway from receptor to nucleus. At first glance the possible complexities involved with such a classification seem overwhelming. However, the clinical prognosis of AML is so variable that such a system may be necessary to accommodate this variability.

REFERENCES

1. Cronkite EP. Analytical review of structure and regulation of hemopoiesis. Blood Cells 1988; 14:313–28.
2. Dexter TM. Regulation of hemopoietic cell growth and development: experimental and clinical studies. Leukemia 1989; 3:469–74.
3. Eaves AC, Eaves C. Maintenance and proliferation control of primitive hemopoietic progenitors in long-term cultures of human marrow cells. Blood Cells 1988; 14:355–68.
4. Ogawa M, Clark SC. Synergistic interaction between interleukin-6 and interleukin-3 in support of stem cell proliferation in culture. Blood Cells 1988; 14:329–37.
5. Graham GJ, Wright EG, Hewick R, et al. Identification and characterization of an inhibitor of hemopoietic stem cell proliferation. Nature 1990; 344:442–4.

6. Metcalf D. The molecular control of cell division, differentiation commitment and maturation in hemopoietic cells. Nature 1989; 339:27–30.
7. Morstyn G, Burgess AW. Hemopoietic growth factors: a review. Cancer Res 1988; 48:5624–37.
8. Cannistra SA, Griffin JD. Regulation of the production and function of granulocytes and monocytes. Semin Hematol 1988; 25 (3):173–88.
9. Bot FJ, van Eijk L, Schipper P, Backx B, Löwenberg B. Synergistic effects between GM-CSF and G-CSF or M-CSF on highly enriched human marrow progenitor cells. Leukemia 1990; 4:325–8.
10. Vadhan-Raj S, Keating M, LeMaistre A, et al. Effects of recombinant human granulocyte-macrophage colony-stimulating factor in patients with myelodysplastic syndromes. Engl J 1987; 317:1545–52.
11. Antin JH, Smith BR, Holmes W, Rosenthal DS. Phase I/II study of recombinant human granulocyte-macrophage colony-stimulating factor in aplastic anemia and myelodysplastic syndrome. Blood 1988; 72:705–13.
12. Ganser A, Völkers B, Greher J, et al. Recombinant human granulocyte-macrophage colony-stimulating factor in patients with myelodysplastic syndromes—a phase I/II trial. Blood 1989; 73:31–7.
13. Griffin J, Löwenberg B. Clonogenic cells in acute myeloblastic leukemia. Blood 1986; 68:1185–95.
14. Fialkow PH, Singer JW, Adamson JW, et al. Acute non-lymphocytic leukemia: heterogeneity of stem cell origin. Blood 1981; 57:1068–73.
15. Keinänen M, James MS, Griffin JD, Bloomfield CD, Machnicki J, de la Chapelle A. Clonal chromosomal abnormalities showing multiple-cell-lineage involvement in acute myeloid leukemia. N Engl J Med 1988; 318:1153–8.
16. Griffin JD, Young D, Hermann F, Wagner K, Wiper D, Sabbath KD. Effects of recombinant human GM-CSF on proliferation of clonogenic cells in acute myeloblastic leukemia. Blood 1986; 67:1448–53.
17. Hoang T, Wong G, Nara N, Clark S, Minden MD, McCulloch EA. Effects of recombinant GM-CSF on the blast cells of acute myeloblastic leukemia. Blood 1986; 68:313–6.
18. Kelleher C, Miyauchi J, Wong G, Clark S, Minden M, McCulloch EA. Synergism between recombinant growth factors, GM-CSF and G-CSF, acting on the blast cells of acute myeloblastic leukemia. Blood 1987; 69:1498–503.
19. Vellenga E, Delwel HR, Touw IP, Lowenberg B. Pattern of acute myeloid leukemia colony growth in response to recombinant granulocyte-macrophage colony-stimulating factor (rGM-CSF). Exp Hematol 1987; 15:652–6.
20. Vellenga E, Young DC, Wagner K, Wiper D, Ostapovicz D, Griffin JD. The effects of GM-CSF in promoting growth of clonogenic cells in acute myeloblatic leukemia. Blood 1987; 69:1771–6.
21. Löwenberg B, Salem M, Delwel R. Effects of recombinant multi-CSF, GM-CSF, G-CSF and M-CSF on the proliferation and maturation of human AML in vitro. Blood Cells 1988; 14:539–49.
22. Cozzolino F, Rubartelli A, Aldinucci D, Sitia R, Torcia M, Shaw A, Guglielmo DR. Interleukin 1 as an autocrine growth factor for acute myeloid leukemia cell. Proc Natl Acad Sci U S A 1989; 86:2369–73.

23. Delwel R, van Buitenen C, Salem M, et al. Interleukin-1 stimulates proliferation of acute myeloblastic leukemia cells by induction of granulocyte-macrophage colony-stimulating factor release. Blood 1989; 74:586–93.
24. Bradbury D, Bowen G, Kozlowski R, Reilly I, Russell N. Endogenous interleukin-1 can regulate the autonomous growth of the blast cells of acute myeloblastic leukemia by inducing autocrine secretion of GM-CSF. Leukemia 1990; 4:44–7.
25. Hoang T, Haman A, Goncalves O, et al. Interleukin 1 enhances growth factor-dependent proliferation of the clonogenic cells in acute myeloblastic leukemia and of normal human primitive hemopoietic precursors. J Exp Med 1988; 168:463–74.
26. Hoang T, Haman A, Goncalves O, Wong GG, Clark SC. Interleukin-6 enhances growth factor-dependent proliferation of the blast cells of acute myeloblastic leukemia. Blood 1988; 72:823–6.
27. Salem M, Delwel R, Touw I, Mahmoud LA, Elbasousy EM, Löwenberg B. Modulation of colony stimulating factor (CSF)-dependent growth of acute myeloid leukemia by tumor necrosis factor. Leukemia 1990; 4:37–43.
28. Hoang T, Levy B, Onetto N, Haman A, Rodriguez-Cimadevilla JC. Tumor necrosis factor α stimulates the growth of the clonogenic cells of acute myeloblastic leukemia in synergy with granulocyte/macrophage colongy-stimulating factor. J Exp Med 1989; 170:15–26.
29. Budel LM, Elbaz O, Hoogerbrugge H, et al. Common binding structure for granulocyte macrophage colony-stimulating factor and interleukin-3 on human acute myeloid leukemia cells and monocytes. Blood 1990; 75:1439–45.
30. Onetto-Pothier N, Aumont N, Haman A, et al. Characterization of granulocyte-macrophage colony-stimulating factor receptor on the blast cells of acute myeloblastic leukemia. Blood 1990; 75:59–66.
31. Budel LM, Touw IP, Delwel R, Löwenberg B. Granulocyte colony-stimulating factor receptors in human acute myelocytic leukemia. Blood 1989; 74:2668–73.
32. Budel LM, Touw IP, Delwel R, Clark SC, Löwenberg B. Interleukin-3 and granulocyte-mononocyte colony-stimulating factor receptors on human acute myelocytic leukemia cells and relationship to the proliferative response. Blood 1989; 74:565–71.
33. Park LS, Waldron PE, Friend D, et al. Interleukin-3, GM-CSF, and G-CSF receptor expression on cell lines and primary leukemia cells: receptor heterogeneity and relationship to growth factor responsiveness. Blood 1989; 74:56–65.
34. Evans JAM, Mire-Sluis AR, Hoffbrand AV, Wickremasinghe RG. Binding of G-CSF, GM-CSF, tumor necrosis factor-α and γ-interferon to cell surface receptors on human myeloid leukemia cells triggers rapid tyrosine and serine phosphorylation of a 75-d protein. Blood 1990; 75:88–95.
35. Begley CG, Metcalf, Nicola NA. Primary human myeloid leukemia cells: comparative responsiveness to proliferative stimulation by GM-CSF or G-CSF and membrane expression of CSF receptors. Leukemia 1987; 1:1–8.
36. Young DC, Griffin JD. Autocrine secretion of GM-CSF in acute myeloblastic leukemia. Blood 1986; 68:1178–81.
37. Young DC, Wagner K, Griffin JD. Constitutive expression of the granulocyte-macrophage colony-stimulating factor gene in acute myeloblastic leukemia. J Clin Invest 1987; 79:100–6.

38. Cheng GYM, Kelleher CA, Miyauchi J, et al. Structure and expression of genes of GM-CSF and G-CSF in blast cells from patients with acute myeloblastic leukemia. Blood 1988; 71:204–8.
39. Young DC, Demetri GD, Ernst TJ, Cannistra SA, Griffin JD. In vitro expression of colony-stimulating factor genes by human acute myeloblastic leukemia cells. Exp Hematol 1988; 16:378–82.
40. Kaufman DC, Baer MR, Gao XZ, Wang Z, Preisler HD. Enhanced expression of the granulocyte-macrophage colony stimulating factor gene in acute myelocytic leukemia cells following in vitro blast cell enrichment. Blood 1988; 72:1329–32.
41. Oster W, Cicco NA, Klein H, et al. Participation of the cytokines interleukin 6, tumor necrosis factor alpha and interleukin 1-beta secreted by acute myelogenous leukemia blasts in autocrine and paracrine leukemia growth control. J Clin Invest 1989; 84:451–7.
42. Griffin JD, Rambaldi A, Vellenga E, Young DC, Ostapovicz D, Cannistra SA. Secretion of interleukin-1 by acute myeloblastic leukemia cells in vitro induces endothelial cells to secrete colony stimulating factors. Blood 1987; 70:1218–21.
43. Murohashi I, Tohda S, Suzuki T, Nagata K, Yamashita Y, Nara N. Autocrine growth mechanisms of the progenitor of blast cells in acute myeloblastic leukemia. Blood 1989; 74:35–41.
44. Ernst TJ, Ritchie AR, O'Rourke R, Griffin JD. Colony-stimulating factor gene expression in human acute myeloblastic leukemia cells is posttranscriptionally regulated. Leukemia 1989; 3:620–5.
45. Stocking C, Löliger C, Kawai M, Suciu S, Gough N, Ostertag W. Identification of genes involved in growth autonomy of hematopoietic cells by analysis of factor-independent mutants. Cell 1988; 53:869–79.
46. Souza LM, Boone TC, Gabrilove J, et al. Recombinant human granulocyte colony-stimulating factor: effects on normal and leukemic myeloid cells. Science 1986; 232:61–5.
47. Nicola NA, Begley CG, Metcalf D. Identification of the human analogue of a regulator that induces differentiation in murine leuekaemic cells. Nature 1985; 314:625–9.
48. Estey EH, Dixon D, Kantarjian HM, et al. Treatment of poor-prognosis, newly diagnosed acute myeloid leukemia with Ara-C and recombinant human granulocyte-macrophage colony-stimulating factor. Blood 1990; 75:1766–9.
49. Buechner T, Hiddemann W, Koenigsmann M, et al. Hematologic and therapeutic effects of recombinant human GM-CSF following chemotherapy (CT) in patients with acute leukemias at higher age or after relapse. Blood 1989; 74 (7, suppl 1:27a).
50. Wolff S, Herzig R, Fay J, et al. High-dose cytarabine and daunorubicin as consolidation therapy for acute myeloid leukemia in first remission: long term followup and results. J Clin Oncol 1989; 7:1260–7.
51. Cannistra SA, Groshek P, Griffin JD. Granulocyte-macrophage colony-stimulating factor enhances the cytotoxic effects of cytosine arabinoside in acute myeloblastic leukemia and in the myeloid blast crisis phase of chronic myeloid leukemia. Leukemia 1989; 3:328–34.

52. Tafuri A, Lemoll RM, Gulati S, Clarkson B, Andreff M. Rationale and limitations of combined cytokine-chemotherapy treatment for acute myeloblastic leukemia (AML). Blood 1989; 74 (7, suppl 1:231a).
53. Miyauchi J, Kelleher CA, Wang C, Minkin L, McCulloch EA. Growth factor influence the sensitivity of leukemic stem cells to cytosine arabinoside in culture. Blood 1989; 73:1272–8.
54. Bhalla K, Birkhofer M, Arlin Z, Grant S, Lutzky J, Graham G. Effect of recombinant GM-CSF on the metabolism of cytosine arabinoside in normal and leukemic human bone marrow cells. Leukemia 1988; 2:810–3.
55. Muhm M, Andreeff M, Geissler K, et al. RhGM-CSF in combination with chemotherapy—a new strategy in the therapy of acute myeloid leukemia. Blood 1989; 74 (7, suppl 1:117a).

13

Interleukin-3: A Review

Razelle Kurzrock, Moshe Talpaz, and Jordan U. Gutterman

University of Texas, M. D. Anderson Cancer Center, Houston, Texas

I. INTRODUCTION

The hematopoietic growth factors are glycoprotein hormones that regulate the proliferation and differentiation of hematopoietic progenitor cells and the function of mature blood cells (1–4). That circulating factors control red cell production was recognized in 1906 by Carnot and Deflandre, who induced erythrocytosis in normal rabbits by infusing them with plasma from anemic animals (5). Then, in the 1960s, Pluznik and Sachs (6) and Bradley and Metcalf (7) developed the semisolid culture systems requisite for the growth of bone marrow progenitor cells in vitro. This led to the discovery of hematopoietic growth factors, originally termed colony-stimulating factors (CSFs) because they stimulated the formation of colonies of cells derived from individual bone marrow progenitors. It is now known that such factors appear to fall into two broad, albeit overlapping, categories: multipotential growth factors and lineage-restricted growth factors. Interleukin-3 (IL-3) exemplifies a multilineage hematopoietin and has therefore also been designated multi-CSF.

The introduction of techniques for the purification of small amounts of proteins, particularly the development of high-performance liquid chromatography and the parallel development of microsequencing methodology, allowed the partial amino acid sequencing of these factors. Finally, recent cloning of the hematopoietin genes has permitted the production of large amounts of purified material suitable for exploitation in the clinical setting (8,9). The preliminary results of trials using these molecules suggest that they are potent inducers of blood cell production in vivo and are therefore likely to revolutionize the manner in which hematologic problems are managed.

II. CELLULAR AND MOLECULAR BIOLOGY

A. Endogenous Sources

A. Interleukin-3 is a product of activated T helper cells that have been stimulated by antigens or lectins (Table 1). This lymphokine can also be obtained from cloned T cell lines. In addition, certain myeloid leukemias (e.g., WEHI-3B) represent pathologic sources of interleukin-3 (reviewed in Ref. 32).

TABLE 1 Characteristics of Interleukin-3[a]

Normal cellular source	T helper lymphocyte (8,10) (CD^{28+} subset) (11)
Chromosomal location	5q23–33 (12)
Progenitor cell targets	CFU-blast, CFU-GEMM, CFU-GM, CFU-G, CFU-M, CFU-Eo, CFU-MEG, CFU-baso, BFU-E (13–21)
Molecular mass	14,000–28,000
Homology between murine and human proteins	29%
Synergy (in vitro) between IL-3 and other hematopoietins (reviewed in Ref. 32)	IL-3 synergizes with:IL-6, G-CSF, and erythropoietin to stimulate the proliferation of hematopoietic stem cells (22–24); erythropoietin, BFU-E (24,25); M-CSF, CFU-M, CFU-GM, (26–28); IL-4, BFU-E, CFU-G, CFU-M, CFU-mast (29,30); IL-1 and IL-5, CFU-Eo (31); hemin, CFU-GEMM (32); GM-CSF and erythropoietin, CFU-MEG (33)
Synergy (in vivo) between IL-3 and other hematopoietins	IL-3 followed by GM-CSF produces synergistic myelomonocytic cell increases in primates and mice (27,34,35); IL-3 followed by erythropoietin enhances the expansion of erythroid progenitors and reticulocytes in primates (36)

[a]BFU-E = burst forming unit erythroid; CFU = colony-forming unit; CFU-baso = colony-forming unit basophil; CFU-Eo = colony-forming unit eosinophil; CFU-G = colony-forming unit granulocyte; CFU-M = colony-forming unit macrophage; CFU-MEG = colony-forming unit megakaryocyte; G-CSF = granulocyte colony-stimulating factor; GM-CSF = granulocyte macrophage colony-stimulating factor; M-CSF = macrophage colony-stimulating factor.

B. Cellular Growth and Function

The hematopoietins interact with blood cells at different levels in the cascade of cell differentiation, from the multipotent progenitor to the circulating mature cell. In general, colony-stimulating factors have several distinct activities: they enhance survival, promote proliferation, induce differentiation, and stimulate functional activation (37–40). IL-3 supports progenitors at early stages of hematopoietic development but needs other factors for the process of terminal differentiation (41). The progenitor cell targets are of multiple cell lineages (Table 1) and include myelomonocytic, erythroid, platelet, and even lymphoid precursors (reviewed in Ref. 32). IL-3 can also induce murine bone marrow elements to differentiate to osteoclastlike cells (42). This molecule can, in addition, provoke the proliferation of pulmonary alveolar macrophages, although not of peritoneal macrophages (43), and can augment phagocytosis by macrophages (44) and eosinophils (45), as well as monocyte fungicidal activity (46). Importantly, some of the proliferative effects of IL-3 on unfractionated, and semipurified bone marrow populations may be indirect and involve accessory cell interactions (47).

In suspension cultures of human bone marrow cells grown in the presence of IL-3, the basophilic, eosinophilic, and neutrophilic myelocytes and macrophages develop within 2 weeks (48). By 3 weeks, however, the majority of nonadherent cells became eosinophilic myelocytes. In contrast to the results seen in mouse bone marrow cell cultures, IL-3 does not induce the differentiation of mast cells in the human system studied by Saito and colleagues (48).

Regulation of megakaryocyte proliferation is an activity of IL-3, and this molecule is obligate for CFU-MEG colony formation and stimulates the proliferation and limited differentiation of megakaryocytes. Full megakaryocyte development requires a synergistic coregulator that influences the characteristics of megakaryocyte maturation, such as number, size, cytoplasmic content, and genetic content in maturity. Indeed, it is also possible that optimum human megakaryocyte formation requires the presence of more than one synergistic regulator (49). Recently, Lotem and coworkers showed that the megakaryocyte-inducing activity of IL-3 may be due to the production of IL-6 in bone marrow cultures (50). It has also been noted that the effect of a suboptimal concentration of IL-6 is additive to that of IL-3 on CFU-MEG (51), a phenomenon postulated to be due to the IL-3-induced expansion of an IL-6-responsive cell (50).

C. IL-3 and Cellular Growth in Human Disease

The effect of IL-3 on bone marrow cultures in certain human diseases has been studied. For instance, Halperin and colleagues (52) noted that IL-3 increased the number and size of the burst forming unit-erythroid (BFU-E) colonies in samples derived from patients with Diamond-Blackfan anemia (a congenital, normochromic macrocytic anemia of infancy characterized by absent reticulocyte response and decreased marrow erythroid cells). Further, these individuals have an impaired dose response to erythropoietin, and IL-3 was able to correct this defect. These experiments suggest the possibility of IL-3 as a therapeutic agent in Diamond-Blackfan anemia.

The effect of IL-3 on blasts cells derived from patients with acute myelogenous leukemia has also been assessed (53). IL-3 was found to be an effective stimulator of blast renewal and terminal divisions, although great patient-to-patient variation was apparent. Whether there is a preferential effect on normal versus leukemic blast cells is not known.

D. Synergy

IL-3 enhances the effects of many other hematopoietins (Table 1). In particular, IL-3 has been shown to be synergistic with IL-6 (22), G-CSF (23), and erythropoietin (24) in supporting proliferation of human hematopoietic stem cells in vitro. IL-3 also potentiates the induction capacity of erythropoietin for erythroid burst colony formation (24). Warren and Moore (31) have demonstrated that there is, in addition, potentiation between IL-3 and IL-1, as well as between IL-3 and IL-5 in the production of eosinophils from primitive precursor elements. Their data suggest that the concatenate action of IL-1, IL-3, and IL-5 is a requirement for the in vitro generation of eosinophils from progenitors (31). Synergism between M-CSF and IL-3 is evident in the regulation of the in vitro proliferation of monocytes and macrophages (26). Similarly, combinations of IL-3 and IL-4 enhance the generation of BFU-E, CFU-G, CFU-M, and CFU-mast (30). Finally, as discussed shortly, in monkey and mouse studies, sequential administration of IL-3 and GM-CSF results in synergistic myeloid responses.

E. Cytokine Induction

IL-3 enhances the endotoxin-associated release of tumor necrosis factor (TNF-α) from monocytes (54). Therefore, IL-3 may stimulate killing indirectly by enhancing the expression of TNF.

F. Receptors

IL-3 ligates to a receptor distinct from that of other colony-stimulating factors and interleukins (55). At the target cell level, however, occupation by one colony-stimulating factor of its receptors downregulates other colony-stimulating factor receptors, a phenomenon known as cross- or trans-modulation (55,56). It is uncertain whether downmodulation in this context leads to inactivation or activation. What is known biologically is that the colony-stimulating factors can interact on the same target cell and produce potentiated responses.

The murine IL-3 receptor is estimated to have a molecular mass of 72,500 (57), and the human IL-3 receptor, 140,000. One laboratory found high-affinity

IL-3 receptors on 13 of 15 acute myelogenous leukemia cases (58). Monocytes from normal individuals can also bind IL-3 (57). In a different study, however, only one of five leukemia cell lines having a monocytic or myelogenous phenotype bound ^{125}I-radiolabeled IL-3 (59), but three cell lines of pre-B cell phenotype did so (59). Nonetheless, cells isolated from patients with acute lymphoblastic leukemia did not bind IL-3 (57).

One group of researchers (60) has estimated that the IL-3 receptor density varies between 2000 and 5000 per cell for different factor-dependent cell lines, whereas another group (61) obtained estimates of only 1000 receptors per cell. Finally, Park and colleagues (62) has suggested that maximum biologic activity can be obtained with only 50% receptor saturation.

G. Structure and Sequence

The human, murine, rat, and gibbon IL-3 genes have been cloned (13,63–70). Expression systems for IL-3 cDNA have consisted of both prokaryotic and mammalian cell lines (13,45,63–70). Recombinant IL-3 produced by bacteria is not glycosylated but still exhibits biologic activities similar to those of naturally produced IL-3 (69,70), an observation that suggests that the carbohydrate moiety present on the molecule, although extensive, is not required for its biologic activity in vivo or in vitro.

Human IL-3 is distinct in structure and sequence from the other colony-stimulating factors. Further, this molecule has only 29% amino acid homology to its murine counterpart (Table 1). There is therefore no cross-species activity between the human and mouse molecules. In contrast, gibbon and human IL-3 share 93% of their sequence.

After removal of the signal peptide, the molecular mass of IL-3 is 14,000–28,000. Common decanucleotide regions (71), which possibly represent transcription-activating signals, lie 5′ to the genes for IL-3, GM-CSF, Il-2 and interferon-γ, all of which are molecules produced coordinately by T lymphocytes after stimulation by lectins (inductive signaling).

H. IL-3 and Tyrosine Kinases

Tyrosine phosphokinase activity is a unique enzymatic property. It is associated with less than 1% of cellular proteins but is nonetheless pivotal in regulating growth and differentiation, as evidenced by its close coupling to the ability of many oncogenes and growth factor receptors to exert their effects.

IL-3 inhibits the tyrosine kinase enzymatic activity (but not the mRNA levels) of viral SRC in murine cell lines infected by this virus (72). Other studies suggest that IL-3-induced coativation of serine/threonine and tyrosine kinase activities may be an important element in IL-3 signal transduction (73). In fact, IL-3 stimulates the tyrosine phosphorylation of a set of proteins distinct from those phosphorylated by IL-2, IL-4, and GM-CSF (74). Finally, Ableson murine leukemia virus infection abrogates the requirement for IL-3 in a variety of cell lineages by a nonautocrine mechanism. Experiments suggest that the IL-3 requirement is eliminated because of high levels of tyrosine phosphorylated proteins in the cells with an active viral-ABL gene (75) or, alternatively, because of induction of the C-MYC protooncogene (76).

I. Signal Transduction

Several signal transduction pathways have been suggested for IL-3. These include activation of protein kinase C (77,78) and fluctuations in cytoplasmic ATP (38), glucose transport (79), or calcium (80).

J. Chromosomal Localization

IL-3 is found on the long arm of chromosome 5 and is closely linked to GM-CSF. Indeed, these two hematopoietins are only 9 kilobases apart (12). Apparently, a cluster of hematopoietic growth factors and their receptors reside in this region of the genome (81). It has been shown that IL-3, as well as other hematopoietins, are often deleted in myelodysplastic patients with a 5q- abnormality (82). Although intriguing, the significance of this finding for the pathogenesis of the disease is unknown.

K. Interleukin-3 and Transformation

Proliferation of normal diploid cells in culture is under the control of growth factors. In the absence of the proper mitogens, cells leave the cell cycle and become reversibly arrested in the G_1/G_0 phase. Transformed cells have relaxed cell cycle control and may reverse the cell cycle in the absence of endogenous growth factors. Lack of growth factor requirement seems to be an important feature of transformed cells and contributes to their defective growth control. There are experimental data that favor the notion that growth factor independence in the autonomous growth of transformed cells may be due to the constitutive expression of any of the controlling elements along the normal mitogenic pathway: the growth factor itself, the membrane receptor serving as a transducer of the extracellular signal, or the intracellular signal system that ultimately leads to the initiation of DNA synthesis (83,84). The constitutively expressed factors that function as transforming proteins in the malignant cell may be encoded by oncogenes, or alternatively, their expression may be under the control of oncogenes. There is already evidence that several oncogenes encode proteins that are identical to growth factors or their receptors. For instance, the SIS oncogene encodes the β chain of the platelet-derived growth factor, and the FMS oncogene encodes the M-CSF receptor. Interleukin-3, to date, has not been found to be related to an oncogene, yet several lines of experimental evidence suggest that aberrant expression of this molecule can cause altered growth patterns and, under certain circumstances, be tumorigenic. On the premise that autocrine stimulation can be a mechanism of transformation (83), Chang and coworkers (85) infected murine marrow cells with a retroviral vector bearing an IL-3 cDNA insert and then transplanted these cells into lethally irradiated syngeneic recipients. Extremely high levels of IL-3 were detected in the sera of these animals, and they developed a myeloproliferative syndrome with extensive neutrophilic infiltration of the spleen, lung, liver, and muscle. The majority of transplanted mice died within 5 weeks. The infected cells did not produce any disease when transplanted into normal or sublethally irradiated secondary recipients. Thus, dysregulated IL-3 expression by normal hematopoietic cells produces a fatal, but nonneoplastic, myeloproliferative syndrome.

Wong and colleagues (86) have shown that infection of fetal liver cells with a recombinant retrovirus containing the IL-3 coding sequence results in the formation of factor-independent colonies composed of various types of hematopoietic cells. Established cell lines could be generated from these mixed hematopoietic colonies. These lines can secrete a growth factor but were not tumorigenic. Similar results were obtained from infection of two factor-dependent cell lines with the IL-3 virus, except that these clones all became tumorigenic. These data indicate that endogenous IL-3 production can support normal differentiation and immortalization of primary hematopoietic cells or, in previously immortalized cells, can lead to tumorigenicity (86).

III. IN VIVO STUDIES

A. Mouse Studies

IL-3 is the only colony-stimulating factor able to stimulate mast cell proliferation; it has a spectacular dose-related effect in elevating splenic levels of mast cells (up to 100-fold), with lower increases occurring in other tissues (70). IL-3 administration to normal animals also greatly augments CFU-S and CFU-E (87,88). Its action on granulocyte-macrophage levels is intermediate between those of G-CSF and GM-CSF.

B. Monkey Trials

Krumwieh and Seiler (34) administered IL-3 daily, by intravenous bolus injection, to cynomolgus monkeys. This molecule alone did not increase neutrophil counts. However, when IL-3 was given for 8 days followed by 5 days of GM-CSF, synergistic myelomonocytic responses were seen. There was also evidence of increased platelet counts. In a different study (89), IL-3 was administered subcutaneously every day for 14 days to rhesus monkeys. There was an increase in basophils and eosinophils, as well as an increase in histamine levels. As in the previous study, interleukin-3 followed by GM-CSF administration resulted in synergistic stimulation of neutrophil counts. However, simultaneous administration of IL-3 and GM-CSF had the same effect as GM-CSF alone.

The effect of IL-3 on chemotherapy-induced myelosuppression has also been tested (90). There was no significant impact on neutrophil recovery, but eosinophils and basophils increased. Concomitant IL-3 and GM-CSF was not better than GM-CSF alone.

C. Human Studies

Investigation of recombinant IL-3 in the human is currently in early phase I stages. The most complete studies are those performed by us and by Ganser and coworkers in Germany (91). The latter group described preliminary findings in nine patients with bone marrow failure treated with subcutaneously administered material (91). IL-3 was injected daily for 15 days at doses ranging from 60 to 500 μg/m^2. Apparently, multilineage responses were seen in all patients. In our trial (92), a 4 h intravenous infusion was used. Patients were treated daily for 28 days at doses ranging from 30 to 1000 μg/m^2. A total of 24 patients have been entered on the study. Their diagnosis included bone marrow failure caused by myelodysplastic syndrome (13 patients), aplastic anemia (8 patients), or prolonged high-dose chemotherapy (3 patients). Modest responses in all lineages have been observed, although the type and degree of response varies tremendously between individuals. Parallel mixed colony culture assays in two patients showed a significant increase in CFU-GM in one patient, but not in a second, between days 1 and 28. Side effects in both our study and the German group's trial have been minimal and consisted mostly of low-grade fever and mild headaches. The maximum tolerated dose has not been reached.

D. Pharmacology

Pharmocokinetic studies in the cynomolgus monkeys suggest a half-life of 5–10 minutes after IV. bolus injection of IL-3 (34). Our trial in humans also indicates a rapid clearance, with a half-life ranging from 13.4 to 23.5 minutes at a dose of 60 μg/m^2; the mean half-life for the 250 μg/m^2 dose was 53 minutes (92). This short half-life suggests that IL-3 should be given by prolonged IV infusion; alternatively, the subcutaneous or intramuscular routes may be useful, as administration of many cytokines in these ways results in prolonged serum levels.

IV. CONCLUSIONS

The medical uses for hematopoietic growth factors may be applied to three general areas: replenishment of iatrogenic or disease-associated hematopoietic dysfunction by raising cell counts from suppressed to normal levels; augmentation of host defenses against infections; and the increased production of effector cells with cytotoxic activities.

The correction of suppressed blood counts is the most clear-cut therapeutic expectation. Granulocytopenia, thrombocytopenia, and anemia are frequent causes of morbidity and mortality after chemotherapy and radiation therapy of cancer patients and often limit the doses of effective therapeutic agents. Furthermore, many disease states, including the myelodysplastic syndrome, acquired immunodeficiency syndrome (AIDS), aplastic anemia, and solid tumors metastatic to the bone marrow, may themselves cause intractable cytopenias. Treatment of anemia with red blood cell transfusions is possible but not without side effects. Platelet transfusions may be a useful temporizing measure, but many patients quickly become resistant to donor platelets. The short half-life of granulocytes makes transfusion of this blood element of limited therapeutic benefit, and many granulocytopenic patients succumb to infection. These theoretical considerations have already prompted clinical trials of some of the hematopoietic growth factors (GM-CSF, G-CSF, and erythropoietin), with extremely encouraging results (93–95). The beneficial effects were accomplished with remarkably few side effects. Ultimately, combinations of different CSFs may be tailored to the needs of individual disease states.

IL-3 is a potent CSF that affects a relatively early progenitor cell in vitro. In the presence of the proper additional factors, these progenitors can mature into elements of neutrophilic, macrophage-monocytic, eosinophilic, megakaryocytic, and erythroid lineages. Hence, IL-3 may have a multiplicity of effects on blood cells in vivo and could be effective at raising granulocyte, monocyte, and platelet counts and alleviating anemia. The therapeutic applications for an agent with such a broad spectrum of hematopoietic effects encompasses disease-related and iatrogenic cytopenias (due to chemotherapy, radiation therapy, or transplantation), AIDS and other immunodeficiency diseases, malignancies, and infectious processes. Human IL-3 has only recently been cloned, and hence its potential salutary properties are only in their most preliminary stages of testing. However, results to date indicate that this molecule has few side effects and is biologically active in both humans and other primates, although its maximum potential may be realized only when it is administered in combination with other hematopoietins.

ACKNOWLEDGMENTS

Research conducted in part by the Clayton Foundation for Research. Dr. Gutterman is a Senior Clayton Foundation Investigator.

REFERENCES

1. Metcalf D. The granulocyte-macrophage colony-stimulating factors. Science 1985; 229:16–22.

2. Clark SC, Kaman R. The human hematopoietic colony-stimulating factors. Science 1987; 236:1229–37.
3. Sieff CA. Hematopoietic growth factors. J Clin Invest 1987; 79:1549–57.
4. Groopman JE, Molina J-M, Scadden DT. Hematopoietic growth factors: biology and clinical applications. N Engl J Med 1989; 321:1449–59.
5. Carnot P, Deflandre C. Sur l'activite hemopoietique des differents organes au cours de la regeneration du sang. CR Hebd Acad Sci 1906; 143:432–5.
6. Pluznik DH, Sachs L. The cloning of normal "mast" cells in tissue culture. J Cell Comp Physiol 1965; 66:319–24.
7. Bradley TR, Metcalf D. The growth of mouse bone marrow cells in vitro. Aust J Exp Biol Med Sci 1966; 44:287–99.
8. Otsuka T, Miyajima A, Brown H, et al. Isolation and characterization of an expressible cDNA encoding human IL-3: induction of IL-3 mRNA in human T-cell clones. J Immunol 1988; 140:2288–95.
9. Dorssers L, Burger H, Bot F, et al. Characterization of a human multilineage colony-stimulating factor cDNA clone identified by a conserved noncoding sequence in mouse interleukin-3. Gene 1987; 55:115–24.
10. Niemeyer CM, Sieff CA, Mathey-Prevot B, et al. Expression of human interleukin-3 (multi-CSF) is restricted to human lymphocytes and T-cell tumor lines. Blood 1989; 73:945–51.
11. Guba SC, Stella G, Turka LA, June CH, Thompson CB, Emerson SG. Regulation of interleukin-3 gene induction in normal human T-cells. J Clin Invest 1989; 84:1701–6.
12. Yang YC, Kovacic S, Kriz R, et al. The human genes for GM-CSF and IL-3 are closely linked in tandem on chromosome 5. Blood 1988; 71:958–61.
13. Yang YC, Ciarletta AB, Temple PA, et al. Human IL-3 (multi-CSF): identification by expression cloning of a novel hematopoietic growth factor related to murine IL-3. Cell 1986; 47:3–10.
14. Leary AG, Yang YC, Clark SC, Gasson JC, Golde DW, Ogawa M. Recombinant gibbon interleukin-3 supports formation of human multilineage colonies and blast cell colonies in culture: Comparison with recombinant human granulocyte-macrophage colony-stimulating factor. Blood 1987; 70:1343–8.
15. Sonada Y, Yang YC, Wong GG, Clark SC, Ogawa M. Analysis in serum-free culture of the targets of recombinant human hematopoietic growth factors: interleukin-3 and granulocyte/macrophage-colony-stimulating factor are specific for early developmental stages. Proc Natl Acad Sci U S A 1988; 85:4360–4.
16. Long MW, Hutchinson RJ, Gragowski LL, Heffner CH, Emerson SG. Synergistic regulation of human megakaryocyte development. J Clin Invest 1988; 82:1779–86.
17. Bruno E, Miller ME, Hoffman R. Interacting cytokines regulate in vitro human megakaryocytopoiesis. Blood 1989; 73:671–7.
18. Metcalf D, Begley CG, Johnson GR, et al. Biologic properties in vitro of a recombinant human granulocyte-macrophage colony-stimulating factor. Blood 1986; 67:37–45.
19. Caracciolo D, Clark SC, Rovera G. Human interleukin-6 supports granulocytic differentiation of hematopoietic progenitor cells and acts synergistically with GM-CSF. Blood 1989; 73:666–70.

20. Hoang T, Haman A, Goncalves O, et al. Interleukin-1 enhances growth factor-dependent proliferation of the clonogenic cells in acute myeloblastic leukemia and of normal human primitive hematopoietic precursors. J Exp Med 1988; 168:463–74.
21. Bruno E, Briddell R, Hoffman R. Effect of recombinant and purified hematopoietic growth factors on human megakaryocyte colony formation. Exp Hematol 1988; 16:371–7.
22. Leary AG, Ikebuchi K, Hirai Y, et al. Synergism between interleukin-6 and interleukin-3 in supporting proliferation of human hematopoietic stem cells: comparison with interleukin-1α. Blood 1988; 71:1759–63.
23. Ikebuchi K, Clark SC, Ihle JN, Souza LM, Ogawa M. Granulocyte colony-stimulating factor enhances interleukin-3-dependent proliferation of multipotential hempoietic progenitors. Proc Natl Acad Sci U S A 1988; 85:3445–9.
24. Migliaccio G, Migliaccio AR, Visser JWM. Synergism between erythropoietin and interleukin-3 in the induction of hematopoietic stem cell proliferation and erythroid burst colony formation. Blood 1988; 72:944–51.
25. Suda J, Suda T, Kubota K, Ihle JN, Saito M, Mirua Y. Purified interleukin-3 and erythropoietin support the terminal differentiation of hemopoietic progenitors in serum-free culture. Blood 1986; 76:1002–6.
26. Chen BD-M, Clark CR. Interleukin-3 (IL-3) regulates the in vitro proliferation of both blood monocytes and peritoneal exudate macrophages: synergism between a macrophage lineage-specific colony-stimulating factor (CSF-1) and IL-3. J Immunol 1986; 137:563–70.
27. Broxmeyer HE, Williams DE, Hangoc G, et al. Synergistic myelopoietic actions in vivo after administration to mice of combinations of purified natural murine colony-stimulating factor I, recombinant murine interleukin-3, and recombinant murine granulocyte/macrophage colony-stimulating factor. Proc Natl Acad Sci U S A 1987; 84:3871–5.
28. Koike K, Stanley ER, Ihle JN, Ogawa M. Macrophage colony formation supported by purified CSF-1 and/or interleukin-3 in serum-free culture: evidence for hierarchical difference in macrophage colony-forming cells. Blood 1986; 67:859–64.
29. Schmitt E, Fassbender B, Beyreuther K, Spaeth E, Schwarzkopf R, Rude E. Characterization of a T-cell-derived lymphokine that acts synergistically with IL-3 on the growth of murine mast cells and is identical with IL-4. Immunobiology 1987; 174:406–19.
30. Rennick D, Yang G, Muller-Sieburg C, et al. Interleukin-4 (B-cell stimulatory factor-1) can enhance or antagonize the factor-dependent growth of hemopoietic progenitor cells. Proc Natl Acad Sci U S A 1987; 84:6889–93.
31. Warren DJ, Moore MAS. Synergism among interleukin-1, interleukin-3, and interleukin-5 in the production of eosinophils from primitive hemopoietic stem cells. J Immunol 1988; 140:94–9.
32. Monette FC. The role of interleukin-3 and heme in the induction of erythropoiesis. Ann N Y Sci 1989; 554:49–58.
33. Teramura M, Katahira J, Hoshino S, Motoji T, Oshimi K, Mizoguchi H. Effect of recombinant hemopoietic growth factors on human megakaryocyte colony formation in serum-free cultures. Exp Hematol 1989; 17:1011–6.

34. Krumwieh D, Seiler FR. In vivo effects of recombinant colony-stimulating factors on hematopoiesis in cynomolgus monkeys. Transplant Pro 1989; 221:2964–7.
35. Donahue RE, Seehra J, Metzger M, et al. Human IL-3 and GM-CSF act synergistically in stimulating hematopoiesis in primates. Science 1988; 241:1820–2.
36. Umemura T, Al-Khatti A, Donahue RE, Papyannopoulou T, Stamatoyannopoulos G. Effects of interleukin-3 and erythropoietin on in vivo erythropoiesis and F-cell formation in primates. Blood 1989; 74:1571–6.
37. Begley CG, Lopez AF, Nicola NA, et al. Purified colony-stimulating factors enhance the survival of human neutrophils and eosinophils in vitro: a rapid and sensitive microassay for colony-stimulating factors. Blood 1986; 68:162–6.
38. Whetton AD, Dexter TM. Effects of hematopoietic cell growth factor on intracellular ATP levels. Nature 1983; 303:629–31.
39. Metcalf D. Clonal analysis of proliferation and differentiation of paired daughter cells: action of granulocyte-macrophage colony-stimulating factor on granulocyte-macrophage precursors. Proc Natl Acad Sci U S A 1980; 77:5327–30.
40. Metcalf D, Burgess AW. Clonal analysis of progenitor cell commitment to granulocyte and macrophage production. J Cell Physiol 1982; 111:275–84.
41. Sonoda Y, Yang Y-C, Wong GG, Clark SC, Ogawa M. Analysis in serum-free culture of the targets of recombinant human hemopoietic growth factors: interleukin-3 and granulocyte/macrophage-colony-stimulating factor are specific for early developmental stages. Proc Natl Acad Sci U S A 1988; 85:4360–4.
42. Barton BE, Mayer R. IL-3 induces differentiation of bone marrow precursor cells to osteoclast-like cells. J Immunol 1989; 143:3211–6.
43. Chen BD-M, Mueller M, Olencki T. Interleukin-3 (IL-3) stimulates the clonal growth of pulmonary alveolar macrophage of the mouse: role of IL-3 in the regulation of macrophage production outside the bone marrow. Blood 1988; 72:685–90.
44. Crapper RM, Vairo G, Hamilton JA, Clark-Lewis I, Schrader JW. Stimulation of bone marrow-derived and peritoneal macrophages by a T-lymphocyte-derived hempoietic growth factor, persisting cell-stimulating factor. Blood 1985; 66:859–66.
45. Lopez AF, To LB, Yang Y-C, et al. Stimulation of proliferation, differentiation, and function of human cells by primate interleukin-3. Proc Natl Acad Sci U S A 1987; 84:2761–5.
46. Wang M, Freidman H, Djeu JY. Enhancement of human monocyte function against *Candida albicans* by the colony-stimulating factors (CSF): IL-3, granulocyte-macrophage-CSF, and macrophage-CSF. J Immunol 1989; 143:671–7.
47. Kannourakis G, Johnson GR. Proliferative properties of unfractionated, purified, and single cell human progenitor populations stimulated by recombinant human interleukin-3. Blood 1990; 75:370–7.
48. Saito H, Hatake K, Dvorak AM, et al. Selective differentiation and proliferation of hematopoietic cells induced by recombinant human interleukins. Proc Natl Acad Sci U S A 1988; 85:2288–92.
49. Long MW. Regulation of human megakaryocytopoiesis. Ann N Y Acad Sci 1989; 554:192–205.
50. Lotem J, Shabo Y, Sachs L. Regulation of megakaryocyte development by interleukin-6. Blood 1989; 74:1545–51.

51. Bruno E, Hoffman R. Effect of interleukin-6 on in vitro human megakaryocytopoiesis: its interaction with other cytokines. Exp Hematol 1989; 17:1038–43.
52. Halperin DS, Estrov Z, Freedman MH. Diamond-blackfan anemia: promotion of marrow erythropoiesis in vitro by recombinant interleukin-3. Blood 1989; 73:1168–74.
53. Miyauchi J, Kelleher CA, Yang Y-C, et al. The effects of three recombinant growth factors, IL-3, GM-CSF, and G-CSF, on the blast cells of acute myeloblastic leukemia maintained in short-term suspension culture. Blood 1987; 70:657–63.
54. Cannistra SA, Vellenga E, Groshek P, Rambaldi A, Griffin JD. Human granulocyte-monocyte colony-stimulating factor and interleukin-3 stimulate monocyte cytotoxicity through a tumor necrosis factor-dependent mechanism. Blood 1988; 71:672–6.
55. Gesner T, Mufson RA, Turner KJ, Clark SC. Identification through chemical cross-linking of distinct granulocyte-macrophage colony-stimulating factor and interleukin-3 receptors on myeloid leukemic cells, KG-1. Blood 1989; 74:2652–6.
56. Walker F, Nicola NA, Metcalf D, Burgess AW. Hierarchical down-modulation of hemopoietic growth factor receptors. Cell 1985; 43:269–76.
57. Urdal DL, Price V, Sassenfeld HM, Cosman D, Gillis S, Park LS. Molecular characterization of colony-stimulating factors and their receptors: human interleukin-3. Ann N Y Acad Sci 1989; 554:167–76.
58. Budel LM, Touw IP, Delwel R, Clark SC, Lowenberg B. Interleukin-3 and granulocyte-monocyte colony-stimulating factor receptors on human acute myelocytic leukemia cells and relationship to the proliferative response. Blood 1989; 74:565–71.
59. Parks LS, Waldron PE, Friend D, et al. Interleukin-3, GM-CSF and G-CSF receptor expression on cell lines and primary leukemia cells: receptor heterogeneity and relationship to growth factor responsiveness. Blood 1989; 74:56–65.
60. Palaszynski EW, Ihle JN. Evidence for specific receptors for interleukin-3 on lymphokine-dependent cell lines established from long-term bone marrow cultures. J Immunol 1984; 132:1872–9.
61. Crapper RM, Clark-Lewis I, Schrader JW. Analysis of the binding of a hemopoietic growth factor, P-cell-stimulating factor, to a cell surface receptor using quantitative absorption of bioactivity. Exp Hematol 1985; 13:941–7.
62. Park LS, Friend D, Gillis S, Urdal DL. Characterization of the cell surface receptor for a multi-lineage colony-stimulating factor (CSF-2a). J Biol Chem 1986; 261:205–10.
63. Fung MC, Hapel AJ, Ymer S, et al. Molecular clonging of cDNA for mouse interleukin-3. Nature 1984; 307:233–7.
64. Yokota T, Lee R, Rennick D, et al. Isolation and characterization of a mouse cDNA clone that expresses mast-cell growth factor activity in monkey cells. Proc Natl Acad Sci U S A 1984; 81:1070–4.
65. Hapel AJ, Fung MC, Johnson RM, Young IG, Johnson G, Metcalf D. Biologic properties of molecularly cloned and expressed murine interleukin-3. Blood 1985; 65:1453–9.
66. Campbell HD, Ymer S, Fung MC, Young IG. Cloning and nucleotide sequence of the murine interleukin-3 gene. Eur J Biochem 1985; 150:297–303.

67. Kindler V, Thorens B, De Kossodo S, et al. Stimulation of hematopoiesis in vivo by recombinant bacterial murine interleukin-3. Proc Natl Acad Sci U S A 1986; 83:1001–5.
68. Gough NM, Gough J, Metcalf D, et al. Molecular cloning of cDNA encoding a murine haematopoietic growth regulator, granulocyte-macrophage colony-stimulating factor. Nature 1984; 309:763–7.
69. Cohen DR, Hapel AJ, Young IG. Cloning and expression of the rat interleukin-3 gene. Nucleic Acids Res 1986; 14:3641–58.
70. Metcalf D, Begley CG, Johnson GR, Nicola NA, Lopez AF, Williamson DJ. Effects of purified bacterially-synthesized murine multi-CSF (IL-3) on hematopoiesis in normal adult mice. Blood 1986; 68:46–57.
71. Stanley E, Metcalf D, Sobieszczuk P, et al. The structure and expression of the murine gene encoding granulocyte-macrophage colony-stimulating factor: evidence for utilization of alternative promoters. EMBO J 1985; 4:2569–73.
72. Watson JD, Jenkins DR, Eszes M, Leung E. Effect of granulocyte-macrophage colony-stimulating factor and interleukin-3 on the v-*src* oncogene. J Immunol 1988; 140:501–7.
73. Ferris DK, Willet-Brown J, Martensen T, Farrar WL. Interleukin-3 stimulation of tyrosine kinase activity in FDC-P1 cells. Biochem Biophys Res Commun 1988; 154:991–6.
74. Morla AO, Schreures J, Miyajima A, Wang JYJ. Hematopoietic growth factors activate the tyrosine phosphorylation of distinct sets of proteins in interleukin-3-dependent murine cell lines. Mol Cell Biol 1988; 8:2214–8.
75. Kipreos ET, Wang, JYJ. Reversible dependence on growth factor interleukin-3 in myeloid cells expressing temperature sensitive v-*abl* oncogene. Oncogene Res 1988; 2:277–84.
76. Cleveland JL, Dean M, Rosenberg N, Wang JYJ, Rapp UR. Tyrosine kinase oncogenes abrogate interleukin-3 dependence of murine myeloid cells through signaling pathways involving c-*myc*: conditional regulation of c-*myc* transcription by temperature-sensitive v-*abl*. Mol Cell Biol 1989; 9:5685–95.
77. Farrar WL, Thomas TP, Anderson WB. Altered cytosol/membrane enzyme redistribution on interleukin-3 activation of protein kinase C. Nature 1985; 315:235–7.
78. Evans SW, Rennick D, Farrar WL. Multilineage hematopoietic growth factor interleukin-3 and direct activators of protein kinase C stimulate phosphorylation of common substrates. Blood 1986; 68:906–13.
79. Dexter TM, Whetton AD, Bazill GW. Haemopoietic cell growth factor and glucose transport. Its role in cell survival and the relevance of this in normal haemopoiesis and leukaemia. Differentiation 1984; 27:163–7.
80. Rossio JL, Ruscetti FW, Farrar WL. Ligand-specific calcium mobilization in IL-2- and IL-3-dependent cell lines. Lymphokine Res 1986; 5:163–72.
81. van Leeuwen BH, Martinson ME, Webb GC, Young IG. Molecular organization of the cytokine gene cluster, involving the human IL-3, IL-4, IL-5, and GM-CSF genes, on human chromosome 5. Blood 1989; 73:1142–8.
82. LeBeau M, Epstein M, O'Brien SJ, et al. The interleukin-3 gene is located on human chromosome 5 and is deleted in myeloid leukemias with a deletion of 5q. Proc Natl Acad Sci U S A 1987; 84:5913–7.

83. Spron MB, Roberts AB. Autocrine growth factors and cancer. Nature 1985; 313:745.
84. Heldin C-H, Westermark B. Growth factors: mechanism of action and relation to oncogenes. Cell 1984; 37:9–20.
85. Chang JM, Metcalf D, Lang RA, Gonda TJ, Johnson GR. Nonneoplastic hematopoietic myeloproliferative syndrome induced by dysregulated multi-CSF (IL-3) expression. Blood 1989; 73:1487–97.
86. Wong PMC, Chung S-W, Nienhuis AW. Retroviral transfer and expression of the interleukin-3 gene in hemopoietic cells. Genes Dev 1987; 1:358–65.
87. Metcalf D, Begley CG, Nicola NA, Johnson GR. Quantitative responsiveness of murine hemopoietic populations in vitro and in vivo to recombinant multi-CSF (IL-3). Exp Hematol 1987; 15:288–95.
88. Naparstek E, Wagner K, Harrison D, Greenberger JS. Hematopoietic effects of continuous intravenous infusion of mice with growth factors produced by the WEHI-3 cell line. Acta Haematol (Basel) 1987; 77:1–5.
89. Mayer P, Valent P, Schmidt G, Liehl E, Bettelhaim P. The in vivo effects of recombinant human interleukin-3: demonstration of basophil differentiation factor, histamine-producting activity, and priming of GM-CSF-responsive progenitors in nonhuman primates. Blood 1989; 74:613–21.
90. Andreeff M, Welte K. Hematopoietic colony-stimulating factors. Semin Oncol 1989; 16:211–29.
91. Ganser A, Lindemann A, Ottmann OG, et al. Effect of recombinant human interleukin-3 in vivo—a phase I trial (abstract). Exp Hematol 1989; 17:484.
92. Kurzrock R, Talpaz M, Estrov Z, Rosenblum MG, Gutterman J. Phase I study of recombinant interleukin-3 in patients with bone marrow failure. J. Clin Oncol 1991; 9:1241–1250.
93. Groopman JE, Mitsuyasu RT, DeLeo MJ, Oette DH, Golde DW. Effect of recombinant human granulocyte-macrophage colony-stimulating factor on myelopoiesis in the acquired immunodeficiency syndrome. N Engl J Med 1987; 317:593–8.
94. Vadhan-Raj S, Keating M, LeMaistre A, et al. Effects of recombinant human granulocyte macrophage colony-stimulating factor in patients with myelodysplastic syndromes. N Engl J Med 1987; 317:1545–52.
95. Eschbach JW, Egrie JC, Downin MR, Browne JK, Adamson JW. Correction of the anemia of end-stage renal disease with recombinant human erythropoietin. N Engl J Med 1987; 316:73–8.

14

Clinical Value of G-CSF: A Critical Review

Gary Spitzer

St. Louis University Medical Center, St. Louis, Missouri

Migeil Bronchud

Oncological Hospital, Barcelona, Spain

I. INTRODUCTION

The establishment of in vitro culture systems from murine and human marrow and blood for hematopoietic progenitor cells has allowed the recognition of many hematopoietic hormones that regulate blood cell production and differentiation. These glycoproteins, known as colony-stimulating factors and interleukins, have been purified from a number of different sources. The initially purified factors were named according to the predominant colony type that they stimulated in vitro. Granulocyte colony-stimulating factor (G-CSF), like macrophage-CSF (M-CSF) and erythropoietin, is generally considered a lineage-specific growth factor. G-CSF acts on committed granulocytic precursors and increases the number and function of neutrophils, but not macrophages, eosinophils, or basophils. G-CSF, M-CSF, and erythropoietin cause proliferation of late committed progenitors; granulocyte-macrophage CSF (GM-CSF) and interleukin-3 (IL-3) act on earlier progenitors and enhance the function of several different types of differentiated cells (1–4). Recent in vitro work by Ogawa's group (5–8) suggests that G-CSF may also act alone or in concert with other cytokines on very early multipotential progenitors. Both G- and GM-CSF increase neutrophil phagocytosis, promote superoxide anion generation in the presence of chemotactic peptides, such as f-met-leu-phe (fMLP), enhance specific binding of fMLP either by increasing receptor numbers or affinity, heighten arachidonic acid release in response to ionophore and multiple chemoattractant agents, increase antibody-dependent cellular cytotoxicity of tumor targets, and increase in vitro survival of neutrophils. GM-CSF, but not G-CSF, increases expression of the surface membrance adhesion molecule Mo-1 and inhibits neutrophil migration (9–19).

G-CSF is produced by monocyte-macrophage cells and by fibroblasts and endothelial cells in response to IL-1, tumor necrosis factor (TNF), and bacteria (20–25), but (unlike GM-CSF) no G-CSF is apparently produced by activated T lymphocytes. G-CSF levels can be detected in normal volunteers, and they increase dramatically during infectious episodes, returning to baseline values on recovery from the acute stage of infection (26).

G-CSF was purified and characterized from a human bladder carcinoma cell line 5637 and then molecularly cloned and expressed in *Escherichia coli* (27,28). Natural human G-CSF is an 19.6 kD glycoprotein with a single polypeptide chain coded for by a gene on chromosome 17qll-21. G-CSF binds to a single-chain receptor molecule of 150,000 kD present only on cells of neutrophil lineage, which is modulated by cell interaction with other growth factors (29–34). Recombinant human G-CSF, expressed in *E. coli,* differs from native G-CSF by the additon of an N-terminal methionine and the absence of glycosylation, resulting in a molecular weight of 18.8 kD. Human G-CFS has also been isolated from a squamous cell carcinoma line CHU-2 and the gene cloned and expressed in monkey COS cells (35). This last molecule contains an additional three codons, resulting in a longer molecule that appears less active in supporting granulocyte colony formation.

II. PRECLINICAL STUDIES

Preclinical in vivo studies confirmed the limited G-CSF action in vitro. Injection of G-CSF in hamsters and nonhuman primates (cynomologus monkeys) produced a dose-dependent increase in neutrophils only (35–38). Neutrophil functional analysis showed an enhanced ability to kill and phagocytose bacteria. G-CSF accelerated recovery after high-dose cyclophosphamide and also after other cytotoxic drugs that produced significant myelosuppression (36). No evidence of depletion of marrow reserve was seen in animals given repeated doses of G-CSF and cycles of chemotherapy.

III. IN VIVO EFFECTS OF G-CSF IN HUMANS

Several studies have evaluated the hematopoietic effects of G-CSF at different doses. Frequently these same patients have received a subsequent cycle of chemotherapy followed by the same dose of G-CSF.

G-CSF was administered at a dose of 1–60 μg/kg body weight to 22 patients with transitional cell carcinoma before chemotherapy as part of a phase I/II study (39,40). A dose-dependent increase in the absolute neutrophil count of 1.8- to 12-fold was seen. An increase in leukocyte alkaline phosphatase, a marker of secondary granule formation, was also seen. In six of eight patients analyzed, an increase in the ratio of bone marrow myeloid to erythroid cells was seen. Day 14 peripheral blood cell-derived CFU-GM increased by day 6 of G-CSF treatment. Circulating levels of eosinophils (unlike the in vivo effects of GM-CSF) and basophils were unchanged; however, a 10-fold increase in monocytes was observed in patients treated at the highest doses. $CD3^+$ lymphocytes showed a small increase in numbers unrelated to dose. Hemoglobin, hematocrit, and platelet count remained near baseline throughout the period G-CSF administration.

A group of 12 patients with small cell bronchogenic cancer (SCBC) were treated with recombinant human G-CSF given by continuous infusion at doses ranging from 1 to 40 μg/kg per day (10,41). Patients received the G-CSF before the start of intensive chemotherapy and after alternate cycles of chemotherapy. G-CSF in vivo was found to have two main effects: (1) an early fall in peripheral neutrophils within the first hour, followed by a rapid influx of mature neutrophils into the circulatory pool, and (2) stimulation of proliferation and differentiation of neutrophil precursors in the bone marrow as shown by a number of observations: an increase in marrow cellularity of 20% with an increase in myeloid-erythroid ratio and a modest increase (8%) in the S phase of colony-forming units, GM (CFU-GM). Despite the increase in the myeloid-erythroid ratio, the CFU-GM/BFU-E (burst-forming unit erythroid) ratio did not change. Morstyn et al. (42) in their phase I studies showed that the majority of the myeloid hypertrophy was at the promyelocyte level. Neutrophils released into the circulation were normal in tests of their mobility and phagocytic activity. This suggests that the major in vivo effect is on later myeloid cells with proliferative potential rather than CFU-GM.

More extensive studies were carried out in two patients with metastatic breast cancer who were treated with G-CSF (43). [3H]thymidine labeling and autoradiography studies were performed on marrow during therapy. Neutrophil migration was evaluated by labeling with [^{99m}Tc-]hexamethylpropyleneamineoxime following the G-CSF infusion. Proliferation increased in all stages of granulopoiesis, but the most increase was from the myeloblast compartment. Labeled cells appearing in the circulation within 1 day compared to the normal 4 to 5 days. The ^{99m}Tc studies demonstrated no sequestration of circulating neutrophils by spleen, lungs, or liver. The half-life of the circulating neutrophils was not significanty changed, and calculations from the flow of labeled cells to the peripheral blood indicated an increase of 3.2 extra amplification divisions during neutrophil development. The dramatic neutrophil response to G-CSF was due to only a modest increase in granulopoietic activity within the morphologically recognizable myeloid compartment (43). There was an increase in serum lactate dehydrogenase (LDH) and, to a lesser extent, alkaline phosphatase in parallel with the rise in neutrophils, but no changes in platelets, hemoglobin, lymphocytes, monocytes, or eosinophils occurred.

Lindemann et al. administered G-CSF (from 1 to 60 μg/kg/day intravenously, IV, over 30 minutes) to 18 patients with advanced refractory malignancy (44,45). There was, as in all studies, a dose-dependent increase in neutrophils with a mean maximum increase of 1.7-fold at 1 μg, 2.7-fold at 3 μg, 5.2-fold at 10 μg, 7.3-fold at 30, and 11.5-fold at 60 μg/kg, with peak counts occurring at 1 week and no further increases or even a slight decrease with continued treatment. Neutrophil counts returned to the pretreatment baseline within 3–6 days after G-CSF was stopped. No effect on reticulocytes was observed. Platelets tended to decrease (an unusual finding in the other phase I studies) by 20–40% relative to pretreatment levels, with a nadir around day 10 and with an increase in mean platelet volume and increased serum platelet factor IV, suggesting accelerated destruction with compensatory increased production and release of young platelets. Interestingly, after this nadir around day 10, there was a spontaneous recovery in platelet counts despite continued therapy. Serum alkaline phosphatase and LDH increased in parallel with the neutrophil count. The only toxicity was mild to moderate bone pain, usually in the low back, sternum, and ribs. In some patients this was transient and occurred during the G-CSF infusion. In others, the bone pain occurred after several days of treatment, several hours after the daily G-CSF infusion, and lasted for several hours. Sweating and fatigue were also observed in some patients at higher dose levels and occurred in association with very high neutrophil counts.

These phase I studies, in summary, showed a dose-dependent increase in granulocytes and, in some studies at higher doses, an increase in monocytes. The marrow myeloid-erythroid ratio is increased with only a small increase in S phase of CFU-GM but without any obvious increase in number within the marrow. Peripheral blood CFU-GM, however, are increased maximally at approximately 5–7 days after beginning the infusion. The side effects in most studies appear to be predominantly bone pain. Other side effects are rare.

IV. MODIFICATION OF CHEMOTHERAPY TOXICITY AT CONVENTIONAL DOSES

A. Problems in the Design of Clinical Studies

All studies except one on the effect of G-CSF on the rate of myeloid recovery after chemotherapy have used historical controls, concurrent controls who refused to participate in the study but received the same chemotherapy, patients treated with the same chemotherapy just before or just after the G-CSF study was performed, or each patient as his or her own control comparing one cycle with and one without the addition of G-CSF. Each of these types of controls is subject to misleading interpretations and selection bias. The patient variables in these types of studies are poorly defined, and the end points of benefit involve newer and different definitions than those used in the interpretation of chemotherapy trials. In the studies discussed in this section and in studies to be described involving more intense therapy, more subtle end points, such as days of hospitalization, days of antibiotics, graphic calculations of days of neutrophils under 1000 or 500 μl, time to next treatment, and mucositis, have been compared between the groups of patients, those receiving G-CSF and those patients who do not receive G-CSF, or alternatively, the hematopoietic toxicity was compared during alternate cycles of chemotherapy with or without factor. The first randomized, double-blind, placebo-controlled trial after the initial cycle introduced a crossover to G-CSF if patients developed fever and were not receiving G-CSF.

Before examining these studies in more detail, it seems that G-CSF significantly shortens the time to 500 and 1000 neutrophils μl^{-1} following conventional chemotherapy and reduces the absolute time under these values. A few studies have shown a decrease in the time to 100 neutrohils μl^{-1}, generally in previously untreated patients receiving chemotherapeutic agents considered to be stem cell sparing. Hospitalizations for fever and neutropenia have been reduced. A study design that has not been tested is a comparison of G-CSF with the best alternative therapy, such as prophylactic antibiotics. An abstract reporting such a study but with GM-CSF showed an increased incidence of documented infections and transfusions in the patients who received GM-CSF. This study may be criticized because the intensity of therapy was greater than usual, inducing severe neutropenia of greater than 4 days in most cycles and to a level of almost zero, a degree of marrow suppression beyond which these growth factors may lose effect because of CFU-GM depletion (46).

Because of lack of information as a result of difficulties with the design and interpretation of clinical trials, an accurate assessment of the impact of G-CSF on the reduction in morbidity as a consequence of the shortening of the hematopoietic toxicity following conventional dose chemotherapy is not straightforward.

B. Reductions in Neutropenia and Morbidity During Alternate Cycles of Chemotherapy and G-CSF

A popular study design to demonstrate the impact of G-CSF on hematopoietic toxicity is to administer the same dose of therapy in alternate cycles with or without G-CSF. There are two studies that have used this approach.

Gabrilove et al. (see Sec. III) first administered the G-CSF as a 30 minute IV infusion daily and found a dose-dependent increase in neutrophils from 1.9-fold at 1 μg/kg to 10.2-fold at 60 μg/kg in 27 patients with transitional cell carcinoma (40). The only toxicity related to the G-CSF was mild to moderate transient bone pain in the low back, sternum, and posterior iliac crests occurring in 72% during G-CSF infusion and in 9% 4–8 after the infusion. Subsequently, in patients who showed a response to G-CSF, G-CSF was given after MVAC [methotrexate (MTX), doxorubicin, vinblastine, and cisplatin] chemotherapy, and the effects were compared to a second cycle of identical therapy without G-CSF in the same patient or to the initial cycle of MVAC therapy in patients who refused to enroll in this same study. The incidence of bone discomfort with G-CSF following chemotherapy was only 20%, suggesting that the discomfort may be related to expansion of neutrophil precursors or release of cytokines. Compared to MVAC without G-CSF, treatment with G-CSF significantly reduced (91%) the number of days per patient on which the absolute neutrophil count was 1000 μl^{-1} or less and reduced the number of days (1 versus 35) on which antibiotics were used to treat fever and neutropenia. Because of the faster and full neutrophil recovery by day 14 after a brief early nadir (day 9 or 10) with G-CSF, the percentage of patients qualified to receive planned chemotherapy with methotrexate and vinblastine on day 14 of the treatment cycle increased from 29 to 100%. The mean cycle length for those without prior pelvic radiation was 29 days with G-CSF compared to 37–38 days without G-CSF. In addition, mucositis in the first cycle was also reduced both in frequency and severity, with grade 2–4 WHO mucositis seen in 10 of 34 without G-CSF compared to 2 of 18 with G-CSF. In 3 patients not receiving G-CSF, mucositis occurred despite absolute neutrophic counts (ANCs) above 1500, suggesting to the authors that the decreased incidence of mucositis may not be simply related to higher neutrophil counts but may involve an additional protective effect on the gastrointestinal epithelium.

There are several concerns with the interpretation of these data. The first criticism is that the G-CSF was administered during the first cycle of therapy. The effects could have been less if administered during the second cycle. For this reason, the protocol was amended to allow some patients who had not previously received G-CSF to be treated with the hormone only during their second cycle of M-VAC chemotherapy. The control group used to compare the hematopoietic toxicity of MVAC in the first cycle are of concern because they are patients who did not participate in the study. Not all patients who were initially treated with G-CSF were entered in the study. Patients were eliminated from study on the basis of an inadequate reponse to G-CSF. However, these were patients who received the lower doses of G-CSF, 1 μg/kg, and had less than a twofold increase in granulocytes. The early introduction of methotrexate and vinblastine on day 14 in this study could enhance the myelosuppression in the second cycle. The therapy itself does not produce very deep and prolonged myelosuppression, and only 2 of 18 control cycles showed an absolute granulacyte count (AGC) of less than 500 μl^{-1} for 3 days or greater, and only 50% of the cycle showing less than 500 AGC at all. Such a transient depression of counts suggests that marrow reserves of CFU-GM and more mature proliferative myeloid precursors are only modestly depressed. Furthermore, such transient depression of granulocytes may in fact be associated with a low incidence of infection. Such an interpretation is suggested by a closer examination of the data. For instance, the recovery is slower with G-CSF in patients with prior pelvic irradiation, demonstrating the importance of marrow reserve. If we examine only the patients entered in the study, not the other controls, febrile episodes are not common. The frequency of febrile episodes in the first cycle was 1 in 18 and in the second cycle only 2 in 18, hardly clinically significant. Even the effect on mucositis could be interpreted differently. The increased incidence in the second cycle could be an early treatment effect of MTX and vinblastine, both drugs that produce mucositis probably independently of neutropenia. The enhancement of hematopoietic recovery is real, but the impact on the reduction in morbidity may be modest and only in patients with noncompromised marrow.

Bronchud et al., in a similarly designed study, showed that 12 of 12 patients with untreated small cell carcinoma of the lung, some of whom had marrow involvement, had 4- to 10-fold dose-dependent increases in absolute neutrophil counts (see Sec. III) in response to a 5 day continuous intravenous infusion of 1–40 μg/kg of G-CSF (41). Of the patients 9 subsequently went on to receive systemic chemotherapy with a combination of intravenous adriamycin, 50 mg/m^2, ifosphamide, 5 g/m^2 by IV infusion, with mesna, 8 g/m^2 on day 1, and etoposide, 120/m^2 on days 1, 2, and 3, also intravenously. The chemotherapy regimen was repeated every 3 weeks, with G-CSF given in alternate cycles as a continuous infusion starting 24 h after the chemotherapy and continued for 14 days. However, in this study patients were randomly assigned to receive the G-CSF in the first or, alternatively, in the second cycle, overcoming some of the criticism of the first study. There was a marked difference in the absolute neutrophil count on day 15 after chemotherapy and G-CSF. Six severe infections occurred during cycles with G-CSF versus none for cycles with G-CSF. No clinical toxicity related to the G-CSF was observed. The absence of any significant musculoskeletal pains clearly related to G-CSF may be because the drug was administered as a continuous IV infusion, thereby minimizing peak levels.

In this study, G-CSF at a dose of only 1 μg/kg by continuous infusion (CI), not bolus, was effective in reducing neutropenia. Despite the similar design, the reduction in febrile episodes appears more impressive than in the Gabrilove group's study. The neutropenia was more severe and protracted in several of the graphic representations, reaching a level of under 100 μl^{-1} and lasting for greater than 4 days. Whether this was related to the patient population or the type of therapy is not clear. The reduction in febrile episodes was reproduced over several alternate cycles. The number of patients, only nine, is small, but a later study continued to show that the frequency of infections is reduced in a slightly increased number of patients (10). Patients with lung cancer may be more susceptible to infection during modest neutropenia than those with other diagnoses because of compromised pulmonary toilet. In this disease recombinant growth factor may be important to reduce the morbidity.

C. Other Studies of G-CSF and Conventional Chemotherapy

In 15 patients with advanced malignancy using twice daily infusions of 1–60 μg/kg of G-CSF for 5 days, Morstyn et al. (42) found dose-dependent increases in neutrophils up to 10-fold. As in studies with GM-CSF, the magnitude of the neutrophil increase was less in patients with prior systemic chemotherapy or extensive radiation. The only toxicity clearly related to treatment was slight bone pain during some infusions. No dose-limiting toxicity was observed, although 1 patient treated with 60 μg/kg died suddenly on day 5 of a probable cardiac event 12 h after the last dose of G-CSF. Patients subsequently received IV melphalan, 25 mg/m^2, followed by G-CSF, which showed dose-dependent acceleration of neutrophil recovery and reduction in the duration of neutropenia. At higher doses of G-CSF, the neutrophil nadir occurred earlier than with low doses. There was a dose-dependent increase in peripheral blood but not bone marrow CFU-GM, both with G-CSF alone and with G-CSF given after IV melphalan, particularly at 30 and 60 μg/kg. By the IV route G-CSF was rapidly cleared from the blood, with a mean half-life of 110 minutes for the second phase.

A second study by the same investigators examined the impact of a prechemotherapy period of G-CSF administration and the effect of varying the timing and duration of postchemotherapy G-CSF (47). Initially, patients received 0.3, 1.0, 3.0, and 10 μg/kg/day subcutaneously on days 1–5 and days 10–18. Melphalan was given on day 9. In the next portion of the study melphalan was administered on day 1 and G-CSF, 10 μg/kg/day, was administered by subcutaneous infusion on five schedules: (1) days 2–13; (2) days 8–13; (3) days 2–18; (4) days 8–18; and (5) days -9 to -2 to 13. G-CSF produced a rapid and sustained elevation in neutrophil levels within 24 h even when started 8 days after melphalan. At doses of 3 μg/kg/day or above, fewer than 1000 granulocytes for greater than 1 day was very rare, particularly in untreated patients. It was not necessary to continue G-CSF for more than 7 days. G-CSF did not consistently alter the course of the thrombocytopenia that followed this dose of melphalan. G-CSF by this route was well tolerated, although mild bone pain occurred and was reduced with acetaminophen. One of 22 patients developed cellulitis at an infusion site. These studies with IV melphalan show the dose-dependent effects of G-CSF and the feasibility of subcutaneous (SC) administration. The concept that pretreatment with growth factor before chemotherapy may protect bone marrow and further enhance myeloid recovery was not borne out in this study.

The concept behind this strategy is initially to enhance the number of early myeloid cells in DNA synthesis by growth factor infusion and then to reduce the proportion of cells in DNA synthesis below steady state at the time of chemotherapy by a rest period of 2–3 days before therapy.

D. A Randomized Study of G-CSF in Small Cell Bronchogenic Carcinoma

The studies reported to date leave many unanswered questions. Does the use of G-CSF increase response rate, decrease mortality, and improve survival? Does the continued administration of G-CSF allow a significant increase in dose intensity or prevent the dose reduction and delay in therapy that occur with repeated cycles of therapy? A properly designed randomized study would answer some of these questions. The nearest study to this ideal is a report by Crawford et al. (48) of an analysis of 207 patients with SCBC. In this study patients were randomized to placebo or treatment with G-CSF as a SC bolus at 2.5–8 μg/kg following 1 day after therapy with CAE (cyclophosphamide, 1 g/m^2; doxorubicin, 50 mg/m^2; and etoposide, 120 mg/m^2 × 3 days) and given to day 17 or until neutrophils exceeded 10×10^3 μl^{-1}. In the first cycle, febrile episodes occurred in 40% of the treated group and 77% of the control group. The duration of granulocytopenia less than 1000 μl^{-1} was 8 days in the control group and only 3.5 days in the treated group. There was a 50% reduction in hospitalization and days of antibiotics during the first cycle. However, if fever developed the code was broken and during the second cycle patients initially treated without G-CSF received identical doses of therapy but with G-CSF and patients who had developed fever on G-CSF had dose reduction with G-CSF for the second cycle. The crossover of the control group who developed febrile episodes eliminated the possibility of resolving the questions of relative dose intensity and tumor response with or without G-CSF. The latter may be a concern, at least theoretically, as receptors for both G-CSF and GM-CSF have been found on SCBC cell lines (49–55). Further, there were a significant proportion of patients with limited disease in this study, yet only a very small number of these patients survive disease free. Could this be because the majority received G-CSF or is it because of the choice of actual therapy, a combination without cisplatin and the absence of local chest irradiation? A second multicenter randomized trial with G-CSF and CAE chemotherapy in SCBC is nearing completion in Europe. In this study, each time febrile neutropenia was observed the study was also unblinded, but control patients did not receive G-CSF in subsequent cycles of chemotherapy. An interim analysis (Trillet et al., 1991 personal communication) confirms a reduction in the incidence of febrile neutropenia and in the requirement for IV antibiotics with no apparent adverse effect of G-CSF on patient survival or tumor response. In both studies, a tendency to develop cumulative thrombocytopenia was observed, and this has been interpreted as a reflection of the more frequent dose reductions in the control arm, although a relative inhibition of megakaryocytopoiesis within the marrow microenvironment cannot yet be ruled out.

E. Use of G-CSF to Increase Dose Intensity

G-CSF should enable the use of higher doses of chemotherapy or more closely coupled cycles of chemotherapy. The increase in dose intensity would have to be shown to improve the response rate and survival compared to conventional treatment without G-CSF.

To evaluate the possible increase in dose intensity G-CSF was given to 17 patients with advanced breast and ovarian cancer (56). Treatment with doxorubicin at doses of 75 mg/m^2 (n = 4 patients), 100 mg/m^2 (n = 5), 125 mg/m^2 (n = 6), and 150 mg/m^2 (n = 2) was followed by infusion of G-CSF for 11 days. G-CSF administration as usual resulted in a return of the absolute neutrophil count to normal or above normal levels within 12–14 days at all dose levels of doxorubicin used and allowed the administration of up to three cycles of high-dose chemotherapy at 14 day intervals. An absolute neutrophil count of 2500 μl^{-1} was not reached until day 19–21 after 75 mg/m^2 of doxorubicin given without G-CSF. At doses of doxorubicin of 125 and 150 mg/m^2 there was marked epithelial toxicity, and despite the enhancement of neutrophil recovery, patients still required admission for febrile episodes. Following doses of 75–100 mg/m^2 every 2 weeks for three cycles, patients started to develop delayed recovery, required red blood cells (4 of 9 patients), and experienced febrile episodes (2 of 9). A dose of 100 mg/m^2 over 4 weeks versus the usual dose of 75 mg/m^2 every 3 weeks represent an approximate 2-fold increase in dose intensity during the first 4 weeks of therapy. At the highest dose intensity, most patients required admission for supportive measures but were able to receive 75 mg/m^2 per week of doxorubicin (a 4.5-fold increase in dose intensity), and all patients responded, with 50% complete responses. To allow more than two to three cycles of chemotherapy and, therefore, a higher total cumulative dose, a ''split'' course might be required to allow sufficient time for epithelial and hematologic recovery after the first two or three cycles. Alternatively, this short intensified approach could be used as good cytoreduction and then proceed to ''consolidation'' therapy (with autologous stem cell support) or, more speculatively, ''maintenance'' therapy with biologic response modifiers. The authors were encouraged by the response rate in patients with advanced breast cancer treated at the higher dose, but the number of patients is too small to draw any conclusions.

The impact of these modest dose escalations and the ability of patients to receive chemotherapy more frequently, at least for a small number of cycles, on response or survival would have to be delineated in a controlled study. Past studies of only severalfold increases in dose in advanced cancer suggest that response rates are increased but not necessarily survival. However, these increases could be significant in micrometastatic disease.

V. IMPACT OF G-CSF ON THE TOXICITY OF HIGH-DOSE THERAPY

Recombinant growth factors are being tested intensively to modify the hematopoietic toxicity of high-dose therapies associated with protracted absolute neutropenia. These therapies vary in their marrow ablative potential, with different spontaneous potentials for trilineage recovery without infusion of marrow. However, a common feature is that CFU-GM or progenitor and more mature proliferative myeloid cells are totally or almost totally depleted for a number of days following the administration of therapy. This means that patients experience prolonged severe neutropenia, and febrile episodes are almost universal.

G-CSF and GM-CSF use following autologous marrow transplantation remarkably enhance the terminal part of granulocyte recovery. However, the febrile episodes are not significantly decreased and days febrile are not marginally different because of the minimal modification of the duration of absolute neutropenia or impact on the time of the first appearance of a neutrophil. The following sections discuss this impact of G-CSF on the toxicity of high-dose therapy both with and without reinfusion of autologous marrow.

A. G-CSF with Autologous Marrow Transplantation

High-dose cyclophosphamide, 6 g/m^2 (Cytoxan); carmustine, 300 mg/m^2 (BCNU); and etoposide (VP-16), 750 mg/m^2 (CBV therapy) with autologous bone marrow transplantation (ABMT) has been shown to be very effective therapy in relapsed Hodgkin's disease (57–59). Complete remission was obtained in 45% of the patients, 75% of these enduring 1 to more than 5 years. The major toxicity of this potentially curative therapy is related to fevers and infections during the neutropenic phase. Most patients (>90%) suffered from febrile episodes; during the period of neutropenia, approximately one-quarter of the patients had radiologic changes consistent with pneumonia, a third or more had documented bacteremia, and approximately one-quarter suffered from severe mucositis (58,59). CBV therapy may therefore be an important model to resolve the impact of recombinant growth factors on toxicity.

We chose for our initial study G-CSF because of its relatively restricted proliferative action to neutrophilic granulocytes alone, without any known in vivo induction of eosinophilia. We initially performed a phase II study employing G-CSF by a 30 minute bolus infusion at a dose of 60 μg/kg/day beginning 24 h after marrow reinfusion in 18 patients with Hodgkin's disease who received CBV

TABLE 1 Hematopoietic Recovery: Bolus Infusion of G-CSF after CBV Chemotherapy

	rhG-CSF	Control	p Value
Neutrophils per μl			
>100	9 (8–19)	13 (7–34)	0.103×10^4
>500	13 (10–31)	21 (10–51)	0.189×10^2
>1000	16 (11–33)	28 (14–61)	0.125×10^5
Platelets			
>50,000 μl^{-1}	32	27.5	0.370

therapy (60,61) and subsequently by continuous infusion at similar and even greater doses in another 21 patients. From Table 1 it is obvious that the difference in recovery to 1000 ANC is remarkably faster (12 days) with G-CSF than control patients. Recovery to 500 ANC is impressive, 9 days faster, and to 100 ANC is 4 days faster. These patterns of recovery are identical to the best recoveries of other studies using either G or GM-CSF after autologous marrow transplantation. However, the febrile episodes were not significantly decreased and days febrile only marginally different.

Sheridan et al. (62) administered G-CSF as a continuous subcutaneous infusion starting at 20 μg/kg/day 24 h after autologous marrow infusion following busulfan, 4 mg/kg/day for 4 days, and cyclophosphamide, 60 mg/kg/day for 2 days (BuCy), to 15 patients with relapsed Hodgkin's and non-Hodgkin's lymphoma, germ cell tumors, and acute lymphocytic leukemia. The median time to an ANC of 500 was similar to that in our study with continuous-infusion G-CSF, 11 days compared to 20 days for historical controls. All patients still had fever in this study, the febrile days were 7 versus 9 days in the historical experience, and positive blood cultures occurred in 53% of treated and 61% of control patients. There were significantly fewer days of parenteral antibiotic therapy, 11 versus 18 days in controls, and less isolation in reverse-barrier nursing, 10 versus 18 days. There was no effect on red cell or platelet recovery, but there was a trend for fewer platelet transfusions in the treated group. No significant toxicity was seen except for localized erythema at 2 of 88 infusion sites, and no significant difference was observed in the incidence of venoocclusive disease of the liver or interstitial pneumonia.

Why are these enhanced dramatic recoveries associated with such subtle differences in days of antibiotics and hospitalization and no reported differences in mortality? Febrile episodes are very much related to the length of time for which patients have less than 100 granulocytes μl^{-1}. The clinical vignette is that within a few days of patients' becoming absolutely neutropenic they develop a fever. The median onset of fever is 4 days after the ABMT that is accompanied by administration or 2 days after developing absolute neutropenia. The proportion of patients with fever rises rapidly thereafter. By the time most patients have recovered to 100 granulocytes μl^{-1}, despite its being hastened with G-CSF, 95% of the patients are already febrile. So, although recombinant G-CSF or GM-CSF dramatically shortens the time needed for full neutrophil recovery, the predominant action, as discussed earlier, is upon morphologically recognizable granulocytic precursors, such as myeloblasts and promyelocytes, rather than stem cells or committed myeloid progenitor cells. Early after transplantation inadequate numbers of progenitors or stem cells exist for adequate neutrophil production with growth factors.

The rapid and impressive recovery to counts of 500 and 1000 ANC could have a major impact if infection did not resolve until neutrophil mass recovered to levels reflected by peripheral blood counts of 500 neutrophils μl^{-1} or more. However, as we explored in other publications, most patients lose their fever before they recover to 100 ANC or almost immediately after, and this reemphasizes the importance of the recovery time to 100 ANC. Of the patients 70–80% resolve their fever by the time an ANC of 100 cells μl^{-1} is measured. The rest lose their fever in the next few days, and a small proportion maintain persistent fevers with adequate neutrophils, probably because of catheter infection. A 500 ANC is not needed to resolve infection, probably only the early immigration of tissue neutrophils. Prolonged severe neutropenia (more than 2 or 3 weeks) without CSF can lead to a higher incidence of opportunistic and fungal infections, however, and clinical experience with G-CSF in this setting suggests a reduction in the incidence of severe fungal or opportunistic infections but no clear change in mortality.

These new clinical benefit end points, such as fewer days of hospitalizaton and days of antibiotics and the occasional reduction in culture-positive febrile episodes without a reduction in the number of febrile episodes, raises obvious questions. Are the design of these studies such that they ensure an invariable positive result for the growth factor? What is the clinical significance of a reduction in culture-positive infection yet no reduction in febrile episodes?

The majority of studies have incorporated clinical protocols that have discharged patients and ceased antibiotics upon patients' achieving a defined ANC of 500 μl^{-1} rather than after the persistent resolution of fever. These clinical practices were established on the basis of publications that incorporated a number of patients, such as leukemia patients, who subsequently did not reestablish hematopoiesis. In these heterogeneous populations, the cessation of antibiotics before a significant neutrophil count was attained was associated with a significant reinfection rate in patients who did not show marrow recovery (63). However, the patients in the studies described here and in similar studies using GM-CSF received ABMT without marrow purging, and almost all will recover neutrophil counts. Recent studies have documented how antibiotics may be terminated before the attainment of a granulocyte count of 500 μl^{-1} without an increased reinfection rate (64). These authors demonstrate, similarly to our data, that most infective episodes resolve with an ANC of less than 125 μl^{-1}. In 75% of the patients a relative monocytosis occurred before the ANC exceeded 100; in the other 25% it occurred with or just after. Of 77 patients discharged before an ANC of 500 μl^{-1}, only 3 of 77 were readmitted with recurrent fever similar to the 2 of 37 patients readmitted following discharge with an ANC already at 500 ANC. There was no mortality related to this policy; the recurrent febrile episodes occurred during adequate granulocyte counts. These new approaches to antibiotic cessation raise the possibility that the effects of recombinant growth factors may have less clinical impact if the clinical design is different. However, it should also be remembered that neutrophil counts below 100–200 μl^{-1} can be unreliable for technical reasons and usually require manual rather than automated cell counting.

B. G-CSF with High-Dose Therapy Without ABMT

Almost a decade ago, we began developing the technique of tandem (double) high-dose chemotherapy (65). This strategy was developed in part because of early skepticism that the dose response of most human solid tumors was steep enough to warrant expectations that a single cycle of high-dose therapy would achieve results significantly different in advanced stages from those of standard chemotherapy. The major combination chemotherapy that we evaluated incorporates cyclophosphamide and etoposide (VP-16), drugs with reversible myeloid toxic effects and, if administered below certain doses, free of serious extramedullary toxicity. We evaluated this combination, along with cisplatinum (CVP), at four dose levels in more than 200 patients; the tumor types of the first 160 patients are shown in Table 2. The therapeutic results with this combination have been impressive in a number of tumors, and there have been a proportion of long-term survivors in patients with metastatic breast cancer (66). The clinical results have been described elsewhere in detail (67). Encouraging clinical outcomes have been confirmed by other investigators (68). These results have

TABLE 2 Patients Treated with CVP

Tumor type	Patient
Breast	117
Lung	26
Gastric	4
Unknown primary	5
Miscellaneous	8

TABLE 3 Duration of Absolute Neutropenia of <100 Cell per μl

Regimen	No. of days
CBV:ABMT	12
CBV:ABMT and G-CSF	7
CVP:no ABMT	12
CVP:ABMT	10
CVP: no ABMT and G-CSF	5.5 Only at 60μg/kg, lesser doses slower
CVP:ABMT and GM-CSF	8
CVP:ABMT and GM-CSF and Mobilized PBSC	8

formed the impetus to examine the modification of hematopoietic toxicity in this approach, as myelosuppresison is CVP's major side effect.

CVP, although severely myelotoxic, is associated with marrow recovery without the reinfusion of marrow. In a randomized study, we compared the hematopoietic recovery of CVP with and without marrow reinfusion. Again because of the significance of neutropenia of less than 100 μl^{-1}, we concentrate on the duration and recovery of this level. Without ABMT the duration is approximately 12 days and with ABMT, 9–10 days (69). Both these periods are significant and are universally associated with febrile episodes (Table 3).

There have now been several reported studies on approaches to modify the toxicity of CVP. Neidhart et al. studied the effect of G-CSF (from 20 to 60 μg/kg/day IV over 30 minutes starting 3 days after the completion of chemotherapy) on hematopoietic recovery after doses of CVP similar to our level 3, cyclophosphamide (5 g/m^2), etoposide (1500 mg/m^2), and cisplatin (150 mg/m^2) at 5 week intervals. The rate of recovery in the 10 treated ptients was compared to a concurrent but nonrandomized control group of 11 patients who received similar treatment but for whom there was inadequate G-CSF and also to a group of 8 patients who received G-CSF for their second cycle of CVP but not their first and thus served as their own controls. At the higher doses only, in small numbers of patients, statistically significant small differences in the duration of absolute neutropenia were noticed compared to a selected number of historical control patients, but the administration of G-CSF as a single IV bolus per day is likely (for biologic and pharmacokinetic reasons) to result in suboptimal neutrophil elevations compared to continuous IV or SC infusions. As in many of the studies with G and GM-CSF, once neutrophil recovery began it was markedly faster than in the control group (70). No information on reduction in febrile episodes or the duration of fever is given. Of importance is that the duration of 6 days in the high-dose G-CSF group and longer in the other patients is a duration in which febrile episodes will still be universal. There was no difference in the duration of thrombocytopenia. Of the 3 patients treated at 40 μg/kg, 2 had severe bone pain requiring morphine when their ANC exceeded 75,000 μl^{-1}. Thereafter, the G-CSF was discontinued when the ANC was ≥75,000 μl^{-1}, and no further episodes of bone pain were observed even at 60 μg/kg. In 3 of 4 patients who did not receive G-CSF with the first cycle and received a second cycle of CVP at the same dose with either 40 or 60 μg/kg of G-CSF, the time to an ANC of 100 μl^{-1} was shortened by only 1 day.

Our studies with GM-CSF and CVP also suggest that even with ABMT we are still confronted with this obstinate, persistent absolute neutropenia of 6–8 days. From our analysis of onset of fever, absolute neutropenia will have to be reduced to approximately 2–3 days to prevent the majority of febrile episodes. Only if we can use growth factors and or stem cells in novel ways to shrink the neutropenic window to this narrow range will morbidity be reduced markedly and hospitalization dramatically reduced.

G-CSF has recently been examined in a randomized study after intensive induction therapy with mitoxantrone and etoposide in relapsed or refractory acute leukemia (71). Recovery to 500 and 1000 ANC μl^{-1} was significantly faster, but the occurrence of febrile episodes remained universal in both groups and the duration of fever insignificantly different, although there were more documented infections in the control group. The authors argue that the enhancement of the late phase of neutrophil recovery prevents documented infections or lessens the severity of an infective episode. It is therefore possible that the impact of G-CSF may be greater in patients who were already neutropenic before high-dose chemotherapy than in those whose counts were normal beforehand.

C. Attempts to Abolish the Absolute Neutropenia of High-Dose Chemotherapy with Growth Factor-Mobilized Peripheral Blood

Early after high-dose therapy with or without marrow transplantation, inadequate numbers of progenitor cells or early myeloid forms exist for adequate neutrophil production with growth factors (60,61).

The number of myeloid progenitors infused after ABMT with G-CSF is still important for very early granulocyte recovery with the use of growth factor (60). To enhance recovery even further, we and others have proposed that it is probably necessary to infuse significantly higher numbers of progenitor cells (71–73). It is important conceptually to understand that the rapidity of early neutrophil recovery is related to the number of CFU-GM infused in autologous marrow. Neutrophil recovery is more rapid when greater numbers of CFU-GM are infused. First, it has been shown in a myeloablative model that a minimal number of GM-CFU are needed to ensure against prolonged and life-threatening neutropenia (1–2 × 104 CFU-GM kg^{-1}) (72). However, the rapidity is not a linear relationship to the number of CFU-GM infused. It is unfortunately a logarithmic-linear relationship (72,73). Because of the limitations on the amount of marrow that can be collected, the usual maximum number of marrow CFU-GM is about 15×10^4 kg^{-1}. These are small increments of CFU-GM in ideal patients over the average (less than 1 log), and it is not surprising that with the use of ABMT with or without growth factor that the shortest duration under 100 ANC is 7–9 days. Approaches besides ABMT and growth factor alone to initiate earlier recovery of granulocytes to the very critical level of 100 μl^{-1} have been a major clinical research interest in the past few years. There has been focus on the concept of harvesting an increasing number of progenitor cells from peripheral blood for subsequent growth factor action after reinfusion.

In limited numbers of patients, impressively rapid hematopoietic recovery is observed with the use of mononuclear cells harvested by pheresis as patients begin a rapid upswing in leukocyte, monocyte, and platelet numbers following the neutropenia of reversible myelotoxic therapy (73,74). This is argued to be related to the collection of increased CFU-GM. Both GM and G have been documented to mobilize progenitors into the peripheral blood (75–77). Of further interest is the suggestion of even faster hematopoietic recovery following collection of peripheral blood cells after administration of both high-dose cyclophosphamide (7 g/m^2) and GM-CSF and its subsequent use with bone marrow (75). Following high-dose melphalan with or without total-body irradiation in patients with no prior therapy, early infusion of marrow and peripheral blood cells can almost totally ameliorate the absolute neutropenia (75). Peters et al. (78) instead collected peripheral blood cells three times following 4 days of G-CSF or GM-CSF and combined this with marrow infusion and growth factor. The duration of the absolute neutropenia was still 7 days, but leukopenia and mortality and morbidity were reduced compared to historical data. Sheridan also added peripheral blood harvested following G-CSF and marrow infusion and demonstrated that neutrophil recovery was identical to the historical experience of marrow and G-CSF without the addition of peripheral blood (the same obstinate 7 days absolute neutropenia), but platelet recovery was enhanced (79).

We conducted a study of somewhat novel design to validate the modifications of peripheral blood in enhancing hematopoietic recovery (80). The data provide some insight into this topical and confusing area. Our recent review of peripheral blood cell transfusions also provides some perspective of this area (81). In our study, peripheral blood cells were collected during the neutrophil upswing following neutropenia induced by cyclophosphamide and Adriamycin at doses of 3 g/m^2 and 50 mg/m^2, respectively, and administration of GM-CSF 1 day following the chemotherapy at doses of 0.6 g/m^2 by continuous infusion over 4 h. Marrow was collected before this from patients and divided into two aliquots. To determine whether peripheral blood cells collected in this fashion hastened the early part of neutrophil recovery, we evaluated its effect on hematopoietic recovery when administered with bone marrow and growth factors. During cycle 1, we gave the patients marrow and GM-CSF following CVP (cyclophosphamide, 5.25 g/m^2; etoposide, 1200 mg/m^2; and cisplatin, 165 mg/m^2). During the second cycle at exactly the same dose, we added peripheral blood to the postchemotherapy marrow infusion and growth factor to see whether it enhanced recovery compared with marrow and growth factor alone. Thus, the first cycle served as an internal control.

In any individual patient the median time of recovery to an ANC of 100 μm^{-1} was not affected by the addition of peripheral blood. That is, the period of early recovery remained 6–8 days long. The terminal part of recovery (to 500 granulocytes μl^{-1}) was shifted minimally, but the difference was of no clinical significance. The overall number of documented infections was not reduced in the second cycle, and patients were febrile for approximately 7 days in each cycle. The median duration of thrombocytopenia (<20,000 and 50,000) was significantly reduced by the peripheral blood cell infusion.

These studies trigger many questions that could be resolved by comparative clinical trial, most important whether GM-CSF or G-CSF indeed adds to the improvement of the quality of the apheresed product over steady state or following the use of chemotherapy alone. What, if any, is the best strategy to harvest enough progenitor cells to regularly reduce the neutropenia period to only the few days' duration needed to prevent most infectious and febrile episodes?

Other techniques in which more progenitor cells might be mobilized remain to be explored. Preclinical models of combinations of growth factors, interleukin-3, and GM-CSF suggest that this approach is either intermediate in efficiency between chemotherapy alone and chemotherapy alone and rhGM-CSF or equivalent to chemotherapy alone. This method causes approximate 50- to 100-fold increases in CFU-GM in the peripheral blood in primates (82). CFU-GM are also impressively increased following interleukin-2 therapy (83). Whether any of these procedures improve the number of the appropriate cell or cells needed for rapid hematopoietic recovery compared to the approaches being used at present will, it is hoped, be carefully evaluated in the next several years.

VI. EFFECTS OF G-CSF IN CYCLIC NEUTROPENIA

Cyclic neutropenia is a poorly understood disorder of stem cell regulation. The disorder can be corrected by transplantation of bone marrow. Nowhere are the results of the different in vivo responses to administration of recombinant growth factors more fascinating than in cyclic neutropenia and congenital neutropenia.

Cyclic hematopoiesis also exists in gray collie dogs. In vitro studies demonstrated that GM-CSF, IL-3, and G-CSF all can stimulate increases in colony formation by canine bone marrow progenitor cells. Because of these results, gray collie dogs were treated with single dose levels of human GM-CSF, IL-3, or G-CSF and also different dose levels of recombinant canine G-CSF subcutaneously to determine if pharmacologic doses of one of these hematopoietic growth factors could alter cyclic production of cells. In vivo IL-3 had no effect on the recurrent neutropenia but was associated with eosinophilia. GM-CSF also did not ameliorate the cycling of hematopoiesis but caused neutrophilia and eosinophilia. However, G-CSF obliterated periodic fluctuation of neutrophil, monocyte, eosinophil, reticulocyte, and platelet counts and caused neutrophilia (84). Other studies of the bone marrow show that the swings in the myeloid-erythroid progenitor cells that are characteristic of this disorder in these dogs are eliminated by G-CSF treatment (84). Recombinant canine G-CSF increased the nadir neutrophil counts and amplitude of fluctuatons at low doses (1 μg/kg/day) and eliminated all cycling of cell counts at high doses (5 and 10 μg/kg/day) (85). The ability only of G-CSF to modify cycling in this model is curious and the mechanism speculative. It suggests a direct or indirect effect on a pluripotent stem cell. The different effects of these growth factors in stimulating increased counts of mature myeloid elements suggest that the response to growth factors of more differentiated progenitor cells is normal.

Six patients with cyclic neutropenia were treated with recombinant human G-CSF for 3–15 months. All had a history of recurrent aphthous stomatitis, pharyngitis, lymphadenopathy, fever, and numerous infections during periods of neutropenia. Daily G-CSF was administered at a dose of 3 to 10 μg/kg/day, either by continuous intravenous infusion or subcutaneously. G-CSF increased the neutrophil counts from a mean of 717 to 9814 μl^{-1}. In five of the six patients, the cycling of blood cell counts continued with increased fluctuations, but the length of the period decreased from 21 to 14 days. The duration of severe neutropenia, defined as less than 200 ANC, decreased from approximately 13 days per month to 1 day. G-CSF therapy reduced the frequency of oropharyngeal inflammation, fever, and infection in these patients. During the first 40 months of treatment, no typical mouth ulcers or bacterial infections occurred; recurrent gingivitis improved (86). The hematopoietic effects in humans, although impressive, do not show the elimination of cycling as in the canine model.

In vitro studies of committed progenitor cells (CFU-GM and BFU-E) in three patients with cyclic neutropenia (two congenital and one acquired) also showed that G-CSF administration did not eliminate the cycling. There was a shortening of the cycle and an increase in the amplitude of variations (from 2- to 3-fold to 10- to 100-fold) in the number of both types of circulating progenitor cells in the two patients with congenital cyclic neutropenia. In the patient with acquired cyclic neutropenia, cycling of both blood cells and progenitors could not be seen. In cultures deprived of fetal bovine serum, erythroid and myeloid bone marrow progenitor cells from untreated patients and from normal subjects differed in growth factor responsiveness. The maximal growth of CFU-GM was induced by

GM-CSF plus G-CSF in the patients, whereas a combination of GM-CSF, G-CSF, and interleukin-3 was required in the normal subjects. Erythropoietin alone induced 4-fold more erythroid bursts from cyclic neutropenic patients than from normal donors (46 versus 11% of the maximal colony number respectively). The growth factor responsiveness of marrow progenitor cells slightly changed during the treatment toward the values observed with normal progenitors (87). These in vitro data demonstrate that the human disease is associated with an abnormal in vivo responsiveness to growth factors and a greater sensitivity to lineage-responsive factors. The disparities between G-CSF-induced effects in canine and human cyclic neutropenia suggest that the pathophysiologic basis for this disorder in the two species may be, at least in part, distinct.

VII. G-CSF IN CONGENITAL NEUTROPENIA

G-CSF has also had impressive activity in congenital agranulocytosis, a disorder characterized by severe neutropenia secondary to a maturational arrest at the level of promyelocytes. G-CSF in doses of 3–60 μg/kg/day was administered to five patients with congenital agranulocytosis. In all five patients, an increase in the number of neutrophils was noted 8–9 days after the initiation of the effective dosage (the dose at which the neutrophil count reached 1000 cells μl^{-1} or more and the bone marrow showed granulocyte maturation beyond the myelocyte stage). The absolute neutrophil counts rose from less than 100 to between 1300 and 9500 cells μl^{-1}. There was a spectrum of responses in these patients ranging from mild to moderate increases in ANC and, with very high doses, dramatic neutrophilia with or without cycles and dysplastic neutrophils. Marrow aspirates obtained after 14 days at the effective dosage showed maturation to the mature neutrophil stage. All five patients have had sustained neutrophil counts of 1000 cells μl^{-1} or more for 9–13 months with subcutaneous maintenance therapy. Preexisting chronic infections resolved, and new infectious episodes and the requirement for intravenous antibiotics decreased (88). Some patients developed mild to moderate splenomegaly following prolonged G-CSF administration without apparent clinical consequence.

Another report contrasts the differential effect of G-CSF and GM-CSF in this condition. Five patients were initially treated with GM-CSF for 42 days and subsequently, 1–3 months later, with G-CSF for 142 days. GM-CSF was administered at a dose of 3–30 μg/kg/day over 30–60 minutes intravenously. In four of the five patients the increase in neutrophil count was due to an increase in eosinophils. Subsequently, all patients received G-CSF at a dose of 3–15 μg/kg/day subcutaneously. In contrast to the GM-CSF effect, all five patients responded to G-CSF with an increase in the ANC to above 1000 μl^{-1} during the first 6 weeks of treatment. This response was maintained during maintenance treatment. No severe bacterial infections occurred during CSF treatment (89).

The effectiveness of G-CSF was also demonstrated in a case of idiopathic neutropenia. G-CSF therapy resulted in normalization of the patient's absolute neutrophil count, healing of chronic oral ulcerations permitting discontinuation of a prophylactic antiobiotic without recurrent infection, and minimal side effects (90).

The distinct responses to G-CSF versus GM-CSF in these congenital neutropenic disorders point to the restricted action of G-CSF and the divergent biologic activities of these two materials.

VIII. EFFECTS ON APLASTIC ANEMIA, MYELODYSPLASTIC SYNDROMES, AND LEUKEMIA

Aplastic anemia is a rare disorder with a very complex and diverse pathophysiology reflecting various types of marrow stem cell malfunction. Champlin et al. (91) treated several patients with aplastic anemia with GM-CSF, and a high proportion responded with increased leukocyte counts, although the duration of these responses was not reported. Nissen et al. (92) failed to demonstrate a useful effect of GM-CSF in severe aplastic anemia, suggesting that the response to CSFs is related to the degree of the intrinsic marrow stem cell defect.

Myelodysplastic syndromes are also a heterogeneous group of disorders of bone marrow function that often lead to severe infectious and hemorrhagic complications. Both G-CSF and GM-CSF have been used in relatively small studies. The majority, but not all these patients, have shown marked but often transient improvements in peripheral neutrophil counts, usually without increases in platelet counts (93–96).

G-CSF probably generated a more persistent neutrophil response with more marked improvements in marrow myeloid maturation, although, again, no careful comparative studies have been reported. Larger prospective studies are required for the long-term safety of both drugs to be established in these conditions and to demonstrate a clear-cut clinical benefit (e.g., in terms of a reduction in antibiotic use or platelet or red blood cell transfusions).

Acute myeloid leukemia was developed by a small number of patients following treatment with CSFs, but it has not yet been ascertained whether these drugs are "leukemogenic" or indeed protect against the development of frank blast transformation by promoting differentiation. Thus, in those patients who demonstrated an increase in peripheral granulocytes following stimulation with G-CSF, it is not altogether clear whether the increase was due to the differentiation and maturation of the myelodysplastic clone or to stimulation of a residual normal clone.

Primary cultures of leukemic or "preleukemic" cells, in general, remain strictly dependent on exogenous CSF for survival and proliferation. McCulloch et al. (97) elegantly demonstrated that the clonogenic blast cells of the acute myeloid leukemias can proliferate and expand in response to IL-3, GM-CSF, or G-CSF (alone or in combination). G-CSF is an effective proliferative stimulus for most chronic myeloid leukemia (CML) and acute myeloid leukemia (AML) populations, but not for acute lymphocytic leukemia (ALL). In cultures of CML with G-CSF, differentiation is complete and colonies contain no clonogenic cells. In AML cultures, morphologic differentiation in the presence of G-CSF is incomplete and usually aberrant. AML blast colony formation is usually stimulated by G-CSF, but autoradiographic studies suggest that a significant proportion of blast cells in any one population lacks G-CSF receptors. If this lack of receptors represents a true subpopulation of blast cells, rather than a limitation of the sensitivity of the assay or a transient phenomenon, then G-CSF would be unable to suppress such a population even if it had effective differentiating powers. In acute promyelocytic leukemias, practically all cells express large numbers of G-CSF receptors (98).

On the other hand, hematopoietic growth factors might be particularly useful for recruiting quiescent leukemic stem cells into the cell cycle, perhaps making them more susceptible to the cytotoxic effects of cycle-specific drugs. Obviously, the dose and scheduling of CSFs in this context might require specific tailoring to the disease (considering the heterogeneous nature of leukemic cells), but their differentiation-inducing activity should be an added bonus, if, indeed, it occurs "in vivo." Stimulation of leukemic blast cells "in vitro" has led to increased cell killing with cytosine arabinoside (99). The preliminary results of an interesting study by Buechner et al. (100) have been recently reported. These authors gave GM-CSF to 30 patients with AML at high risk of early death (patients above the age of 65 or patients with early or second relapse) starting on day 4 after the end of chemotherapy. The median recovery time of blood neutrophils was reduced by 6–9 days compared to historical controls. A marked leukemic regrowth observed in 2 patients was apparently reversible in 1 patient and appeared GM-CSF independent in the second patient. Neutrophil recovery was also speeded up (by about 1 week) in a heterogeneous group of acute leukemic patients treated with G-CSF by Ohno et al. (71), but the incidence of febrile episodes was not significantly different. A total of 108 patients with relapsed or refractory acute leukemia were studied prospectively and randomized to either G-CSF or no G-CSF begun 2 days after the end of the chemotherapy and continued until neutrophil recovery. There was no evidence that G-CSF accelerated the growth of leukemic cells, and the rate of relapse was almost the same in the two groups.

A separate study, looking at the effects of GM-CSF on circulating blast count, thymidine incorporation, and ara-CTP formation in 18 patients with newly diagnosed AML, was recently reported (101). Chemotherapy (daunorubicin and Ara-C) was given when the circulating blast count rose above 50,000 or after 7 days of GM-CSF treatment (whichever came first). GM-CSF resulted in an increase in thymidine incorporation and ara-CTP formation in patients with newly diagnosed AML, suggesting that the stimulus induces more proliferation than differentiation. No similar study has been reported with G-CSF, but despite its probably greater differentiation-inducing ability, it seems likely that one basic problem will remain—the defect in the balance between self-renewal and differentiation that leads to perpetuation of the leukemia.

IX. CONCLUSION

G-CSF is currently being used to support neutrophil recovery after chemotherapy with or without bone marrow transplantation, enhance stem cell harvest, and increase neutrophil counts in chronic neutropenias, aplastic anemia, and myelodysplastic syndrome. Other potential uses not covered here include its application in acquired immunodeficiency syndrome patients and as an adjunct to antibiotics in patients with infection or burns. A number of large ongoing randomized trials should help precisely delineate the indications of G-CSF, and future investigations will incorporate G-CSF as a component of combination growth factor therapy.

REFERENCES

1. Cannistra SA, Griffin JD. Regulation of the production and function of granulocytes and monocytes. Semin Hemat 1988; 25:173–88.
2. Metcalf D. The colony stimulating factors. Discovery, development, and clinical applications. Cancer 1990; 65:2185–95.
3. Moore MAS, Welta K, Gabrilove J, Souza LM. Biological activities of recombinant human granulocyte colony-stimulating factor (rhG-CSF) and tumor necrosis factor: in vivo and in vitro analysis. Hematol Blood Trans 1987; 31:210–20.
4. Lee MT, Kaushansky K, Ralph P, Ladner MB. Differential expression of M-CSF, G-CSF, and GM-CSF by human monocytes. J Leukoc Biol 1990; 47:275–82.
5. Ikebuchi K, Clark SC, Ihle JN, Souza LM, Ogawa M. Granulocyte colony-stimulating factor enhances interleukin 3 dependent proliferation of multipotential hemopoietic progenitors. Proc Natl Acad Sci U S A 1988; 85:3445–9.
6. Ikebuchi K, Ihle JN, Hirai Y, Wong GG, Clark SC, Ogawa M. Synergistic factors for stem cell proliferation: further studies of the target stem cells and the mechanism of stimulation by interleukin-1, interleukin-61 and granulocyte colony-stimulating factor. Blood 1988; 72:2007–14.
7. Kishi K, Ellingsworth LR, Ogawa M. The suppressive effects of type beta transforming growth factor (TGFbeta) on primitive murine hemopoietic progenitors are abrogated by interleukin-6 and granylocyte colony-stimulating factor. Leukemia 1989; 3:687–91.
8. Ogawa M. Effects of hemopoietic growth factors on stem cells in vitro. Hematol Oncol Clin North Am 1989; 3:453–64.
9. Nathan CF. Respiratory burst in adherent human neutrophils: triggering by colony-stimulating factors CSF-GM and CSF-G. Blood 1989; 73:301–6.

10. Bronchud MH, Potter MR, Morgenstern G, et al. In vitro and in vivo analysis of the effects of recombinant human granulocyte colony stimulating factor in patients. Br J Cancer 1988; 58:64–9.
11. Wang JM, Chen ZG, Colella S, et al. Chemotactic activity of recombinant human granulocyte colony stimulating factor. Blood 1988; 72:1456–60.
12. Ohsaka A, Kitagawa S, Sakamoto S, et al. In vivo activation of human neutrophil functions by administration of recombinant human granulocyte colony-stimulating factor in patients with malignant lymphoma. Blood 1989; 74:2743–8.
13. Kaplan SS, Basford RE, Wing EJ, Shadduck RK. The effect of recombinant human granulocyte macrophage colony-stimulating factor on neutrophil activation in patients with referactory carcinoma. Blood 1989; 73:636–8.
14. Peters WP, Stuart A, Affronti ML, Kim CS, Coleman RE. Neutrophil migration if defective during recombinant human granulocyte-macrophage colony-stimulating factor infusion after autologous bone marrow transplantation in humans. Blood 1988; 72:1310–5.
15. Kitagawa S, Yuo A, Souza LM, et al. Recombinant human granulocyte colony-stimulating factor enhances superoxide release in human granulocytes stimulated by the chemotactic peptide. Biochem Biophys Res Commun 1987; 144:1143–6.
16. Baldwin GC, Fuller ND, Roberts RL, Ho DD, Golde DW. Granulocyte- and granulocyte-macrophage colony-stimulating factors enhance neuturophil cytotoxicity toward HIV-infected cells. Blood 1989; 74:1673–7.
17. Wing EJ, Magee DM, Whiteside TL, Kaplan SS, Shadduck RK. Recombinant human granulocyte/macrophage colony-stimulating factor enhances monocyte cytotoxicity and secretion of tumor necrosis factor and interferon in cancer patients. Blood 1989; 73:643–6.
18. Buckle AM, Hogg N. The effect of IFN-gamma and colony-stimulating factors on the expression of neutrophil cell membrane receptors. J Immunol 1989; 143:2295–301.
19. Gamble JR, Rand TH, Lopez AF, Clark-Lewis I, Vadas MA. Heterogeneity of recombinant granulocyte-macrophage colony-stimulating factor-mediated enhancement of neutrophil adherence of endothelium. Exp Hematol 1990; 18:897–902.
20. Zsebo KM, Wypych J, Yuschenkoff VN, et al. Effects of hematopoietin-1 and interleukin-1 activities on early hematopoietic cells of the bone marrow. Blood 1988; 71:962–8.
21. Zsebo KM, Yuschenkoff VN, Schiffer S, et al. Vascular endothelial cells and granulopoiesis: interleukin-1 stimulates release of G-CSF and GM-CSF. Blood 1988; 71:99–103.
22. Fibbe WE, Van Damme J, Billiau A, et al. Human fibroblasts produce granulocyte-CSF, macrophage-CSF, and granulocyte-macrophage-CSF following stimulation by interleukin-1 and poly(rl)•poly(rC). Blood 1988; 72:860–6.
23. Broudy VC, Kaushansky K, Segal GM, et al. Tumor necrosis factor type alpha stimulates human endothelial cells to produce granulocyte/macrophage colony stimulating factor. J Immunol 1987; 139:464–8.
24. Fibbe WE, Daha MR, Hiemstra PS, et al. Interleukin-1 and poly(rC)•poly(rC) induce production of granulocyte CSF, macrophage CSF, and granulocyte-macrophage CSF by human endothelial cells. Exp Hematol 1989; 17:229–34.

25. Broudy VC, Kaushansky K, Harlan JM, Adamson IW. Interleukin-1 stimulates human endothelial cells to produce granulocyte-macrophage colony-stimulating factor and granulocyte colony-stimulating factor. J Immunol 1987; 139:464–8.
26. Kawakami M, Tsutsumi H, Kumakawa T, et al. Levels of serum G-CSF in patients with infections. Blood 1990; 76:1962–4.
27. Souza LM, Boone TC, Garrilove J, et al. Recombinant human granulocyte colony-stimulating factor: Effects on normal and leukemic myeloid cells. Science 1986; 232:61–5.
28. Zsebo KM, Cohen AM, Murdock DC, et al. Recombinant human granulocyte colony stimulating factor: molecular and biological characterization. Immunobiology 1986; 172:176–84.
29. Nicola NA. Hemopoietic cell growth factors and their receptors. Annu Rev Biochem 1989; 58:45–77.
30. Nicola NA, Peterson L. Identification of distinct receptors for two hemopoietic growth factors (granulocyte colony-stimulating factor and multipotential colony-stimulating factor) by chemical cross-linking. J Biol Chem 1986; 12:384–9.
31. Begley CG, Metcalf D, Nicola NA. Binding characteristics and proliferative action of purified granulocyte colony-stimulating factor (G-CSF) on normal and leukemic human promyelocytes. Exp Hematol 1988; 16:71–9.
32. Nicola NA, Peterson L, Hilton DJ, Metcalf D. Cellular processing of murine colony-stimulating factor (multi-CSF, GM-CSF, G-CSF) receptors by normal hemopoietic cells and cell lines. Growth Factors 1988; 1:41–9.
33. Walker F, Nicola NA, Metcalf D, Burgess AW. Hierarchical down-modulation of hemopoietic growth factor receptors. Cell 1985; 43:269–76.
34. Nicola NA, Vadas MA, Lopez AF, Down-modulation of receptors for granulocyte colony-stimulating factor on human neutrophils by granulocyte-activating agents. J Cell Physiol 1986; 128:501–9.
35. Nagata S, Tsuchiya M, Asano S, et al. Molecular cloning and expression of CDNA for human granulocyte colony-stimulating factor. Nature 1986; 319:415–8.
36. Welte K, Bonilla MA, Gillio AP, et al. Recombinant human granulocyte colony-stimulating factor. Effects on hematopoiesis in normal and cyclophosphamide-treated primates. J Exp Med 1987; 165:941–8.
37. Welte K, Bonilla MA, Gabrilove JL, et al. Recombinant human granulocyte-colony stimulating factor; in vitro and in vivo effects on myelopoiesis. Blood Cells 1987; 13:17–30.
38. Gillio AP, Bonilla MA, Potter GK, et al. Effects of recombinant human granulocyte-colony stimulating factor on hematopoietic reconstitution after autologous bone marrow transplantation in primates. Transplant Proc 1987; 19:153–6.
39. Gabrilove JL, Jakubowski A, Fain K, et al. Phase I study of granulocyte colony-stimulating factor in patients with transitional cell carcinoma of the urothelium. J Clin Invest 1988; 82:1454–61.
40. Gabrilove JL, Jakubowski A, Scher H, et al. Effects of granulocyte colony-stimulating factor on neutropenia and associated morbidity due to chemotherapy for transitional-cell carcinoma of the urothelium. N Engl J Med 1988; 318:1414–22.

41. Bronchud MH, Scarffe JH, Thatcher N, et al. Phase I/II study of recombinant human granulocyte colony-stimulating factor in patients receiving intensive chemotherapy for small cell lung cancer. Br J Cancer 1987; 56:809–13.
42. Morstyn G, Campbell L, Souza LM, et al. Effect of granulocyte colony stimulating factor on neutropenia induced by cytotoxic chemotherapy. Lancet 1988; 1:667–72.
43. Lord BI, Bronchud MH, Owens S, et al. The kinetics of human granulopoiesis following treatment with granulocyte colony-stimulating factor in vivo. Proc Natl Acad Sci U S A 1989; 86:9499–503.
44. Hermann F, Schulz G, Lindemann A, et al. Hematologic responses in patients with advanced malignancy treated with recombinant human granulocytemacrophage colony-stimulating factor. J Clin Oncol 1989; 7:159–67.
45. Lindemann A, Herrmann F, Oster W, et al. Hematologic effects of recombinant human granulocyte colony stimulating factor in patients with malignancy. Blood 1989; 74:2644–51.
46. Rodriguez M, Swan F, Hagemeister F, et al. High dose ESAP with GM-CSF vs. prophylactic antibiotics. Blood 1990; 76:370 abstract 1469, suppl. 1.
47. Morstyn G, Campbell L, Lieschke G, et al. Treatment of chemotherapy-induced neutropenia by subcutaneously administered granulocyte colony-stimulating factor with optimization of dose and duration of therapy. J Clin Oncol 1989; 7:1554–62.
48. Crawford J, Ozer H, Stoller R, et al. Granulocyte colony reduction by stimulating factor: of fever and neutropenia induced by chemotherapy in patients with small-cell lung cancer. N Engl J Med 1991; 325:164–170.
49. Baldwin GC, Gasson JC, Kaufman SE, et al. Nonhematopoietic tumor cells express functional GM-CSF receptors. Blood 1989; 73:1033–7.
50. Avalos BR, Gasson JC, Hedvat C, et al. Human granulocyte colony-stimulating factor: biologic activities and receptor characterization on hematopoietic cells and small cell lung cancer cell lines. Blood 1990; 75:851–7.
51. Nachbaur D, Denz H, Zwierzina H, Schmalzl F, Huber H. Stimulation of colony formation of various human carcinoma cell lines by rhGM-CSF and rhIL-3. Cancer Lett 1990; 50:197–201.
52. Dedhar S, Gaboury L, Galloway P, Eaves AC. Human GM-CSF is a growth factor on a variety of cell types of non-hemopoietic origin. Proc Natl Acad Sci U S A 1988; 85:9253–7.
53. Berdel WE, Danhauser S, Steinhauser G, Winton EF. Various human hematopoietic growth factors (IL-3, GM-CSF, G-CSF stimulate clonal growth of non-hematopoietic tumor cells. Blood 1989; 73:80–3.
54. Salmon SE, Liu R. Effects of GM-CSF on in-vitro growth of human solid tumors. J Clin Oncol 1989; 7:1346–50.
55. Vellenga E, Biesama B, Meyer C, Wagteveld L, Esselink M, de Vries EGE. The effects of five hemopoietic growth factors on human small cell lung carcinoma lines: interleukin 3 enhances the proliferation in one of the eleven cell lines. Cancer Res 1991; 51:73–6.
56. Bronchud MH, Howell A, Crowther D, Hopwood P, Souza L, Dexter TM. The use of granulocyte colony-stimulating factor to increase the intensity of treatment with doxorubicin in patients with advanced breast and ovarian cancer. Br J Cancer 1989; 60:121–5.

57. Spitzer G, Dicke KA, Litam J, et al. High-dose combination chemotherapy with autologous bone marrow transplantation in adult solid tumors. Cancer 1980; 45:3075–85.
58. Jagannath S, Armitage JO, Dicke KA, et al. Updated results of CBV and autologous bone marrow transplantation for Hodgkin's disease. In: Dicke KA, Spitzer G, Jagannath S, eds. *Proceedings of the third international symposium on autologous bone marrow transplantation.* Houston: University of Texas Press 1987; 217–21.
59. Jagannath S, Dicke KA, Armitage JO, et al. High-dose cyclophosphamide, carmustine, etoposide, and autologous bone marrow transplantation for relapsed Hodgkin's disease. Ann Intern Med 1986; 104:163–8.
60. Taylor K, Jagannath S, Spitzer G, et al. Recombinant human granulocyte colony-stimulating factor hastens granulocyte recovery after high-dose chemotherapy and autologous bone marrow transplantation in Hodgkin's disease. J Clin Oncol 1989; 7:1791–9.
61. Spitzer G, Ventura G, Jagannath S, et al. Use of recombinant human hematopoietic growth factors and autologous bone marrow transplantation to attenuate the neutropenic trough of high-dose therapy. Int J Cell Cloning 1990; 8:249–61.
62. Sheridan WP, Morstyn G, Wolf M, et al. Granulocyte colony-stimulating factor and neutrophil recovery after high-dose chemotherapy and autologous bone marrow transplantation. Lancet 1989; 2:891–5.
63. Pizzo PA, Robichaud KJ, Wesley R, et al. Fever in the pediatric and young adult patient with cancer: a prospective study of 1001 episodes. Medicine (Baltimore) 1982; 61:153–65.
64. Mullen CA, Buchanan GR. Early hospital discharge of children with cancer treated for fever and neutropenia: identification and management of the low-risk patient. J Clin Oncol 1990; 8:1998–2004.
65. Dunphy FR, Spitzer G, Dicke KA, Buzdar AU, Hortobagyi GN. Tandem high-dose chemotherapy as intensification in stage IV breast cancer. Bone marrow transplantation: current controversies. *UCLA Symp Mol Cell Biol New Series* 1988; 87:245–51.
66. Dunphy FR, Spitzer G, Buzdar AU, et al. Treatment of estrogen receptor-negative or hormonally refractory breast cancer with double high-dose chemotherapy intensification and bone marrow support. J Clin Oncol 1990; 8:1207–16.
67. Spitzer G. An update of autologous stem cell transplantation in solid tumors. Cancer Bull (In Press).
68. Neidhart J, Kohker W, Stidley C, et al. Phase I study of repeated cycles of high-dose cyclophosphamide, etoposide and cisplatin administered without bone marrow transplantation. J Clin Oncol 1990; 8:1728–38.
69. Huan SD, Yau JC, Dunphy FR, et al. Impact of autologous bone marrow infusion on the hematopoietic recovery following high dose cyclophosphamide, etoposide and cisplatin. Submitted.
70. Neidhart J, Mangalik A, Kohler W, et al. Granulocyte colony-stimulating factor stimulates recovery of granulocytes in patients receiving dose-intensive chemotherapy without bone marrow transplantation. J Clin Oncol 1989; 7:1685–92.
71. Ohno R, Tomonga M, Kobayashi T, et al. Effect of granulocyte colony-stimulating factor after intensive induction therapy in relapsed or refractory acute leukemia. N Engl J Med 1990; 323:871–7.

72. Spitzer G, Verma DS, Fisher R, et al. The myeloid progenitor cell—its value in predicting hematopoietic recovery after autologous bone marrow transplantation. Blood 1980; 55:3075–85.
73. Gianni AM, Bregni M, Siena S, et al. Rapid and complete hemopoietic reconstitution following combined transplantation of autologous blood and bone marrow cells. A changing role for high dose chemo-radiotherapy. Hematol Oncol 1989; 7:139–48.
74. To LB, Dyson PG, Branford AL, et al. Peripheral blood stem cells collected in very early remission produce rapid and sustained autologous hemopoietic reconstitution in acute non-lymphoblastic leukaemia. Bone Marrow Transplant 1987; 2:103–8.
75. Gianni AM, Bregni M, Stern AK, et al. Granulocyte-macrophage colony-stimulating factor to harvest circulating hemopoietic stem cells for autotransplantation. Lancet 1989; 2:580–4.
76. Socinski MA, Cannistra SA, Elias A, Antman KH, Schnipper L, Griffin JD. Granulocyte-macrophage colony stimulating factor expands the circulating hemopoietic progenitor cell compartment in man. Lancet 1988; 1:1194–8.
77. Duhrsen U, Villeval J, Boyd J, Kannourakis G, Morstyn G, Metcalf D. Effects of recombinant human granulocyte colony-stimulating factor on hematopoietic progenitor cells in cancer patients. Blood 1988; 72:2074–81.
78. Peters WP, Kurtzberg J, Kirkpatrick G, et al. GM-CSF primed peripheral blood progenitor cells coupled with autologous bone marrow transplantation will eliminate leukopenia following high dose chemotherapy. Blood 1989; 74:50.
79. Sheridan WP, Juttner C, Szer J, et al. Granulocyte colony-stimulating factor (G-CSF) in peripheral blood stem cell and bone marrow transplantation. Blood 1990; 76:2251.
80. Ventura CJ, Spitzer G, Hester J, et al. A controlled trial of mobilized peripheral blood progenitor cells; does their addition to autologous bone marrow transplant and growth factor cause faster hematopoietic recovery? Pro ASCO 1990; 9:9.
81. Spitzer G, Hester J. What advantages are there to using peripheral blood collection over autologous bone marrow in modifying the toxicity of high-dose therapy? In: Henon P, Wunder E, eds. Peripheral blood stem cell autografts. Heidelberg: Springer-Verlag; in press.
82. Geissler K, Valent P, Mayer P, et al. Recombinant human interleukin-3 expands the pool of circulating hemopoietic stem cells in primates-synergism with recombinant human granulocyte/macrophage colony-stimulating factor. Blood 1990; 75:2305–10.
83. Schaafsma MR, Fibbe WE, Van Der Harst D, et al. Increased number of circulating hematopoietic progenitor cells after treatment with high-dose interleukin-2 in cancer patients. Br J Hematol 1990; 76:180–5.
84. Hammond WP, Boone TC, Donahue RE, Souza LM, Dale DC. A comparison of treatment of canine cyclic hematopoiesis with recombinant human granulocyte-macrophage colony-stimulating factor (GM-CSF), G-CSF interleukin-3, and canine G-CSF. Blood 1990; 76:523–32.
85. Lathrop CD, Warren DJ Jr, Souza LN, Jones JB, Moore MAS. Correction of canine cyclic hematopoiesis with recombinant human granulocyte colony-stimulating factor. Blood 1988; 72:1324–8.
86. Hammond WP IV, Price TH, Souza LM, Dale DC. Treatment of cyclic neutropenia with granulocyte colony-stimulating factor. N Engl J Med 1989; 320:1306–11.

87. Migliaccio AR, Migliaccio G, Dale DC, Hammond WP. Hematopoietic progenitors in cyclic neutropenia: effect of granulocyte colony-stimulating factor in vivo. Blood 1990; 75:1951–9.
88. Bonilla MA, Gillio AP, Ruggeiro M, et al. Effects of recombinant human granulocyte colony-stimulating factor on neutropenia in patients with congenital agranulocytosis. N Engl J Med 1989; 320:1574–80.
89. Welte K, Zeidler C, Reiter A, et al. Differential effects of granulocyte-macrophage colony-stimulating factor and granulocyte colony-stimulating factor in children with severe congenital neutropenia. Blood 1990; 75:1056–63.
90. Jakubowski AA, Souza L, Kelly F, et al. Effects of human granulocyte colony-stimulating factor in a patient with idiopathic neutropenia. N Engl J Med 1989; 320:38–42.
91. Champlin RE, Nimer SD, Ireland P, et al. Treatment of refractory aplastic anemia with recombinant human granulocyte-macrophage colony-stimulating factor. Blood 1989; 73:694–9.
92. Nissen C, Tichelli A, Gratwohl A, et al. Failure of recombinant human granulocyte-macrophage colony-stimulating factor therapy in aplastic anemia patients with very severe neutropenia. Blood 1988; 72:2045–7.
93. Ganser A, Volkers B, Greher J, et al. Recombinant human granulocyte-macrophage colony-stimulating factor in patients with myelodysplastic syndromes—a phase I/II trial. Blood 1989; 73:31–7.
94. Herrmann F, Lindemann A, Klein H, et al. Effect of recombinant human granulocyte-macrophage colony-stimulating factor in patients with myelodysplastic syndromes with excess blasts. Leukemia 1989; 3:335–8.
95. Negrin RS, Hacuber DH, Nagler A, et al. Treatment of myelodysplastic syndromes with recombinant human granulocyte colony-stimulating factor. Ann Intern Med 1989; 110:976–84.
96. Kobayashi Y, Okabe T, Ozawa K, et al. Treatment of myelodysplastic syndromes with recombinant human granulocyte colony-stimulating factor: a preliminary report. Am J Med 1989; 86:178–81.
97. McCulloch EA, Minden MD, Miyauchi J, Kelleher CA, Wang C. Stem cell renewal and differentiation in acute myeloblastic leukaemia. J Cell Sci Suppl 1988; 10:267–81.
98. Metcalf D. The molecular control of blood cells. Cambridge MA: Harvard University Press, 1988.
99. Tafuri A, Hegewisch S, Souza L, et al. Stimulation of leukemic blood cells in vitro by colony stimulating factors and interleukin-3: evidence of recruitment and increased cell killing with cytosine arabinoside (abstract). Blood 1990; 72(suppl. 1):105.
100. Buechner T, Hiddemann W, Koenigsmann M, et al. Recombinant human GM-CSF following chemotherapy versus chemotherapy alone in patients with high-risk AML (abstract). Blood 1990; 76(suppl. 1):135.
101. Estey E, Kantarjian H, Keating M, et al. Use of GM-CSF prior to chemotherapy of AML: effects on circulating blast counts, thymidine incorporation and ara-CTP formation (abstract). Blood 1990; 76(suppl. 1):142.

15

Erythropoietin in Hematologic Malignancies

Felicia Mechtild Rosenthal, Albrecht Lindemann, Friedhelm Herrmann, and Roland Mertelsmann

University of Freiburg Medical Center, Freiburg, Germany

Wolfgang Oster

Behringwerke AG, Marburg, Germany

I. INTRODUCTION

Erythropietin (EPO) is one of the human hematopoietic growth factors that has already established its role in the treatment of anemia associated with chronic renal failure. As the primary regulator of erythropoiesis in mammals, it promotes the proliferation and differentiation of erythroid progenitor cells to mature erythrocytes (1). In 1977, Goldwasser and colleagues succeeded in the purification of human EPO from the urine of patients with aplastic anemia (2). It took almost another 10 years until, after structural characterization, the human EPO gene was isolated, cloned, and expressed, thus making sufficient quantities available for clinical application (3,4).

II. BIOLOGY

EPO is a relatively heat- and pH-stable acidic sialylated glycoprotein. Molecular weight determination by sodium dodecyl sulfate (SDS) gel electrophoresis yields a molecular mass in the range of 34–39 kD. The protein moiety is built up by a single chain of 166 amino acids, containing four cysteine molecules and at least two disulfide bonds. From the primary amino acid sequence a relative molecular mass of 18.4 kD of the recombinant polypeptide backbone was deduced. The carbohydrate residues, which contribute nearly 50% to the mature hormone, have been shown to be important for in vivo biologic activity. The asialylated EPO undergoes rapid hepatic extraction from the circulation and thus loses almost all activity (3).

Although during fetal and early neonatal periods the liver is the primary site of EPO production, in the adult this function is assumed by the kidneys (5). In the adult only 10–20% of plasma EPO is produced by the liver (6). Structural and functional aspects of fetal circulation result in a relative hypoxia of the hepatic tissue and may be involved in the liver being the major EPO-producing organ in the fetus (7). Controversy still exists about the cells responsible for the formation of EPO in the adult. Some investigators support the idea that the producer cells are peritubular interstitial cells and capillary endothelial cells found mainly in the inner renal cortex (8,9); others have demonstrated that kidney tubular cells can produce EPO in response to hypoxia (10,11).

The major target cells for EPO have been identified as committed erythroid cells (colony-forming unit erythroid, CFU-E) and to a lesser extent more primitive erythroid progenitor cells, the burst forming unit erythroid (BFU-E). The action of EPO does not seem to be restricted to the erythroid lineage only, as data have also shown an increase in myeloid (GFU-GM) and megakaryocytic (CFU-MK) bone marrow progenitor cells after stimulation with EPO (12–15). This marrow expansion is also accompanied by an increase in respective progenitor cells in the peripheral blood (16–18).

Megakaryocyte development is believed to be controlled by the interaction of several growth factors: thrombopoietin, erythropoietin, interleukin-1 (IL-1), IL-3, and granulocyte-macrophage colony-stimulating factor (GM-CSF) (19). Unlike other hematopoietic growth factors, EPO does not regulate the functional activities of the mature progeny of its target cells.

By in situ hybridization the human EPO gene has been localized to chromosome 7q11–q22 (4). The EPO mRNA is encoded by at least five exons. The entire coding region is contained in a 5.4 kb *Hind*III-*Bam*HI fragment. The recombinant form produced by CHO cells (Chinese hamster ovary cells) does not differ structurally, functionally, or immunogenetically from the native hormone.

The rate of EPO production is primarily controlled at the level of transcription. In response to hypoxia, cobalt, nickel, or manganese, specific mRNA is accumulated and EPO synthesis induced (20). Experiments with cycloheximide show that protein synthesis is required for gene activation. Convincing evidence has been presented that the oxygen sensor is a heme protein (21). Peripheral catabolism of EPO does not seem to play a role in the regulation of EPO plasma levels.

Most recently also the gene for the human EPO receptor has been cloned and localized to chromosome 19p (22,23). The receptor has a region of sequence that is similar to that found in other hematopoietic receptors: the β subunit of the IL-2 receptor, the IL-3, IL-4, IL-6, and GM-CSF receptors (24–28). This region of similarity, located on the extracellular domain, is characterized by four cysteine residues at the amino acid terminus and a conserved Trp-Ser-X-Trp-Ser motif, located just upstream from the transmembrane region. The predicted structural relationship between members of this new hematopoietic receptor family suggests that these receptors interact with similar proteins leading to similar signal transduction pathways.

III. CLINICAL APPLICATIONS

With the availability of recombinant EPO, large-scale clinical studies could be initiated to test EPO efficacy in correcting different types of transfusion-dependent anemias.

Pathogenetically these different types of anemias can be divided into two major groups: anemias with EPO deficiency and those with normal EPO levels. In EPO deficiency states, chronic renal failure being the classic example, clinical studies have clearly documented the effectiveness of EPO to restore hemoglobin levels to normal (29–32). Although hypertension has been seen in some patients, renal function was not affected.

Anemias not primarily characterized by EPO deficiency are a more heterogeneous group; most often multiple factors contribute to low hemoglobin values (33). Anemia of chronic disease, seen in chronic inflammatory (e.g., rheumathoid arthritis) (34,35), infectious (e.g., human immunodeficiency virus, HIV, infection) (36), or neoplastic disease has a characteristic disturbance of iron metabolism caused by the defective release of iron from such cells as macrophages, hepatocytes, and intestinal epithelial cells. Also, erythrocyte survival is reduced as a result of damage by presumed toxic metabolites and increased phagocytosis by activated macrophages. More important, there appears to be an additional defect in EPO secretion. For the degree of anemia EPO levels have been found to be inappropriately low (37,38). Also, the normal inverse linear relation between EPO level and hemoglobin level is impaired, which suggests a defect in the normal feedback mechanism. The cause of the inadequate EPO response remains unclear. A lack of erythroid progenitor cells or their unresponsiveness to EPO does not appear to contribute to the anemia of tumor patients, as in vitro experiments have shown (39).

Erythropoiesis in malignancy is additionally impaired when there is evidence of neoplastic marrow infiltration. The mechanisms of suppression of erythropoiesis is probably partially cytokine mediated, and hematopoiesis is intrinsically normal (40). In hairy cell leukemia (HCL) it has been shown that high levels of tumor necrosis factor α (TNF-α), produced either by local tumor cells or by bone marrow stromal cells, contribute to hematopoietic failure (41). Supraphysiologic doses of EPO might be able to shift the disturbed balance in favor of erythropoiesis. In mice, suppression of erythropoiesis by TNF-α was reversible by exogenous administration of EPO (42). As yet, in the human only trials exist using recombinant human granulocyte or granuolyte-macrophage colony-stimulating factor (G-CSF) to overcome myelosuppression by TNF-α in HCL (43,44). These findings suggest that replacement with EPO may be useful in the therapy of anemic tumor patients.

First experience with EPO in the treatment of anemia caused by cancer has been gained from patients with bone marrow infiltration by multiple myeloma (MM) and low-grade non-Hodgkin's lymphoma (l g NHL) (45–47). In our trial, EPO therapy was preceeded by a 2 week placebo application. EPO was given for at least 6 weeks as an intravenous (IV) bolus injection at a dose of 150 U/kg body weight twice a week. Nonresponders (patients who did not achieve an increase in hemoglobin > 1 g/dl) received the double dose of 300 U/kg for another 4 weeks. In nonresponse, further escalation to 450 U/kg was performed. A significant response of hemoglobin levels was observed in five of six patients. The rise in hemoglobin was accompanied by a reduction in serum ferritin levels. Also, the requirement for red blood cell transfusion was abolished and the platelet transfusion requirement reduced in some patients. One patient with MM showed an increase in platelet counts by >75% above the baseline level. The stimulation of erythro- and thrombopoiesis was maintained for at least 3 months after EPO discontinuation. Our results have been confirmed by other investigators (48).

Other types of anemia in which EPO therapy might prove beneficial are iatrogenically induced anemias following chemo- or radiotherapy, including autologous and allogeneic bone marrow transplantation (49–51). In these settings other hematopoietic growth factors, such as GM- and G-CSF, have already shown efficacy in stimulating myelopoiesis (52–58). In a recently published case report we showed a significant and sustained increase in reticulocyte count, hemoglobin, and hematocrit with EPO given twice weekly as a bolus injection at an escalating dose schedule (150–300 U/kg body weight) (59). An interesting finding was that stimulation of erythropoiesis lasted under continued EPO treatment, although another identical course of chemotherapy was administered: erythrocytes and platelets did not drop to such low levels as reached before. This finding is consistent with other reports (60,61).

One might expect that anemia in patients with MDS (myelodysplastic syndrome), in which dyserythropoiesis is the cause of the anemia, may be more difficult if not impossible to overcome by EPO substitution. Most of these patients have much higher serum EPO levels compared to patients with lg NHL. However EPO serum levels do not correlate with the patients' hemoglobin (62). Also, it cannot be predicted by pretreatment EPO levels which patients are likely to respond to exogenous administration of the growth factor (62,63). Of 10 MDS patients we have treated thus far with EPO, only minor responses have been seen in 4 patients.

Other clinical conditions associated with anemia in which recombinant human EPO might be of therapeutic value include the anemias in premature infants, aplastic anemias or pure red cell anemias, and congenital dyserythropoietic anemias (64,65). In conditions of iron excess, a in hemochromatosis, EPO might help to mobilize body iron stores and increase the tolerance to repeated phlebotomies. In patients scheduled for elective surgery it has been demonstrated that EPO can increase the amount of preoperatively collected autologous blood (66).

In contrast to the adverse events reported for patients with end-stage renal disease, in all other clinical trials no discernible acute toxicities directly related to EPO administration have been noted. This difference may possibly be explained by a predeposition of patients with renal disease to vascular complications and their lack of functioning kidneys to regulate fluid balance. Doubts about possible tumor cell growth stimulation could be dispelled.

As preclinical studies and clinical trials have shown, subcutaneous (SC) administration of EPO seems to have advantages over intravenous injections. Serum half-life is significantly prolonged, and a faster increase in hemoglobin and hematocrit has been documented (Ref. 67 and unpublished results). Also, the maintainance dose of EPO is lower with the SC route.

EPO therapy has clearly demonstrated benefits for most patients with suppressed erythropiesis due to neoplastic bone marrow infiltration (e.g., MM, CML, and NHL) or chemotherapy. Transfusion requirement and related risks of infection, cytotoxic antibody formation, and iron overload were reduced and the quality of life improved. In patients with dyserythropoietic anemias like MDS, EPO offers measurable advantage in only the minority.

Although EPO-induced expansion of the CFU-GM compartment has been described, peripheral neurophil count was not increased in any of our patients. This may be related to the dose and schedule used in these trials. The increase in platelet counts seen in some patients underscores that the potential role of EPO as a thrombopoietic growth factor awaits further evaluation, possibly in combination with other hematopoietic growth factors.

REFERENCES

1. Spivac JL. The mechanism of action of erythropoietin. Int J Cell Cloning 1986; 4:139–66.
2. Miyake T, Kung CK-H, Goldwasser E. Purification of human erythropoietin. J Biol Chem 1977; 252:5558–64.
3. Jacobs K, Shoemaker C, Rudersdorf R, et at. Isolation and characterisation of genomic and cDNA clones of human erythropoietin. Nature 1985; 313:806–10.
4. Law ML, Cai C-H, Lin F-K, et al. Chromosomal assignment of the human erythropoietin gene and its DNA polymorphism. Proc Natl Acad Sci U S A 1986; 83:6920–4.

5. Zanjani ED, Poster J, Burlington H, Mann LI, Wasserman LR. Liver as the primary site of erythropoietin formation in the fetus. J Lab Clin Med 1977; 89:640–4.
6. Fried W. The liver as a source of extrarenal erythropoietin production. Blood 1972; 40:671–7.
7. Zanjani Ed, Ascensao JL, McGlave PB. Studies on the liver to kidney switch of erythropoietin production. J Clin Invest 1981; 67:1183–8.
8. Koury ST, Bondurant MC, Koury MJ. Localization of erythropoietin synthesizing cells in murine kidneys by in situ hybridization. Blood 1988; 71:524–7.
9. Lacombe C, DaSilva JL, Bruneval P, et al. Peritubular cells are the site of erythropoietin synthesis in the murine hypoxic kidney. J Clin Invest 1988; 81:620–3.
10. Maxwell AP, Lappin TRJ, Johnston CF, Bridges JM, McGeown MG. Erythropoietin production in kidney tubular cells. Br J Heamatol 1990; 74:535–9.
11. Rich IN, Noe G, Vogt C, Lemke C. Erythropoietin is produced in the tubules of the renal cortex. Blood 1990; 76(suppl 1:639A).
12. Dessypris EN, Graber SE, Krantz SB, Stone WJ. Effects of recombinant erythropoietin on the concentration and cycling status of human marrow hematopoietic progenitor cells in vivo. Blood 1988; 72:2060–2.
13. Dessypris EN, Gleaton JH, Armstrong OL. Effect of human recombinant erythropoietin on human marrow megakaryocyte colony formation in vitro. Br J Haematol 1987; 65:265–9.
14. Ishibashi T, Koziol JA, Burstein SA. Human recombinant erythropoietin promotes differentiation of murine megakaryocytes in vitro. J Clin Invest 1987; 79:286–9.
15. Clark DA, Dessypris EN. Effects of human recombinant erythropoietin on murine colony formation on vitro. J Lab Clin Med 1986; 108:423–9.
16. McDonald TP, Cottrell MB, Clift RE, Cullen WC, Lin FK. High doses of recombinant erythropoietin stimulate platelet production in mice. Exp Hematol 1987; 15:719–21.
17. Ganser A, Bergmann M, Voelkers B, Gruetzmacher P, Scigalla P, Hoelzer D. In vivo effects of recombinant human erythropoietin on circulating human haematopoietic progenitor cells. Exp Hematol 1989; 17:433–5.
18. Geissler K, Stockenhuber F, Kabrna E, Hinterberger W, Balcke P, Lecher K. Recombinant human erythropoietin and haematopoietic progenitor cells in vivo. Blood 1989; 73:2229.
19. Long MW, Hutchinson RJ, Gragowski LL, Heffner CH, Emerson SG. Synergistic regulation of human megakaryocyte development. J Clin Invest 1988; 82:1779–86.
20. Caro J, Schuster S, Ramirez S, Badiavas EV, Costa-Giomi P, Weinmann R. Transcriptional activation of the erythropoietin gene in response to hypoxia or cobalt. Blood 1989; 32A.
21. Goldberg MA, Dunning SP, Bunn HF. Regulation of the erythropoietin gene: evidence that the oxygen sensor is a heme protein. Science 1988; 242:1412–5.
22. Winkelmann JC, Penny LA, Deaven LL, Forget BG, Jenkins RB. The gene for the human erythropoietin receptor: analysis of the coding sequence and assignment to chromosome 19p. Blood 1990; 78:24–30.
23. Jones SS, D'Andrea AD, Haines LL, Wong GG. Human erythropoietin receptor: cloning, expression, and biologic characterisation. Blood 1990; 76:31–5.

24. D'Andrea AD, Fasman GD, Lodish HF. Erythropoietin receptor and interleukin-2 receptor β-chain: a new receptor family. Cell 1989; 58:31–5.
25. Itoh N, Yonehara S, Schreurs J, et al. Cloning of an interleukin-3 receptor gene: a member of a distinct receptor gene family. Science 1990; 247:324.
26. Mosley B, Beckmann MP, March CJ, et al. The murine interleukin-4 receptor: molecular cloning and characterization of secreted and membrane bound forms. Cell 1989; 59:335.
27. Urdal DL, Idzerda RL, Beckmann MP, Cosman D, March CK, Park LS. Receptors of hematopietic growth factors. In: Mertelsmann R, Herrmann F, eds. Hematopoietic growth factors in clinical applications. New York: Dekker. 1990; 63–87.
28. Gearing DP, King JA, Gough NM, Nicola NA. Expression cloning of a receptor for human granulocyte-macrophage colony-stimulating receptor. EMBO J 1989; 8:3667.
29. Adamson JW. The promise of recombinant human erythropoietin. Semin Hematol 1989; 26:5–8.
30. Eschbach JW, Egrie JC, Downing MR, Browne JK, Adamson JW. Correction of the anemia of end-stage renal disease with recombinant human erythropietin. N Engl J Med 1987; 316:73–80.
31. Lim VS, DeGowin RL, Zavala D, et al. Recombinant human erythropoietin treatment in predialysis patients. Ann Intern Med 1989; 110:108–14.
32. Eschbach JW, Kelly MR, Haley R, Abels RI, Adamson JW. Treatment of the anemia of progesssive renal failure with recombinant human erythropoietin. N Engl J Med 1989; 321:158–62.
33. Lee GR. The anemia of chronic disease. Semin Hematol 1983; 29:61–80.
34. Means RT, Olsen NJ, Krantz SB. Treatment of the aenmia of rheumatoid arthrithis with recombinant human erythropoietin: clinical and in vitro studies. Arthritis Rheum 1989; 32:638–42.
35. Pincus T, Olsen NJ, Russell IJ, et al. Multicenter study of recombinant human erythropoietin in correction of anemia in rheumatoid arthritis. Am J Med 1990; 89:161–8.
36. Fischl M, Galpin JE, Levine JD, et al. Recombinant human erythropoietin for patients with AIDS treated with zidovudine. N Engl J Med 1990; 322:1488–93.
37. Miller CB, Jones RJ, Piantodosi S, Abeloff MD, Spivak JL. Decreased erythropoietin response in patients with the anemia of cancer. N Engl J Med 1990; 24:1689–92.
38. Cox R, Musial T, Gyde OHB. Reduced erythropoietin levels as a cause of anaemia in patients with lung cancer. Eur J Cancer Clin Oncol 1986; 22:511–4.
39. Dainiak N, Kulkarni V, Howard D, Kalamati M, Dewey M, Hoffman R. Mechanisms of abnormal erathropoiesis in malignancy. Cancer 1983; 51:1101–6.
40. Faquin WC, Schneider TJ, Goldberg MA. Effects of inflammatory cytokines on erythropoietin production in Hep3B cells. Blood 1990; 76(suppl 1:560A).
41. Lindemann A, Ludwig WD, Oster W, Mertelsmann R, Herrmann F. High level secretion of TNF-alpha contributes to hematopoietic failure in hairy cell leukemia. Blood 1989; 73:880–4.

42. Johnson CS, Cook CA, Furmanski P. In vivo suppression of erythropoiesis by Tumor necrosis factor-alpha (TNF-alpha): reversal with exogenous erythropoietin (EPO). Exp Hematol 1990; 18:109–113.
43. Lindemann A, Herrmann F, Mertelsmann R, Gamm H, Rumpoldt AH. Slenic hematopoiesis following GM-CSF therapy in a patient with hairy cell leukemia. Leukemia 1990; 4:606–7.
44. Glapsy JA, Baldwin GC, Robertson PA, et al. Therapy for neutropenia in hairy cell leukemia with recombinant human granulocyte colony-stimulating factor. Ann Intern Med 1988; 109:789–95.
45. Oster W, Herrmann F, Gamm H, et al. Erythropoietin (EPO) for the treatment of anemia of malignancy associated with neoplastic bone marrow infiltration. J Clin Oncol 1990; 8:956–62.
46. Ludwig H, Fritz E, Kotzmann H, Höcker P, Gisslinger H, Barnas U. Erythropoietin treatment for the chronic anemia of malignancy. Blood 1989; 73(suppl:16A).
47. Pedrazzini A, Bernasconi-Zapf M, Zucca E, Kern H, Goldhirsch A, Cavalli F. Erythropoietin in the treatment of anemia in multiple myeloma. Blood 1990; 76(suppl 1:629A).
48. Ludwig H, Fritz E, Kotzmann H, Höcker P, Gisslinger H, Barnas U. Erythropoietin treatment of anemia associated with multiple myeloma. N Engl J Med 1990; 322:1693–9.
49. Ebell W, Bucsky P, Dietrich H, et al. Use of recombinant human erythropoietin after bone marrow transplantion. Mol Biotherm 1989; 1:53A.
50. Ayash L, Elias A, Demetri G, et al. Recombinant human erythropoietin (EPO) in anemia associated with autologous bone marrow transplantation (ABMT). Blood 1990; 76(suppl 1:513A).
51. Medenica R, Huschart T. Erythropoietin prevents anemia in chemotherapy cancer patients. Blood 1990; 76(suppl 1:608A).
52. Herrmann F, Wieser M, Schulz G, Lindemann A, Oster W, Mertelsmann R. Single daily subcutaneous administration of rhGM-CSF ameliorates hematopoietic toxicity of chemotherapy in outpatients. Blood 1988; 72:390A.
53. Link H, Freund M, Kirchner H, et al. Enhancement of autologous bone marrow transplantation with recombinant granulocyte-macrophage colony-stimulating factor (rhGM-CSF). In: Berger HG et al., eds Cancer therapy. Berlin: Springer-Verlag, 1989; 96–102.
54. Antman KS, Griffin JD, Elias A, et al. Effect of recombinant human granulocyte-macrophage colony-stimulating factor of chemotherapy-induced myelosuppression. N Engl J Med 1988; 319:593–8.
55. Peters WP. The effect of recombinant human colony-stimulating factors on hematopoietic reconstitution following autologous bone marrow transplantation. Semin Hematol 1989; 26:18–23.
56. Gabrilove JL, Jakubowski A, Scher H, et al. Effect of granulocyte colony-stimulating factor on neutropenia and associated morbidity due to chemotherapy or transitional cell carcinoma of the urothelium. N Engl J Med 1988; 318:1414–22.
57. Lindemann A, Herrmann F, Oster W, et al. Hematologic effects of recombinat human granulocyte colony-stimulating factor in patients with malignancy. Blood. 1989; 74:2644–51.

58. Sheridan W, Morstyn G, Wolf M, et al. Granulocyte colony-stimulating factor and neutrophil recovery of the high-dose chemotherapy and antologous bone marrow transplantation. Lancet 1989; 8668:891–5.
59. Oster W, Herrmann F, Cicco A, et al. Erythropoietin prevents chemotherapy-induced anemia. Blut 1989; 59:1–5.
60. Henry DH, Rudnick SA, Bryant E, et al. Preliminary report of two double-blind, placebo-controlled studies using human recombinant erythropoietin in the anemia associated with cancer. Blood 1989; 74(suppl 1:6A).
61. Miller CB, Platanias LC, Ratain MJ, et al. A phase I/II trial of erythropoietin (EPO) in the treatment of chemotherapy-induced anemia. Blood 1990; 76(suppl 1:615A).
62. Besa EC, Nathan F, Sylvester L, Catalano P. Erythropoietin response of severely transfusion-dependent patients with myelodysplastic syndrome to recombinant human erythropoietin (EPO) does not correlate with baseline serum EPO levels. Blood 1990; 76(suppl 1:521A).
63. van Kamp H, Prinsze-Postema TC, Kluin PM, den Ottolander GJ, Willemze R, Fibbe WE. Effect of subcutaneously-administered human erythropoietin on erythropoiesis in patients with myelodysplasia. Blood 1990; 76(suppl 1:671A).
64. Rhondeau SM, Christensen RD, Ross MP, Rothstein G, Simmons MA. Responsiveness to recombinant human erythropietin of marrow erythroid progenitors from infants with "anemia of prematurity." J Pediat 1988; 112:935.
65. Tischler HJ, Leblanc S, Brune H, Welte K, Poliwoda H, Link H. Recombinant human erythropoietin in the treatment of pure red cell anemia. Blut 1989; 59:340A.
66. Goodnough LT, Rudnick S, Price TH, et al. Increased preoperative collection of autologous blood with recombinant human erythropoietin therapy. N Engl J Med 1990; 321:1163–8.
67. Bommer J, Ritz E, Weinreich T, Bommer G, Ziegler T. Subcutaneous erythropietin. Lancet 1988; 13:406.

Future Directions in Biological Therapy

Moshe Talpaz and Razelle Kurzrock

University of Texas, M. D. Anderson Cancer Center, Houston, Texas

The speculative exercise of predicting future directions in biological therapy may perhaps benefit from the critical assessment of past events. Looking into these past events, we would dare to say that the most influential event in the development of biological therapies as a "legitimate" clinical discipline in cancer management has been the rapid exploitation of recombinant DNA technology for large-scale production of cytokines.

While many of these peptides are under various stages of development and assessment, it appears that several therapeutic possibilities for their usage are emerging:

1. Supportive therapies to ameliorate toxicity, primarily by facilitating recovery of tissues injured by other cancer treatment modalities, i.e., chemotherapy and radiotherapy.
2. Modifiers of tumor cell responses to established forms of treatment, i.e., biologic peptides as chemotherapy or radiation therapy sensitizers.
3. Tumor growth inhibitors.
4. Enhancers of the host's immune response.

Within the context of these therapeutic possibilities, several treatment modalities, such as myeloid growth factors, are already used to support bone marrow recovery; and interferons are being used as antitumor agents in hematologic malignancies. However, these represent only the beginning. New therapies will undoubtedly emerge at a rapid pace.

A great deal of attention was recently directed toward hematopoietic growth factors such as granulocyte colony stimulating factor (G-CSF), granulocyte monocyte colony stimulating factor (GM-CSF), interleukin-3 (IL-3), erythropoietin (EPO), and macrophage colony stimulating factor (M-CSF). In hematologic malignancies, these agents are being used to promote recovery of normal hemopoiesis after high doses of chemotherapy with and without bone marrow transplantation. Attempts to use these growth factors to stimulate the growth of the myeloid leukemic cells, and thereby alter their responsiveness to chemotherapeutic agents, are under way as well (1,2). Similar therapeutic concepts will be addressed with novel growth factors, such as the stem cell growth factor, interleukin-1 (IL-1), and others.

In many ways, interferon-α (IFN-α) has been the prototype of cytokines with direct antitumor activities. Its mode of action remains somewhat obscure, but recent findings provide information on the ability of growth-inhibitory cytokines to modulate either the production or the effect of growth-promoting cytokines. In the case of IFN-α, such mechanisms may reflect activity at various levels (regulation of message stability, alteration of receptors, and interruption of signal transduction) (3–5). In this regard, it is of interest that many of the hematopoietic malignancies produce cytokines in an aberrant fashion, and that these cytokines may participate in tumor promotion or progression through autocrine or paracrine networks (3, 6–10). Therefore, disruption of the activity of endogenous growth factors may well be the major mode of action of interferons.

Further clinical trials may use such observations in order to design rational and novel therapeutic strategies. For example, IL-4 has recently been shown to inhibit growth of myelomonocytic, myeloid, and lymphoid leukemias, probably through the interruption of the production of growth factors such as IL-1 and IL-6 (11–14,15,16). IL-4 is now entering clinical trials in lymphomas and myelomas, conditions in which excessive production of IL-6 has already been demonstrated. Other therapeutic strategies directed specifically toward depletion of excessive growth factors may include the usage of cytokine-neutralizing monoclonal antibodies or cytokine-soluble receptors, such as naturally occurring soluble receptors to IL-4, IL-6, TNF-α, or truncated receptors to IL-1(9). Competitive inhibitors to various cytokines, either naturally occurring or synthetic, provide another means for modulating growth factor activity. For example, interleukin-1 receptor antagonist (IL-1RA), a natural monocyte-generated protein, which inhibits myeloid leukemias in vitro (9), is currently being evaluated in myeloid leukemias. Genetically engineered construction of a toxin combined with the receptor-binding domain of a growth factor is yet another potential therapeutic vehicle to exploit dependence of a malignancy on a certain growth factor (17).

Finally, certain genes (oncogenes) that are involved in the normal cellular process of growth and maturation, when perturbed, lead to a malignant phenotype. Genes possessing a transformation-inhibitory potential, which is lost when the structural integrity of the gene is disrupted (tumor suppressor genes), have also been described. The specific defects in these genes provide a target for innovative gene-directed therapies. Examples of gene-directed therapy include (1) the use of all-*trans* retinoic acid in acute promyelocytic leukemia, a disease characterized by a translocation-mediated disruption of the retinoic acid receptor-alpha gene (18); and (2) the development of antisense oligomers to prevent translation of the aberrant bcr-abl protein generated by the Philadelphia translocation in chronic myelogenous leukemia (19). Because it is now apparent that genetic abnormalities in cancer often involve the alteration of growth factors, growth factor receptors, or their signal transduction pathways, a biologic approach to modulation of these defects holds enormous promise for the future.

REFERENCES

1. Miyauchi J, Kelleher CA, Wang C, Minkin S, McCulloch EA. Growth Factor influence—the sensitivity of leukemic stem cells to cytosin arabinoside of culture. Blood 1989; 73:1272–8.
2. Cannistra SA, Groshek P, Griffin JD. Granulocyte-macrophage colony-stimulating factor enhances the cytotoxic effects of cytosine arabinoside in acute myeloblastic leukemia and in the myeloid blast crisis phase of chronic myeloid leukemia. Leukemia 1989; 3:328–34.
3. Heslop HE, Bianchi ACM, Cordingley FT, Turner M, DeMel WCP, Hoffbrand AV, Brenner MK. Effects of interferon-α on autocrine growth factor loops in B lymphoproliferative disorders. J Exp Med 1990; 172:1729–34.
4. Pfeffer LM, Donner DB, and Tamm I. Interferon-alpha downregulates insulin receptors in lymphoblastoid (Daudi) cells. Relationship to inhibition of cell proliferation. J Biol Chem 1987; 262:3665–70.
5. Fish EN and Banerjee K. Growth control: Characterizations of the antagonism between growth factors and interferon. J Interferon Res 1989; 9:2–7 (abstract).
6. Carter A, Merchav S, Silvian-Draxler I, Tatarsky I. The role of interleukin-1 and tumour necrosis factor-α in human multiple myeloma. Br J Haematol 1990; 74:424–31.
7. Kawano H, Hirano H, Matsuda T, Taga T, Horii Y, Iwato K. Asaoku H, Tang B, Tanabe O, Tanaka H, Kuramoto A, Kishimoto T. Autocrine generation and requirement of BSF-2/IL6 for human multiple myelomas. Nature 1988; 332:83–5.
8. Biondi A, Rossi V, Bassan R, Barbui T, Bettoni S, Sironi M, Mantovani A, Rambaldi A. Constitutive expression of the Interleukin-6 gene in chronic lymphocytic leukemia. Blood 1989; 73:1279–84.
9. Estrov Z, Kurzrock R, Wetzler M. Kantarjian H, Blake M, Harris D, Gutterman JU, Talpaz M. Suppression of chronic myelogenous leukemia colony growth by

IL1 receptor antagonist and soluble IL-1 receptors: A novel application for inhibitors of IL-1 activity. Blood 1991; 78(6):1476-1484.

10. Wetzler M, Kurzrock R, Taylor K, Spitzer G, Kantarjian H, Ku S, Gutterman JU, Talpaz M. Constitutive and induced expression of growth factors in cultures of normal and chronic phase CML Ph[1] bone marrow stroma. Blood 1989; 74–333 (abstract).
11. Herrmann F, Andreeff M, Gruss H-J, Brach MA, Lubbert M, Mertelsmann R. Interleukin-4 inhibits growth of multiple myelomas by suppressing Interleukin-6 expression. Blood 1991; In Press.
12. Taylor CW, Grogan TM, Salmon SS. Effects of interleukin-4 on the in vitro growth of human lymphoid and plasma cell neoplasm. Blood 1990; 75:1114–8.
13. Hart PH, Vitti GF, Burgess DR, Whitty GW, Piccoli DS, Hamilton JA. Potential antiinflammatory effects of interleukin-4: Suppression of human monocyte tumor necrosis factor alpha, interleukin-1, and prostaglandin E. Proc Natl Acad Sci USA 1989; 86:3803–7.
14. Standiford TJ, Strieter RM, Chensue SW, Westwick J, Kasahara K, Kunkel SL. Il-4 inhibits the expression of IL-8 from stimulated human monocytes. J Immunol 1990; 145:1435–9.
15. Imai Y, Nara N, Tohda S, Nagata K, Suzuki T, Nagasawa M, Murohashi I, Aoki N. Antiproliferative and differentiative effects of recombinant interleukin-4 on a granulocyte colony-stimulating factor-dependent myeloblastic leukemic cell line. Blood 1991; 78:471–8.
16. Akashi K, Shibuya T, Harada M, Takamatsu Y, Uike N, Eto T, Niho Y. Interleukin-4 suppresses the spontaneous growth of chronic myelomonocytic leukemia cells. J Clin Invest 1991; 88:223–30.
17. Kiyokawa T, Shirono K, Hattori T, Nishimura H, Yamaguchi K, Nichols JC, Strom TB, Murphy Jr, and Takatsuki K. Cytotoxicity of interleukin-2 toxin toward lymphocytes from patients with adult T-cell leukemia. Cancer Res 1989; 49:4042–6.
18. de The H, Lavau C, Marchio A, Chomienne C, Degos L, Dejean A. The PML-RARα fusion mRNA generated by the t(15;17) translocation in acute promyelocytic leukemia encodes a functionally altered RAR. Cell 1991; 66:675–84.
19. Szczylik C, Skorski T, Nicolaides NC, Manzella L, Malaguarnera L, Venturelli D, Gewirtz AM, Calabretta B. Selective inhibition of leukemia cell proliferation by BCR-ABL antisense oligodeoxynucleotides. Science 1991; 253:562–5.

Index